NEUROLOGY FOR THE SPECIALTY BOARDS

BOARD REVIEW SERIES

NEUROLOGY FOR THE SPECIALTY BOARDS

David S. Gloss
Leon A. Weisberg

Lippincott Williams & Wilkins
a Wolters Kluwer business
Philadelphia · Baltimore · New York · London
Buenos Aires · Hong Kong · Sydney · Tokyo

Acquisitions Editor: Frances DeStefano
Managing Editor: Julia Seto
Marketing Manager: Kim Schonberger
Production Editor: Fran Gunning
Manufacturing Coordinator: Kathleen Brown
Design Coordinator: Risa Clow
Compositor: Scribe, Inc.
Printer: Data Reproductions Corp.

Copyright © 2007 by David S. Gloss, M.D.

530 Walnut Street
Philadelphia, PA 19106

All rights reserved. This book is protected by copyright. No part of this book may be reproduced in any form or by any means, including photocopying, or utilized by any information storage and retrieval system without written permission from the copyright owner.

The publisher is not responsible (as a matter of product liability, negligence, or otherwise) for any injury resulting from any material contained herein. This publication contains information relating to general principles of medical care that should not be construed as specific instructions for individual patients. Manufacturers' product information and package inserts should be reviewed for current information, including contraindications, dosages, and precautions.

Printed in the United States of America

First Edition, 2007

Library of Congress Cataloging-in-Publication Data

Gloss, David S., 1969–
 Neurology for the specialty boards / David S. Gloss, Leon A. Weisberg.
   p. ; cm.
 Includes index.
 ISBN 13: 978-1-4051-0481-4
 ISBN 10: 1-4051-0481-3
 1. Neurology—Examinations, questions, etc. I. Weisberg, Leon A.,
1941– II. Title.
 [DNLM: 1. Nervous System—Examination Questions. 2. Nervous System Diseases—Examination Questions. 3. Neurology—Examination Questions. WL18.2 G563n 2006]
  RC356.G58 2006
  616.80076—dc22   2006027319

The publishers have made every effort to trace the copyright holders for borrowed material. If they have inadvertently overlooked any, they will be pleased to make the necessary arrangements at the first opportunity.

To purchase additional copies of this book, call our customer service department at **(800) 638-3030** or fax orders to **(301) 824-7390**. International customers should call **(301) 714-2324**.

Visit Lippincott Williams & Wilkins on the Internet: http://www.LWW.com. Lippincott Williams & Wilkins customer service representatives are available from 8:30 am to 6:00 pm, EST.

06 07 08
1 2 3 4 5 6 7 8 9 10

We dedicate this book to Dr. Carlos Garcia, a beloved member of the department who worked tirelessly with residents. He passed away during its writing.

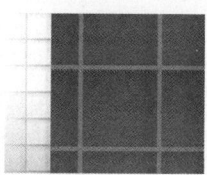

Contents

Contributors ix
Preface xi
Acknowledgments xiii

SECTION I SCIENTIFIC UNDERPINNINGS
1. Development 1
2. Anatomy I: Structural Anatomy 8
3. Anatomy II: Vascular Anatomy 27
4. Physiology and Neurophysiologic Testing 35
5. Pathology 59
6. Pharmacology 83

SECTION II CLINICAL NEUROLOGY
7. Cerebrovascular Disease 95
8. Cerebellum 108
9. Spinal Cord 114
10. Peripheral Nerves 122
11. Demyelination 131
12. Muscle 141
13. Movement Disorders 151
14. Infection 163
15. Neoplasm 169
16. Headache and Pain 181
17. Epilepsy 192
18. Cognitive and Emotional Alteration 200
19. Pediatrics 209
20. Neuroradiology 224
21. Sleep 241
22. Neuroophthalmology 248
23. Neurosurgery for the Neurologist 253
24. Internal Medicine for the Neurologist 260

25. Neuropsychiatry   267
26. Vertigo and Dizziness   275
27. Autonomic Nervous System and Hypothalamus   281
28. Special Senses   288
29. Final Exam   295

Index   313

Contributors

Tulane Neurology Faculty
Crabtree, Elizabeth, M.D.
Elliot, Debra, G., M.D.
Garcia, Carlos A., M.D.
Seltzer, Benjamin, P., M.D.

Tarulli, Andrew, W., M.D.
Beth Israel Deaconess Medical Center Neurophysiology Fellow,
Harvard Medical School Clinical Fellow in Neurology

Tulane Residents
Gump, William, M.D.
Martin-Schild, Sheryl, M.D., Ph.D.
Michell, Vincent, M.D.
Suros, Jose, M.D.
Wible, Elissa, M.D.
Wilcox, Amy, M.D.

Mahoney, Brent, M.D., Ph.D.
Virginia Commonwealth University's Massey Cancer Center Resident

Preface

The specialty board exam is fraught with peril: 40 percent of those who attempt it each year do not pass. In addition, those who have passed it are required to take a recertification exam every ten years.

This book is a resource for those studying for this exam or the annual in-service exam or those who will take the surprisingly neurology-laden specialty board in psychiatry. We made no attempt to be comprehensive; we made every attempt to be correct and to focus on high-yield materials. We believe that sometime during their residency, every resident should read a complete resource from cover to cover to give them the complete details that this short resource could not possibly attempt to provide. And this book is probably not enough to pass the exam: there are entire books devoted to the subjects of each of these chapters.

Some sections are intended specifically for residents. We have included, for example, a page or so of each of the commonly encountered neurophysiological modalities with enough detailed knowledge to allow a resident to start working with them. The knowledge here, combined with some practical knowledge obtained during residency, is probably enough to answer the relevant questions encountered on the boards.

Our strategy is threefold. First, we have written an extensive basic science section as a way to review as well to help prospective test-takers score extra points where a few extra points could tip the balance in their favor. We have tried to make the basic science section relatively comprehensive without getting bogged down in unimportant details. Seond, we have written a sketch of the clinical knowledge, focusing on the most important information that readers might encounter on the boards. Having a strong science background and a basis on the clinical side will allow readers to focus their additional studies on the clinical side without missing the easy points from basic science or areas that might be lacking in their residency. We have made pediatrics the largest clinical chapter, since pediatrics questions are frequently asked. Third, we have written an extensive section of questions that are approximately at the level of the boards. We have intentionally made them slightly easier; if readers cannot answer these questions, this is a signal that they have not adequately prepared for the test, and hopefully they will have enough time to do something about it!

We wish all the test takers luck and hope that this book might make some small impact on the large number of residents unable to pass the boards every year. We also hope that this book will save time for prospective test takers by providing a helpful and accurate source of basic information that will serve as a jumping-off point for more advanced readings.

David S. Gloss
Leon A. Weisberg

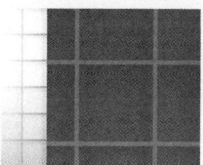

Acknowledgments

We would like to thank the residents and faculty of Tulane University School of Medicine for contributing either directly or indirectly to this book. Particularly, we would like to thank Doctors P. Sarala and J. Venuti for their reviews of particular chapters, Doctor P. Rosel for his help with images, Jennifer Smith for graphic design, and Marilee Hanemann for her anatomic drawings.

SECTION I

SCIENTIFIC UNDERPINNINGS

CHAPTER 1

Development

I. Nervous System: Embryonic and Fetal Development

A. **Develops from the neural plate** (ectoderm)
  1. Notochord and mesoderm induce formation of neural plate through transforming growth sphincter paralysis factor β (TGF-β).

B. **Neural plate differentiates** neural crest, neural tube by invagination.
  1. **Neurulation** (neural tube formation) begins day 22, junction spinal cord and brain (fourth somite)
  2. **Neural tube nonfusion** five specific sites ⇒ spina bifida, anencephaly, craniorachischisis
  3. **The lumen of the neural tube is the neural canal.** Anterior neuropore closes day 25, posterior day 27. The neural canal of the neural tube forms the ventricular system and the central canal of the spinal cord.
      a. Failure of anterior neuropore to close during fourth week = **anencephaly**
          i. **Meroanencephaly:** rudimentary brainstem, most common serious anomaly, always acrania, extrauterine life is impossible, risk in future pregnancies is about 6%
          ii. **Holoanencephaly:** no recognizable organized brain with large cavity
      b. Partial closure of anterior neuropore = **encephalocele**
          i. **Hernia of brain and its coverings** through a midline skull defect
          ii. **Frontal hernia:** risk of meningitis, some children are normal, more common in Asia/Africa
          iii. **Posterior hernia:** severe often, grave deficits, more common in Western hemisphere
      c. Failure of posterior neuropore to close = **myeloschisis** = **spinal cord cleft**

1

i. **Diastematomyelia:** spinal cord in halves connected by bone or connective tissue
ii. **Spina bifida occulta:** L5 or S1, affects 10% of normals, often small dimple or tuft of hair arising; dimple shows region of closure of posterior neuropore end of fourth week
iii. **Spinal dermal sinus:** under dimple, can connect to dura
iv. **Spina bifida cystica:** Sac with fluid/meninges—meningocele, if spinal cord, nerves—meningomyelocele and neurologic deficit; if sphincter paralysis ⇒ saddle region anesthesia

d. **Meckel-Gruber syndrome**
i. **Rare:** autosomal recessive, lethal malformation with occipital encephalocele and includes polycystic kidneys, pancreas, or liver, hexa/heptadactyly of all four limbs

e. **Chiari malformation** (also called Arnold-Chiari but Arnold contributed much less)
i. **Type I:** cerebellar ectropion, can be with a kinked cervical cord; presents with headache (often suboccipital), nystagmus, and other brain stem dysfunction, including weakness and ataxia. Treatment: surgery within 2 years
ii. **Type II:** medulla, fourth ventricle herniation into cervical region, brain malformations, myelomeningocele, syringomyelia, diastematomyelia. Symptoms: neurogenic stridor, neurogenic dysphagia, apneic spells. Treatment: surgery when any of three symptoms appears
iii. **Type III:** meningomyelocele, cerebellar herniation into cervical cord, none survive
iv. **Type IV:** cerebellar hypoplasia

f. **Neural tube defects** (NTDs)
i. **Diagnosis:** α-fetoprotein (AFP) and acetylcholinesterase elevations at 15 to 16 weeks, confirmation by ultrasound; blood contamination can be a source of false positive for AFP
ii. **Prevention:** folic acid given before 28th day of pregnancy
   (a) Folic acid 0.4 mg qd for all women of childbearing age or folic acid 4.0 mg qd if diabetes, on anticonvulsant therapy, or previous neural tube defect (NTD) from 1 month before trying to 3 months after pregnant (1).
   (b) Some medications antagonize folic acid: methotrexate, valproate (VPA), carbamazepine (CBMZ), trimethoprim (TMP).
iii. **Risks:** Recurrence: 2% to 3%, Diabetes 1%, VPA or CPMZ 1%, close relative 0.7%. Risk in general population about 1 in 700 to 1,000.

C. **Brain**
1. The brain forms from the neural tube rostral to the fourth pair of somites.
2. Fusion of the rostral neuropore forms the three primary brain vesicles.
   a. **Forebrain**—prosencephalon divides fifth week to (anterior) telencephalon, (posterior) diencephalon
   b. **Midbrain**—mesencephalon
   c. **Hindbrain**—rhombencephalon; this divides into the metencephalon and myelencephalon
3. **Forebrain.** Closure anterior neuropore, optic vesicles appear, form retinae and optic nerves
   a. **Second pair vesicles** soon appear: cerebral vesicles become cerebral hemispheres, lateral ventricles. Telencephalon includes cerebral vesicles. Both telencephalon, diencephalon contribute to third ventricle. Choroid plexus forms in choroid fissure. Hemispheres expand and meet, mesenchyme trapped, becomes falx cerebri
      • Microcephaly, or small brain, calvarium with a normal-sized face results in severe mental retardation. Etiologies: radiation, alcohol abuse, cytomegalovirus (CMV), rubella, or toxoplasma
      • Failure of forebrain midline cleavage = holoprosencephaly + telencephalon is a single ventricular cavity. Associated arrhinencephaly. Etiology: alcohol abuse, trisomy 13
      i. **Corpus striatum** is swelling of cerebral hemisphere floor. Floor expands slower than hemisphere, resulting in C shape of hemispheres. Corpus striatum is divided by internal capsule into caudate, lentiform nuclei. C-shape of caudate conforms to lateral ventricle

ii. The connections between the hemispheres are few.
   (a) Lamina terminalis forms corpus callosum. As corpus callosum grows, extends beyond lamina. Lamina becomes optic chiasm and septum pellucidum.
   (b) Agenesis of the corpus callosum: asymptomatic or seizures, mental deficiency. Diagnosis ⇒ bat-wing third/lateral ventricles, electroencephalographic (EEG) asynchrony. Seen in Aicardi syndrome (X-linked dominant, neuronal migration defects, chorioretinopathy; asynchronous burst suppression of sleep spindles), Andermann syndrome, nonketotic hyperglycinemia
   (c) The anterior commissure connects the olfactory bulbs.
   (d) The hippocampal commissure connects the hippocampal formations.
  b. **Diencephalon:** The lateral walls of the third ventricle form into three nodules, which become the epithalamus, thalamus, and hypothalamus.
     i. Epithalamus pineal body, habenula, post commissure, choroid plexus third ventricle
     ii. Thalami grow rapidly and fuse in 70% forming the mass intermedia, a gray-matter bridge across the third ventricle. The subthalamus (ventral thalamus) forms the subthalamic nucleus, zona incerta, fields of Forel; neuroblasts create the globus pallidus.
     iii. Hypothalamus gives rise to mammillary bodies. Pituitary gland is formed from multiple parts. Neurohypophyseal bud projects into floor of diencephalon and forms pars nervosa, infundibular stem, median eminence. Hypophyseal (Rathke) pouch projects upward from stomodeum (primitive mouth cavity). Anterior pouch proliferates becomes pars distalis. Extension of the anterior pouch grows around infundibular stem becoming pars tuberalis. Posterior part of pouch does not proliferate, becomes pars intermedia.
        (a) Remnants of Rathke pouch can become craniopharyngioma: 3% of intracranial tumors occur in sella turcica, suprasellar cistern, or third ventricle. Two types: adamantinomatous and papillary. The adamantinomatous type far more common. On magnetic resonance imaging, heterogenous, moderately enhancing tumor with well-defined cystic component bright on T1 and T2; can be calcified. Papillary type is found in adult, not calcified
        (b) Remnants of the Rathke pouch rise to incidental Rathke cleft cysts (11% at autopsy), which are small and almost always asymptomatic. They do not enhance.
4. **Midbrain**
   a. **Mesencephalon:** neural canal narrows, becomes cerebral aqueduct; alar plates migrate to form inferior and superior colliculi; basal plates form tegmentum and substantia nigra; the cerebral peduncles arise from descending fibers from other parts of the brain.
5. **Hindbrain**
   a. **Metencephalon:** dorsal alar plates form cerebellum; intermediate alar plate forms cerebral cortex; alar plates form pontine, cochlear, vestibular, and trigeminal sensory nuclei.
   b. **Myelencephalon:** this forms the medulla including the cuneate, gracile, and olivary nuclei; pyramids; and parts of the vagus, hypoglossal, and glossopharyngeal nerves.

D. **Spinal cord**
   1. Spinal cord forms from the neural tube caudal to the fourth pair of somites.
   2. The neural tube is pseudostratified columnar epithelium.
   3. The neural tube differentiates into three layers (from inner to outer).
      a. **Ventricular** zone forms the neuroblasts and the macroglia.
      b. **Intermediate** or mantle zone forms neuroblasts from ventricular zone and forms neurons.
      c. **Marginal** zone inside the external limiting membrane (ELM) becomes white matter.
      d. The **microglia** forms later when blood vessels develop.
      e. The **ELM** is surrounded by mesenchyme, which becomes the meninges.
         i. Initially it condenses to form the primordial meninx.
         ii. The external layer thickens to form the dura.

4 SECTION I SCIENTIFIC UNDERPINNINGS

       iii. The inner layer remains thin and forms the leptomeninges with neural crest cells.
       iv. The leptomeninges forms the pia and arachnoid, connected by arachnoid trabeculae.
  4. **Growth of neural tube** forms alar plate and basal plate separated by sulcus limitans.
    a. **Alar plate** forms the dorsal (gray) horns.
    b. **Basal plate** forms ventral and lateral (gray) horns, separated by ventral median fissure.
  5. **Embryonic spinal cord** extends entire length of spinal canal; nerve roots exit at level of origin.
    a. The spinal canal and dura grow more rapidly than spinal cord.
       i. Newborn conus medullaris at L2-3, adult inferior border of L1.
       ii. This level in an adult actually ranges from T12 to L3.
       iii. The dura and arachnoid end at S2 in adult; the pia continues as the filum terminale.
  6. **Myelination** begins late fetal, continues through first years, largely finished by second year, but reticular formation, thalamic radiations, cerebral commissures, and intracortical association areas continue to develop until about 10th year.
    a. Central nervous system (CNS) myelin oligodendrocytes. Sensory first, motor next, then association areas
    b. Myelin sheaths of peripheral nerves from Schwann cells, derived from neural crest; sensory before motor; this myelination starts before CNS myelination begins

E. **Neural crest**
  1. Forms the **dorsal root ganglion**. Initially bipolar neuroblasts, become unipolar neurons.
  2. **Also forms** cranial nerve ganglia, somatic and visceral sensory cells of the peripheral nervous system, autonomic ganglia, pia, arachnoid, Schwann cells, preganglionic sympathetics, melanocytes, chromaffin cells of the adrenal medulla, and odontoblasts
    a. Failure of neural crest cells to migrate to the colon causes agenesis of Auerbach plexus and resulting Hirschsprung disease = congenital megacolon
    b. Odontoblasts are often contained in molar teeth; this is why all unerupted molars should be taken out, as they can otherwise form dentigerous cysts

II. Postnatal Development

A. **Reflexes**
  1. Present **at birth** (when disappears, month)
    a. **Moro** (3 to 6 months)—drop back head 3 cm, extension, abduction of arms, opening of palms
    b. **Suck** (4 to 6 months)—sucks when object placed in mouth
    c. **Grasp**—grasps object with hand with hand stimulation or foot with foot stimulation, disappears 6 months (hand) and 10 months (foot); why don't ask to squeeze fingers with GCS (Glasgow Coma Score)
    d. **Galant** (2 to 6 months—if suspended prone, stroking paravertebral region causes truncal concavity toward stroked side
    e. **Tonic labyrinthine supine** (6 to 9 months)—extend neck while prone and this causes tonic extension of neck and legs with shoulder retraction and adduction
    f. **Tonic labyrinthine prone** (6 to 9 months)—flex neck while supine and this causes flexion of trunk and protraction of shoulders
    g. **Asymmetric tonic neck** (4 to 10 months)—rotate head laterally >45 degrees while supine and get extension of limbs ipsilateral to chin and flexion contralateral
    h. **Babinski** (10 months)—great toe dorsiflexion on stroking lateral foot; actually several Babinski reflexes, so clearer to say extensor plantar response
  2. Present **after birth** (when appears/when disappears).
    a. **Landau** (3 months/24 months)—ventral suspension ⇒ extension head, neck, hips; knee flexion
    b. **Parachute** (9 months/persists)—prone suspension thrust down, arms extend, fingers spread

      c. Symmetric tonic neck (5 months/8 to 9 months/not present in most normals)—extend/flex head while sitting causes extension of arms and flexion of legs/vice versa

B. **Average milestones** (month, year)
  1. **1 month:** smiles spontaneously, head up 45 degrees
  2. **3 months:** regards own hand, follows 180 degrees, squeals, sits up head steady, rolls over
  3. **6 months:** feeds self, passes cube, imitates speech sounds, sits with no support
  4. **9 months:** waves bye-bye, pincer grasp, says dada/mama, pulls to stand
  5. **1 year:** drinks from cup, puts block in cup, dada/mama specific, stands alone
  6. **18 months:** removes garment, tower of four cubes, six words besides mama/dada, runs
  7. **2 years:** puts on clothing, tower of six cubes, speech half understandable, jumps up
  8. **4 years:** prepares cereal, copies +, names four colors, hops
  9. **DQ** (development quotient) = development age/chronological age x 100; refer to development neuropsychiatrist for DQ <70, diagnostic of developmental delay.

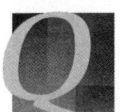# STUDY QUESTIONS FOR CHAPTER 1

Directions: Each of the numbered items or incomplete statements in this section is followed by answers or by completions of the statement. Select the ONE lettered answer or completion that is BEST in each case.

1. What part of the embryonic brain becomes the substantia nigra?

(A) Prosencephalon
(B) Mesencephalon
(C) Metencephalon
(D) Myelencephalon

2. A 22-year-old woman is treated with valproic acid for generalized tonic clonic seizures. She has had no seizures in the last year, but prior to treatment, had two to three seizures per month. Although she reports that she is not currently pregnant, she does plan on trying to conceive in the next few years. What changes should you make to her medical regimen?

(A) Discontinue anticonvulsants
(B) Add folic acid, 0.4 mg per day
(C) Add folic acid, 1 mg each day
(D) Add folic acid, 4 mg each day
(E) Dissuade her from becoming pregnant

3. A normal 2 year, 1 month old would be diagnosed with developmental delay if he could not do which of the following?

(A) Use a fork
(B) Know two words besides mama/dada
(C) Draw a square
(D) Make a tower of four cubes

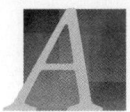 # ANSWERS AND EXPLANATIONS

1. B. Mesencephalon forms cerebral aqueduct, colliculi, substantia nigra. Prosencephalon (A) forms cerebral hemispheres, hypothalamus, thalamus. Metencephalon (C) forms pons and cerebellum. Myelencephalon (D) forms medullar oblongata.

2. D. Folic acid, 4 mg each day, is recommended for women of childbearing age who take anticonvulsants. Doses of 0.4 mg and 1 mg per day are insufficient. Discontinuing her anticonvulsants is not a good idea, as her seizures were difficult to control, and the risk of seizures to a fetus is greater than the risk of anticonvulsants. The rate of neural tube defects in women with epilepsy who take anticonvulsants is about 10% and can be lowered by taking folic acid. Dissuading this patient from becoming pregnant is wrong.

3. B. 50th percentile is 16.5, so DQ is 66, developmentally delayed. In A, 50th percentile is 22 months, DQ is 22/25 = 88. C is expected of 4 1/2 year old, indicates a gifted child. Child should also be referred to receive appropriate services. In D, 50th percentile is 23, so a DQ of 92.

CHAPTER 2

Anatomy I: Structural Anatomy

I. Sensation and Perception

A. Somatic sensation
  1. **General somatic afferent** = temperature, nondiscriminative touch (erotic), pressure, and pain. All have survival value.
     a. **Peritrichial (bare) nerve endings:** epidermis of skin and cornea of eye, unmyelinated
     b. **Merkel disks:** glabrous (i.e., hairless) skin, touch-sensitive regions of body, associated with skin epithelial cells called Merkel cells, for light touch
     c. **Meissner corpuscles:** tactile discrimination, especially for edges/points, three to four myelinated nerve endings encapsulated; glabrous hand, foot, lip, nipple, tongue
     d. **Pacinian corpuscle:** pressure, touch, vibration, digits of hand, breasts, joints
     e. **Ruffini endings:** stretch/pressure in skin and nail beds
     f. **Krause end bulbs:** involved in temperature, papillary region of dermis
     g. **Golgi tendon organs:** interface of tendon and muscle, force, proprioception, group IB axon synapses to spinal cord inhibitory interneuron of corresponding alpha motor neuron.
     h. **Neuromuscular spindle:** skeletal muscle, detect length change, used for proprioception, group IA axon
     i. **Thermoreceptors:** three kinds—warmth, cold, nociceptors; can detect 2°C change
     j. **Nociceptors:** three types—extreme heat/cold, mechanical, transmitters like bradykinin
  2. **Peripheral nerves** enter the dorsal root. The area of skin innervated by a dorsal root is a dermatome. Dermatomes overlap: pain < nondiscriminatory tactile
     a. C6 supply thumb, C7 second and third digits, C8 fourth and fifth digits
     b. L4 medial malleolus; L5 medial digits, top foot; S1 lateral malleolus and digits, heel
  3. **The spinal gray matter** is divided into 10 lamellae defined by cytoarchitecture (Figure 2-1)
     a. **Laminae I–VI** comprise dorsal horn, VIII and IX ventral horn
     b. **Lamina I** (marginal zone) pain/temperature sensory relay
     c. **Lamina II** (substantia gelatinosa) integrates afferents then projects back to lamella I. This is functionally the most important, acting as a sensory gate
     d. **Laminae III–VI** (nucleus proprius) sensory integration and descending pathways
     e. **Lamina VII** (Clarke nucleus and the intermediolateral nucleus) thoracic, lumbar spine only as part of spinocerebellar pathway. Clarke: limb position and movement, projects to the cerebellum. Interomediolateral nucleus: autonomic preganglionic neurons
     f. **Lamina VIII** skeletal muscle interneurons
     g. **Lamina IX** motor nuclei
     h. **Lamina X** surrounds central canal and functions similar to I and II
  4. Discriminative touch, vibration, limb proprioception are conveyed by large afferents, and lamellae III and IV ipsilaterally synapse dorsal column nuclei in caudal medulla. They subsequently decussate in internal arcuate fibers of medulla and project to ventral posterolateral thalamus (VPL) through medial lemniscus and finally to primary somatic

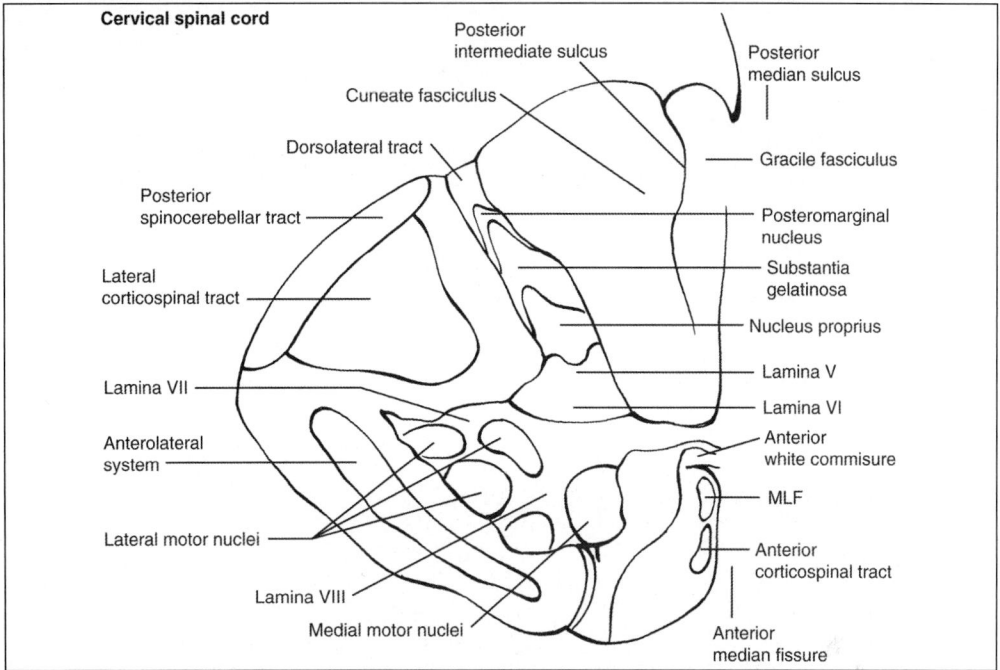

Figure 2-1 Axial drawing of the cervical spinal cord.

sensory cortex (SSC) through internal capsule. Thus, lesions below medulla will be ipsilateral to deficits, whereas above will be contralateral to deficit.
5. **Pain and temperature:** synapse in dorsal root ganglion and decussate in few segments, causing contralateral deficit. Ascends spinoreticular, mesencephalic, and thalamic tracts. Spinoreticular tract synapses reticular formation in medulla and pons, then to thalamus. Spinomesencephalic tract synapses tectum of midbrain, superior colliculus, or mesencephalic periaqueductal gray. Spinothalamic, spinoreticular tract project to three areas of thalamus: VPL (which in turn projects to SSC), intralaminar nuclei (projects to cortex, basal ganglia), and posterior nuclei (projects to parietal lobe). Please review the pons, midbrain, and medulla where these projections are located (Figures 2-2–2-5), as they will be frequently encountered throughout the chapter.
6. **The primary sensory cortex** (postcentral gyrus and central sulcus) projects to the secondary sensory cortex (upper lateral sulcus), which projects to the insula and back to the primary sensory cortex. Both primary and secondary cortices project to motor cortex.

B. Vision
  1. **Retina** has 10 layers from external to choroid to level of optic nerve:
     a. **Retinal pigmented epithelium**—attached to Bruch membrane, blood retinal barrier, rod and cone tips surrounded by cell extensions ⇒ site of retinal detachment
     b. **Rods (dim light, rhodopsin), cones (bright light, iodopsin)**—one of red, green, or blue
     c. **Outer limiting membrane**—zonula adherents between Müller cells and photoreceptors
     d. **Outer nuclear layer**—nuclei of rods and cones
     e. **Outer plexiform layer**—synapses between photoreceptors and other neurons, including bipolar cells; interneurons use glutamate, same inhibition as ganglion cells (see subsequent text)
     f. **Inner nuclear layer**—nuclei of other neurons besides rods and cones
     g. **Inner plexiform layer**—dendrites project to ganglion cells from photoreceptors
     h. **Ganglion cell layer**—cell bodies of large ganglion neurons, which fire in response to circular zone of light and inhibit firing of neurons in circular zone of nearby neurons; this detects weak color contrasts and changes the appearance of objects due to background.

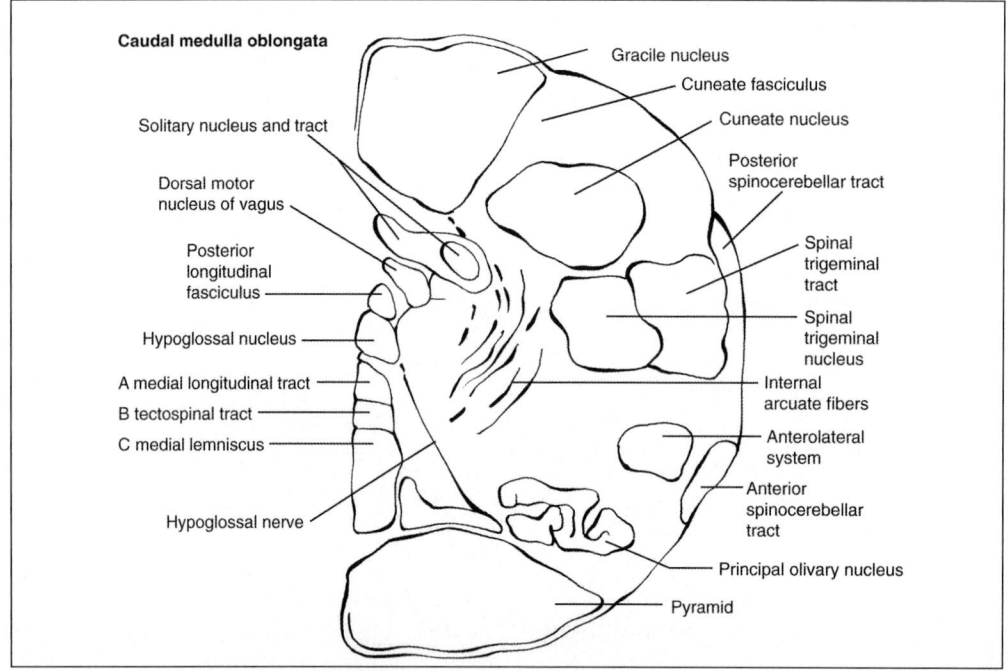

Figure 2-2 Axial drawing of the caudal medulla.

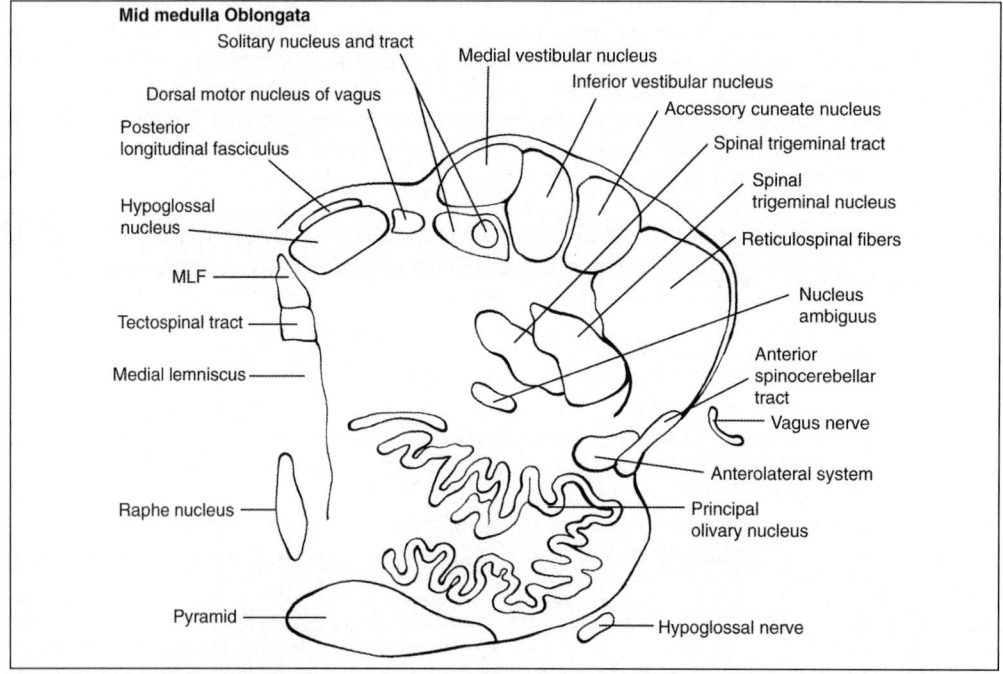

Figure 2-3 Axial drawing of the rostral mid-medulla.

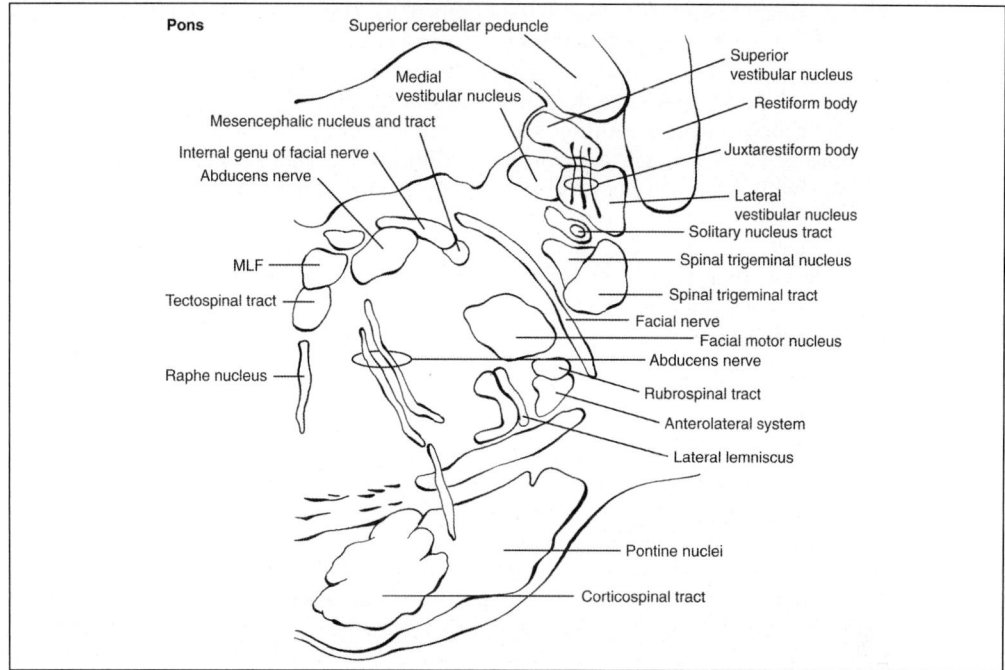

Figure 2-4 Axial drawing of the pons.

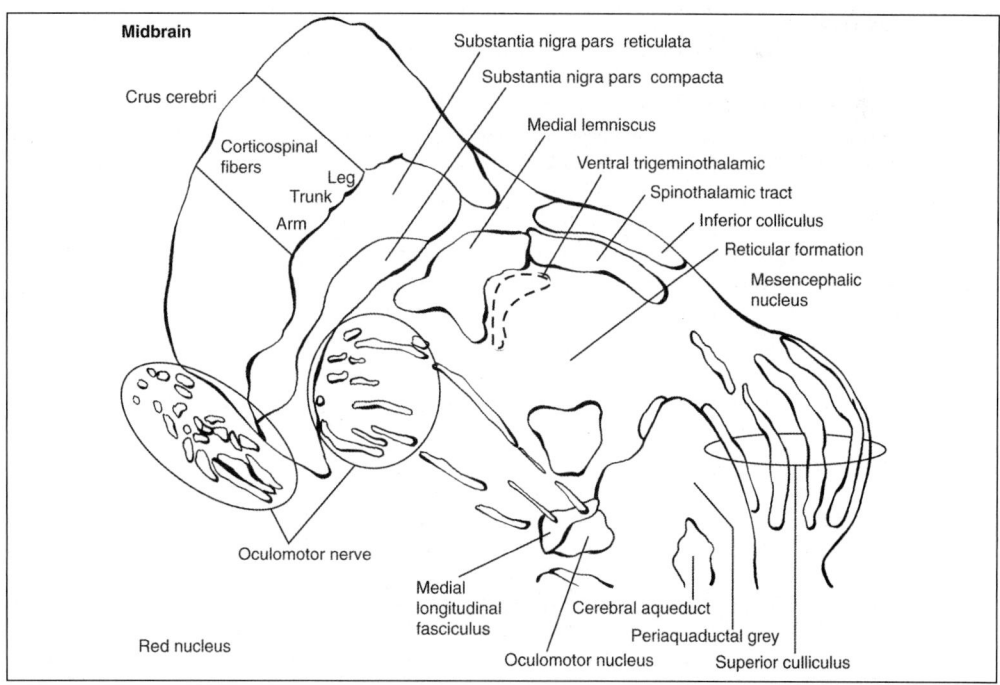

Figure 2-5 Axial drawing of the midbrain.

This is thought to be the biologic basis of much art. During full adaptation to darkness, ganglion cells lose their surround inhibition and become light detectors.
  i. The ganglion cells are of two major types: those that are stimulated when light is increased and those that are stimulated when light is decreased.
  ii. The ganglion cells are further subdivided into M cells with large cell bodies (M for magnocellular), which are concerned with gross features, and more numerous P cells with small cell bodies (P for parvocellular), which are concerned with color detail and are thought to be concerned with fine detail.
  iii. Few cells with unknown function; some respond to overall light intensity
 i. **Optic nerve fiber layer**—unmyelinated ganglion cell axons pierce the sclera, after which the axons becomes myelinated
 j. **Inner limiting membrane**—basal laminae of Müller cells
2. **Fovea** is area where proximal neural elements shifted away giving least light distortion
3. **Optic nerve** includes 1 million nerves; >30 times more than auditory nerve
  a. When light enters the eye, it is inverted.
  b. The left hemivisual field projects to the medial (or nasal) hemiretina on the left eye and the lateral (or temporal) hemiretina on the right eye.
  c. There is a crescent-shaped temporal region where vision is monocular.
  d. Visual impulses travel in the optic nerve.
  e. At the level of the optic chiasm, the nasal hemiretinal fibers decussate.
  f. **The left optic tract** contains the entire right hemifield of vision and vice versa. The left optic tract projects to three areas: left lateral geniculate nucleus (LGN), left pretectal midbrain (pupillary reflexes), and superior colliculus (eye movements)
    i. The ganglion cells related to ambient light intensity project to pretectal midbrain. Pretectal neurons project bilaterally to the preganglionic parasympathetic neurons in Edinger-Westphal nucleus and travel via cranial nerve (CN) III to innervate ciliary ganglion.
    ii. The superior colliculus controls saccadic eye movements.
  g. **Left LGN** has visuotopic representation with fovea occupying half of visual field. Six layered: ventral layers 1, 2 (magnocellular layers) receive visual input from M ganglion cells; dorsal layers 3–6 (parvocellular layers) receive input from P ganglion cells
    i. 1, 4, 6 receive input from the ipsilateral nasal hemiretina
    ii. 2, 3, 5 receive input from the contralateral temporal hemiretina
  h. **LGN** projects to six-layered visual cortex (V1) via the optic radiations. Inferior retina projects via Meyer loop in temporal lobe to inferior bank of calcarine fissure.
    i. Layer 4 is subdivided into 4A, 4B, 4Ca, 4Cb
    ii. M cells terminate in 4Ca and P cells terminate in 4Cb. 4Ca projects to 4B. Both 4B and 4Cb project to layers 2, 3 as does intralaminar nuclei of the LGN. These then project to visual association areas and layers 5, then 6.
    iii. V1 has three classes of cells: simple cells, complex cells, and blobs
    iv. Simple cells have oriented rectilinear activation zones, surrounded by rectilinear inhibition zone; therefore, activation of simple cell in outer zone will cause inhibition.
    v. Complex cells have larger oriented activation zones.
    vi. Blobs are the only cells that react to tiny points of light and are important for color vision. Only P cells project to blobs.
    vii. The simple and complex cells decompose a visual image into line segments.
    viii. V1 is subdivided into columns; each subserves an axis about 10 degrees apart.
    ix. All the columns are divided into two regions, called ocular dominance columns, one devoted to the left eye and the other to the right, and are involved in depth perception.
    x. The tip of the calcarine cortex subserves the macula. This is why a typical posterior cerebral artery infarction is macula sparing.
  i. **Visual agnosias** (agnosia is defined as a loss of ability to recognize the meaning of sensory stimuli) and affected Brodmann areas
    17 = V1, 18 = V2 + 3, 19 = V4 + 5 (V5 = middle temporal area)

i. Object agnosia left 18, 20, 21
   ii. Outlines/drawings agnosia right 18, 20, 21
   iii. Prosopagnosia bilateral 20, 21
   iv. Color agnosia right 18
   v. Color anomia could be speech zone or 18, 37 connections
   vi. Achromatopsia 18, 37
   vii. Visual spatial agnosia right 18, 37
   viii. Movement agnosia temporoparietal occipital junction
  j. **Motion perception** has a special neural system.
   i. Only primates and humans can react to nonmoving objects
   ii. Simple vertebrates (including dinosaurs) do not see nonmoving objects
   iii. Motion is broken up into simple axis movements by neurons in V1 + 5 and pattern of movement by neurons solely in V5.

C. **Hearing**
  1. **Hearing** is the sensation of the frequency of vibrations in the air.
  2. **Vibrations** are transmitted through external auditory meatus to tympanic membrane causing vibrations on it. Malleus attached to tympanic membrane, then incus, and finally stapes attached to oval window. Round window equalizes pressure.
   a. The cochlea spirals around the modiolus 2 1/2 times. The organ of Corti rests on the basilar membrane connecting the scala media and the scala tympani.
   b. Within the organ of Corti are hair cells, which detect vibration. Different regions of the cochlea respond to different frequencies of sound.
   c. The hair cells release a neurotransmitter and activate bipolar neurons of the spiral ganglia in the modiolus.
  3. Nuclei of auditory neurons in cochlear nucleus, which is located on the inferior cerebellar peduncle of the pons. The cochlear nucleus projects via three pathways.
   a. The dorsal and intermediate acoustic stria decussate to the lateral lemniscus
   b. Synapse in superior olivary nucleus projects ipsilaterally through the lateral lemniscus, projects contralaterally via trapezoid body to contralateral lateral lemniscus
  4. These **neurons** synapse in the inferior colliculus of the midbrain and again in the medial geniculate nucleus (MGN) of the thalamus.
  5. Finally, they **synapse** in the primary auditory cortex of the superior temporal gyrus.
  6. The **auditory cortex** is divided into separate areas for frequency, localization, speech.

D. **Balance**
  1. The **inner ear**, or labyrinth, is the location of the organs of balance.
  2. Separated into bony labyrinth and membranous labyrinth. Bony labyrinth houses the membranous labyrinth and is bounded by the petrous portion of the temporal bone.
  3. The **vestibular division** of the membranous labyrinth has two portions—a pair of otolith organs and three perpendicular semicircular canals.
   a. The membranous labyrinth is filled with endolymph similar to intracellular fluid. (Excessive endolymph production can cause Ménière disease.) This labyrinth is surrounded by perilymph similar to cerebrospinal fluid (CSF), which drains into CSF by the perilymphic duct.
  4. The **otolith organs** detect linear acceleration and are housed in the utricle.
   a. The **utricle** has a thickened portion with hair cells called the macule.
   b. The **macule** is covered by a jellylike substance. Calcium carbonate crystals called otoliths are embedded in this substance. When the head is erect, the macula is horizontal.
   c. The saccule also contains a macule oriented vertically.
  5. The **semicircular canals** detect angular acceleration.
   a. Semicircular canals begin and end at utricle; each has enlarged region near utricle called the ampule.
   b. Inside the ampule is the ampullary crest, an epithelial hillock on top of which resides vestibular hair cells surrounded by the cupula, a jellylike substance.
   c. With rotation of the head, the cupula displaces the hair cells.

6. **Hairs of each cell:** one large cilia (kinocilium) and about 50 tapering stereocilia.
7. **Hair cells** excite nerve fibers, which have their cell bodies in vestibular ganglion, each having a superior and inferior division. Inferior division innervates posterior semicircular canal and posterior part of saccular macule. Superior division innervates all other regions.
8. The **axons** form the vestibular portion of the vestibulocochlear nerve and run through internal auditory meatus with facial nerve. They synapse at four different sites, each with a different function: lateral vestibular nucleus (LVN), medial vestibular nucleus (MVN), superior vestibular nucleus (SVN), and inferior vestibular nucleus (IVN)
    a. **Ventral LVN** is innervated by utricular macule and semicircular canals. Dorsal LVN is innervated by cerebellum and spinal cord and projects to lateral vestibulospinal tract (LVT), which allows for baseline tone in leg extensors and arm flexors, giving upright posture. Purkinje cells of cerebellar vermis inhibit dorsal nucleus. Decerebrate rigidity is caused by unopposed excitation of the LVN.
    b. **MVN** is innervated by the semicircular ducts and projects to medial vestibulospinal tract, which terminates in cervical spinal cord in motor synapses controlling neck muscles. It controls reflexive head movements correlated with the eyes.
    c. **Both MVN and SVN** project to medial longitudinal fasciculus and participate in vestibulooculomotor reflexes.
    d. **IVN** receives input from the components of the vestibular nerve and cerebellar vermis. It projects to the vestibulospinal and vestibuloreticular pathways.

E. **Smell and taste**
  1. **Smell**
      a. **Olfactory epithelium** lay in 5 cm² region of posterior nasal cavity over superior, medial turbinates. Bipolar neurons projecting through cribriform plate onto olfactory bulb in groups of 10 to 100. Each group synapses on tufted cells and one mitral cell in olfactory bulb. New olfactory epithelium is formed every 60 days.
      b. **Mitral cells** project to inhibitory periglomerular cells. These cells control habituation of smells; that is, a person wearing perfume does not smell the perfume after a while, but everyone else does.
      c. **Mitral, tufted cells** project to five areas: anterior olfactory nucleus (AON), olfactory tubercle, pyriform cortex, cortical nucleus of amygdala (CNA), entorhinal area (EA).
          i. AON projects to contralateral olfactory bulb through anterior commissure.
          ii. Olfactory tubercle projects to medial dorsal nucleus (MDN) of thalamus via stria medullaris, then orbitofrontal cortex. This and MDN mediate perception of odors.
          iii. The pyriform cortex projects to the CNA and EA.
          iv. CNA and EA are thought to be involved in the affective component of odors. This is supposed, in part, due to the projection of the EA to the hippocampus.
  2. **Taste**
      a. **Taste receptor cells** located on tongue; taste buds located in three types of papillae.
          i. Several hundred fungiform papillae on anterior two thirds of tongue contain one to five taste buds.
          ii. Foliate papilla on posterior edges of tongue degenerate by second or third year of life.
          iii. Eight to 12 large circumvallate papilla located just anterior to the sulcus terminalis.
          iv. There are about 3,000 taste buds. Each contains 50–150 receptor cells. Average lifespan is 10 days; therefore, it takes about 10 days to recover taste when you burn your tongue.
      b. **There are four (probably five) primary tastes:** sweet at tip of tongue, salty at frontal half along sides, sour along sides, and bitter along back. L-Glutamate is the fifth taste.
      c. **Taste innervation:**
          i. **Anterior two thirds** of tongue (fungiform papillae)—chorda tympani branch of CN VII with cell bodies in the geniculate ganglion.
          ii. **Posterior one third** (fungiform and circumvallate)—lingual branch of CN IX with cell bodies in the petrosal ganglion.
          iii. **Palate**—greater petrosal branch of CN IX, cell bodies in the petrosal ganglion

iv. **Epiglottis and esophagus**—superior laryngeal branch of CN X with cell bodies in the nodose ganglion
  d. All **taste innervation synapses** in rostral lateral solitary nucleus in medulla gustatory nucleus. They project to parvocellular portion of ventral posterior nucleus (VPN) of thalamus and then to gustatory region of postcentral gyrus and frontal operculum and insula. A few neurons of gustatory nucleus project to pontine parabrachial nuclei.

F. **Pain**, the most common presenting complaint
  1. More than **2 million** adult Americans are unable to work because of chronic pain.
  2. **Pain is conscious unpleasant sensation** originating from specific part of body. Nociception is nervous signal of nociceptors that may be experienced as pain.
  3. **Confusing** aspects of pain
    a. **Hyperalgesia** is primary (due to the original injury) and secondary (spread of hyperalgesia to regions not including the original injury)
    b. **Deafferentation pain** caused by hyperactivity of dorsal horn neurons without afferent input, as is seen in phantom limb pain
    c. **Thalamic pain** syndrome is pain anywhere in the body, usually due to involvement of ventrobasal thalamus
  4. **Nociceptors** may be thinly myelinated (Aδ) and unmyelinated C fibers
    a. **Dorsal horn neurons** are divided into two broad classes: nociceptive specific neurons and wide dynamic range, which receive signals from both nociceptors and mechanoreceptors.
    b. **Aα and Aβ mechanoreceptor fibers** synapse in laminae V, VI, and I
    c. **Aδ and C nociceptors** synapse in the dorsal horn and travel up and down a few spinal segments in the tract of Lissauer before synapsing.
    d. **Aδ nociceptors** synapse in lamina V and lamina I
    e. **C nociceptors** synapse in lamina II, which project to lamina I
    f. Somatic, visceral components project to same neurons on dorsal horn ⇒ referred pain.
    g. Nociceptors release glutamate and peptides including substance P
  5. There are **five major pathways for pain transmission**
    a. **Spinothalamic tract**—Laminae I and V–VII decussate in spinal cord, travel in anterolateral system (ALS), and synapse in central lateral nucleus (CLN) of thalamus. It then synapses in postcentral gyrus and association cortex.
      i. CLN has two groups of nuclei: the medial nuclear group from laminae VI, VII, VIII and the lateral nuclear group from laminae I and V
    b. **Spinoreticular tract**—Laminae VII, VIII most, but not all, decussate in spinal cord and all travel up the ALS. They synapse in the reticular formation of the pons and medulla and then project to CLN; this follows the same pathway as the spinothalamic tract.
    c. **Spinomesencephalic tract**—Laminae I and V decussate and synapse on the mesencephalic reticular formation (lateral periaqueductal gray). These connect to hypothalamus and then to limbic system.
    d. **Spinocervical tract**—Few neurons in laminae III, IV project to lateral cervical nucleus of upper cervical cord, then decussate, travel via medial lemniscus to the VPL and posterior medial nuclei (PM).
    e. **Dorsal column**—Lamina III, IV synapse on gracile and cuneate nuclei of medulla.
  6. **Periaqueductal gray neurons** descend, synapse in nucleus raphe magnus, nucleus paragigantocellularis of medulla, and then via dorsolateral furunculus to synapse in laminae I, II, V as inhibitory connections.

II. Movement

A. **Voluntary movement**
  1. **Primary motor cortex** (MI) = Precentral gyrus = Brodmann 4
    a. Each motor cortex is organized somatotopically

b. **Supplementary motor cortex** (MII) = superior and medial hemisphere anterior to precentral gyrus = Brodmann 6. Stimulation causes movement on both sides of body.
   c. **Premotor cortex** = lateral hemisphere anterior to precentral gyrus also Brodmann 6. Stimulation causes movement of more than one joint.
   d. **Cingulate gyrus** Brodmann 24 is an additional premotor area.
 2. **Projections** in and among the various areas
   a. Each of MI, MII, and premotor cortex project to each other.
   b. MI projects to cerebellum; this projects to caudal ventral lateral nucleus of thalamus (VLc), rostral part of ventral posterolateral nucleus of thalamus (VPLr), and nucleus X of thalamus. VLc and VPLr reciprocally interconnect with MI.
   c. MII projects to striatum; this projects to globus pallidus, subsequently to rostral ventral lateral nucleus of thalamus (VLr), and ventral anterior nucleus (VA).
   d. The premotor cortex and nucleus X of the thalamus reciprocally interconnect.
 3. What do we know about movement?
   a. MI encodes both degree and acceleration of force.
   b. The direction of force is provided by the vector sum of a group of neurons, each providing impulse and direction. During movement, MI receives updated information about muscle coordinates and motion.
   c. Purposeful movements originate in MII and premotor areas. Complex movement and bilateral movement are planned in MII, but executed with the premotor areas.
   d. The posterior parietal lobe Brodmann 5, 7, 39, 40 coordinates movement with sight.

B. **Spinal reflexes**
 1. **Afferent receptors** (encapsulated)
   a. **Muscle spindles** are located parallel to muscle fibers. They are innervated by group I (large, thickly myelinated) fibers and group II (small, myelinated) fibers.
     i. Each spindle has muscle fibers called **intrafusal fibers** (regular fibers are extrafusal); these do not contribute to force contraction. There are three different kinds of intrafusal fibers.
     ii. **Nuclear chain fibers** have nuclei in parallel.
     iii. **Nuclear bag fibers** have nuclei in their center. There are static and dynamic versions of nuclear bag fibers. Each muscle spindle has one of each.
     iv. Two types of sensory endings terminate on muscle spindles. One group (Gr) Ia axon terminate on all intrafusal fibers (primary ending). Primary endings are sensitive to rate of change of muscle length, muscle length. They reset their basal firing with a new static length, remaining sensitive to velocity. One group II axon terminates on one chain, static bag intrafusal fibers (secondary ending). Secondary endings are sensitive to muscle length.
     v. **Muscle spindles** are innervated by two types of gamma motor neurons and some collaterals of alpha motor neurons (which normally innervate only extrafusal fibers). Firing of these efferents causes shortening of intrafusal fibers and increased rate of firing of sensory afferents. A gamma motor neuron called static motor neurons causes increased firing during static conditions of both primary and secondary endings. Static motor neurons innervate nuclear chain and static bag fibers. Another type, called dynamic motor neurons, markedly increases firing of primary endings during change of muscle length. These innervate dynamic nuclear bag fibers.
     vi. During contraction, **gamma motor neurons** stimulate intrafusal fibers to maintain tension. Motor cortex stimulation causes simultaneous activation of both alpha and gamma motor neurons.
   b. **Golgi tendon organs** are located between muscle and tendon and innervated by group I fibers.
     i. **Collagen** that connects to tendon and the extrafusal fibers surrounding the Golgi tendon organ forms a capsule. Collagen bundles are braided inside Golgi tendon organ.

ii. A single Gr Ib afferent enters capsule, loses its myelination, and branches into multiple fine endings that innervate collagen bundles. When tendon is stretched, afferent increases firing. Even a single motor unit twitch is registered by the afferent.
2. Stretch reflexes
   a. Gr Ia transmit muscle stretch to spinal cord through dorsal roots. Some afferents make excitatory connections with same muscle and others excite inhibitory neurons of antagonist motor units. Thus, muscle reflexes are both monosynaptic and bi-synaptic.
   b. **Muscle tone** is regulated by stretch reflexes. Normal tone maintained by corrections applied to counterbalance changes. Muscle spindles enhance feedback responsiveness.
   c. Larger corrections are seen in increased tone with stretch reflexes causing the overcorrection. This makes for oscillating movements like clonus of the ankle extensors with applied dorsiflexion in spasticity causing a 4-Hz oscillation of ankle extensors.
   d. **Stretch reflexes** help maintain smooth response with rapid movement. Without the stretch reflexes, such changes are neither smooth nor symmetric.
3. **Spinal coordination** is allowed by inhibitory interneurons.
   a. There are **three major types of spinal inhibitory interneurons**:
      i. **Gr Ia inhibitory interneurons** coordinate reciprocal muscles.
      ii. **Renshaw cells** located in ventral horn form a negative feedback loop in which increased muscle firing causes increased inhibition of motor neurons of muscles that send afferents to it, increased inhibition of neurons that innervate synergistic muscles, and disinhibition of Gr Ia interneurons of antagonist muscles.
      iii. **Gr Ib inhibitory interneurons** are innervated by Golgi tendon organs, Ia afferents, cutaneous and joint afferents, and descending central pathways. The Gr Ib inhibitory interneurons innervate same muscle as Golgi tendon organ and modulate fine motor control.
   b. **Flexion withdrawal** is a protective graded reflex where limb flexes due to flexor muscle activation and extensor muscle inhibition with strength proportional to noxious stimulus. This activates crossed extensor reflex where, in contralateral limb, extensors activated flexors inhibited. The purpose of crossed extensor reflex is to enhance postural stability with flexor withdrawal; this helps maintain fluidity during voluntary movements.
   c. **Walking** is a series of steps. It can be done automatically because the coordination takes place in the spinal cord, as part of reflex behavior.
      i. In animals, stimulation of several nuclei will produce walking. *N*-methyl-D-aspartate (NMDA) receptors play some role. Balance requires intact vestibular system and brainstem functioning.
      ii. Afferent input improves coordination and compensates for external disturbances. An example is the stumble corrective action, which produces brisk flexion on cutaneous stimulation of the bottom of the foot (in cats).

C. Posture
   1. **Posture is maintained by two major mechanisms.** Anticipatory mechanisms predict changes and have programmed responses to correct for the changes. They are improved by experience. Compensatory mechanisms are rapid stereotyped movements evoked by sensory changes following loss of balance.
      a. These mechanisms are graded to maintain stable posture.
      b. Muscle proprioceptors, vestibular receptors, and visual changes all activate them.
      c. Anticipatory and compensatory mechanisms are used during standing and walking.
      d. While moving an external object, postural muscles contract before movement is executed to maintain stability. In fact, movement is delayed until the postural response.
      e. Vestibular reflexes arise from head position changes and neck reflexes from neck position changes. They maintain head position while moving.
         i. When the neck moves backward there is reflex arm, leg extension, forward flexion.
         ii. Left arm rotation produces extension of left extremities and flexion of right extremities.

2. **Pathways**
   a. **Vestibulospinal:** Semicircular canals, otolith organs project to medial, lateral, vestibular nucleus (only otolith) of medulla. Lateral vestibular nucleus projects ipsilaterally via lateral vestibular tract to all spinal segments: excites extensors and inhibits flexors. Medial vestibular nucleus projects bilaterally through medial vestibulospinal tracts to cervical, thoracic segments innervating back, neck motor units, and interneurons.
   b. **Corticospinal and reticulospinal:** Premotor, motor, and sensory cortex project to pontine reticular formation (PRF). Some neurons synapse there. More synapsing occurs at medullary reticular formation (MRF). PRF projects ipsilaterally through medial reticulospinal tract. MRF projects bilaterally through lateral reticulospinal tract. MRF inhibits spinal reflexes. PRF facilitates spinal reflexes.
      i. These reflexes coordinate posture and movement. Loss increases use of compensatory mechanisms to maintain posture.
      ii. Destruction of the brainstem above the vestibular nuclei and below the red nucleus causes decerebrate rigidity. Vestibulospinal and reticulospinal pathways become tonically activated, causing activation of extensor motor units. Destruction of the vestibular nerves reduces decerebrate rigidity by decreasing tonic activation of vestibular nuclei.
   c. **Lesions of premotor cortex or pathway** produce spasticity with a similar activation pattern as decerebrate rigidity.
   d. **Decorticate rigidity**, or leg extension and arm flexion, is seen with intact brainstem and large cortical lesions. This happens, in part, because the rubrospinal tract projects to the cervical cord, counteracting the vestibulospinal influence on arm but not leg.

D. **Cerebellum**
   1. The cerebellum has more than 50% of brain neurons.
   2. It is composed of gray matter, white matter, and three pairs of deep nuclei: fastigial, interposed, and dentate. White matter courses through cerebellum, branching like a tree. Smallest branching and its surrounding gray matter is called a folia (leaf-like pattern).
      a. Primary fissure divides cerebellum into anterior and posterior lobes. The posterolateral fissure divides posterior lobe from flocculonodular lobe. Smaller fissures divide anterior and posterior lobes into lobules.
   3. There are **ten lobules** from anterior and making an arc around the cerebellum: lingula, central, culmen (primary fissure), declive, folium (horizontal fissure), tuber, pyramis, uvula (medially) and tonsil (laterally), (posterolateral fissure) nodulus (medially), and flocculus (laterally)
      a. **Cerebellum** is divided by two longitudinal furrows into vermis and two hemispheres. Each hemisphere is divided into lateral and intermediate regions.
      b. Histologically, **cerebellum has three layers**.
         i. **Outermost layer**: molecular layer, mainly composed of granule cell axons running parallel to folium. Also interneurons (stellate and basket cells), dendrites of Purkinje cells.
         ii. **Middle layer** is Purkinje cell layer; this contains Purkinje cells in a single layer. They are inhibitory, use γ-aminobutyric acid (GABA) as their neurotransmitter, are sole output of cerebellum.
         iii. **Innermost layer** is granular layer; contains cell bodies of granular cells. Their number exceeds the number of neurons in cerebral cortex. Also, cerebellar glomeruli where granule cells receive contacts from afferent mossy afferents. Golgi cells suppress mossy fiber excitation of granule cells by decreasing period of excitation.
      c. The **afferent input** to cerebellum is of **four different types**.
         i. **Mossy fibers** are projections of brainstem nuclei; form spinocerebellar tracts. Each granule cell excites row of Purkinje cells. Surrounding this is a row of inhibition originating from basket cell activation. Summation of many granule cell excitations will produce a single action potential (simple spike).
         ii. **Climbing fibers** originate in inferior olivary nucleus. Each one contacts from one to five Purkinje cells and each Purkinje cell only has connections from a single

climbing fiber. A single firing will produce a large amplitude action potential followed by a high frequency series of smaller action potentials (complex spike).
  iii. The **raphe nuclei** terminates on both the granular and molecular layers with serotonergic neurotransmission transmission.
  iv. The **locus ceruleus** terminates on all three layers with noradrenergic neurotransmission.
  d. The **cerebellum** has **three different functional divisions**.
      i. The **spinocerebellum** is the vermis and the intermediate hemispheres. This receives afferents from spinal cord, with vermis receiving midline information and intermediate hemispheres from periphery. They also receive somatotopically organized auditory, vestibular, and visual afferents.
      ii. **Somatic sensory afferent projections** to spinocerebellum are four: dorsal spinocerebellar tract for peripheral sensation in the trunk and legs; ventral spinocerebellar tract provides information about interneuron activity; cuneocerebellar and rostral spinocerebellar tracts provide information about the neck and arms
      iii. The **spinocerebellar cortex** seems to have two somatotopic maps of the body, one each in the anterior and posterior lobes, oriented opposite one another. These somatotopic maps show fractured somatotopy: a sharply demarcated peripheral area sends afferents to a sharply demarcated area in the spinocerebellar cortex, but adjacent regions of the cortex can receive information from quite separate parts of the body.
  e. The **vermis** projects somatotopically to fastigial nuclei, which project bilaterally to lateral vestibular nuclei, reticular formation, and crossed projections to ventrolateral thalamus (VL). These synapse on a different population of neurons as the globus pallidus. The information to VL is projected to MI. The intermediate hemispheres project to interposited nuclei. The interposited nuclei project via superior cerebellar peduncle to contralateral magnocellular part of red nucleus. Some projections from superior cerebellar peduncle change direction and synapse in the VL, which projects to limb areas of the motor cortex. The spinocerebellum controls ongoing limb movement.
  f. The **intermediate hemispheric projections** to contralateral rubro- and corticospinal tracts decussate in the superior cerebellar peduncle. These tracts themselves decussate before projecting to spinal cord. This means that as they cross twice, lesions in the intermediate hemisphere produce ipsilateral deficits.
  g. The **spinocerebellum** controls movement execution and maintenance of basal muscle tone. Spinocerebellar lesions cause great reduction in gamma motor neuron activity, which in turn causes a strong reduction in afferent activity from muscle spindles.
4. The **cerebrocerebellum** is the lateral hemispheres. It receives input from pontine cortical relays of primary sensory, motor, premotor, and posterior parietal cortices and projects to the dentate nucleus. The dentate nucleus projects to the motor cortex and thalamus, which projects back to the premotor cortex (Brodmann 6) and parvocellular part of the red nucleus. This part of the red nucleus projects back to the cerebellum via the ipsilateral inferior olivary nucleus. It functions in planning, timing, and initiation of movement. Lesions cause five dysfunctions: terminal tremor, overshooting of rapid movements (hypermetria), repetition of simple but fast tapping movements, delays in starting and ending movements, and inability to determine length of time elapsed.
5. The **vestibulocerebellum** is the flocculonodular lobe. It receives afferent input from medullary vestibular nuclei and sends reciprocal efferent output. It controls fluidity of body and eye movement during standing and walking.
6. The **cerebellum** is necessary for learning motor skills.

E. **Basal ganglia**
  1. Controls movement through **five nuclei:** caudate, putamen, globus pallidus, subthalamic nucleus, and substantia nigra.
  2. The **neostriatum** (caudate and putamen), receives afferent input of basal ganglia, which comes from the intralaminar nuclei of the thalamus and the cerebral cortex. Both are

topographically organized. The most important connection is the corticostriatum, which receives input from the entire cerebral cortex.
- a. The **putamen** functions in motor control.
- b. **Caudate** has three functions. Body involved in eye movements, projects to superior colliculus, and thalamus to control saccadic eye movements (oculomotor circuit). Dorsolateral caudate has projections from dorsolateral prefrontal cortex; involved with memory of spatial orientation (dorsolateral prefrontal circuit). Ventromedial caudate has projections from lateral orbitofrontal cortex; is involved in behavior (lateral orbitofrontal circuit).
- c. **Neostriatum** projects to globus pallidus through striatopallidal pathway and substantia nigra through striatonigral pathway.
3. The **globus pallidus** is divided into internal segment (GPi), external segment (GPe). GPe projects to subthalamic nucleus. GPi, substantia nigra pars reticulata (SNpr) projects to ventral lateral, ventral anterior, and mediodorsal nuclei of thalamus. The GPi projects to centromedian nucleus of thalamus.
4. The **substantia nigra** (SN) has two parts: SNpr and pars compacta (SNpc). The SNpr is the ventral pale zone that resembles the GPi. The SNpc is the dorsal dark zone containing dopamine.
5. **Subthalamic nucleus** (STN) projects to GPi. Lesions of STN produce hemiballismus.
6. Disorders of the motor system
   - a. Parkinson's disease destroys more than 90% of SN dopaminergic neurons before patient shows signs. Degeneration of noradrenergic neurons of locus ceruleus, serotonergic neurons of raphe nuclei occurs. Main treatments are dopamine replacement and enhancement of dopamine reception.
   - b. Huntington disease destroys the intrastriatal cholinergic and GABAergic neurons. Loss of inhibitory GABA transmission causes dyskinesias.

F. Ocular motor system
1. Eye muscles
   - a. In **floor of fourth ventricle**, CN VI (abducens nucleus) projects to lateral rectus muscle. Lateral rectus muscle abducts eye. Abducens lesion will cause diplopia on lateral gaze.
   - b. At **level of superior colliculus in midbrain**, oculomotor nucleus projects to medial, inferior, and superior recti, and inferior oblique muscles. Medial rectus muscle adducts eye. Inferior rectus moves eye down and out. Superior rectus moves eye up and in. Inferior oblique moves eye up and out. Oculomotor lesion causes mydriasis, ptosis, inability to move past midline. Downward movement is only possible if eye moves down and in.
   - c. At the **level of the inferior colliculus in the midbrain**, the trochlear nucleus innervates the superior oblique muscle. This muscle moves the eye down and in. A lesion causes skew deviation and patients often turn their head toward the paretic side, tilting their head.
2. The eye is kept on target by **five control systems**.
   - a. The **vestibuloocular system** keeps an image stable during brief head rotation using afferents from the vestibular system. There is specific control of semicircular canals on eye muscles; for example, horizontal semicircular canal activates ipsilateral medial rectus and contralateral lateral rectus and inhibits contralateral medial rectus and ipsilateral lateral rectus. When head is still, a tonic signal is sent. When the head is moved in canal's plane, signal increases and away from plane causes decreased signal. It should be no surprise that lesions in the vestibular system cause nystagmus, with both eyes driven to one direction by the imbalance and then jerked back by the functioning canal.
   - b. The **optokinetic** keeps an image stable during sustained head rotation. It complements the vestibuloocular system by using visual information.
     - i. The **optokinetic reflex** uses this—here one expects saccades when a vertically striped drum is slowly moved because the eye tracks the stripe.
     - ii. The **optokinetic** interprets visual motion as head motion. This is the source for all kinds of optical illusions.

iii. Both the **optokinetic and vestibuloocular reflexes** are under voluntary control and can learn from experience. This modulation requires the cerebellum.
   c. **Saccadic eye movements** shift an image rapidly from periphery to central vision. Horizontal saccades are created by paramedian pontine reticular formation. Vertical saccades are created by rostral interstigial nucleus of medial longitudinal fasciculus in the mesencephalic reticular formation.
   d. The **pursuit movements** keep the image of a moving target. It is voluntary and requires concentration. For pursuit to be smooth, pons, cerebellum, and cerebral cortex have to be functioning.
   e. The **vergence movements** move eyes in opposite directions to adjust for depth vision. It is controlled by neurons near midbrain oculomotor nucleus.

III. Integration of Motor and Sensory Systems

A. **Cranial nerves**
  1. **Functional classification of cranial nerves**—neuroscientists have given up classification, but it is still in relatively common use among neurologists, so worth reviewing.
     a. **General somatic afferent**—temperature, pain, touch, and proprioception of the skin, muscles of the head and neck, and mouth CN V, VII, IX, X
     b. **Special somatic afferent**—hearing, balance, vision with cochlea, vestibular organ, retina CN II, VIII
     c. **General visceral afferent**—mechanical, pain, temperature, and proprioception of pharynx, larynx, gut, cardiac, smooth muscle CN V, VII, IX, X
     d. **Special visceral afferent**—olfaction and taste CN I, VII, IX, X
     e. **General somatic efferent**—control of somatic skeletal muscles CN III, IV, XI, XII
     f. **General visceral efferent**—control of autonomic effectors CN III, VII, IX, X
     g. **Special visceral efferent**—control of branchiomeric skeletal muscles CN V, VII, IX, X, XI
  2. **Cranial nerves and their pathways** have been covered in sufficient detail. Here, we will give the location of each nuclei and other important structures, as having a three-dimensional (3D) understanding will aid in localization (Figures 2-2–2-4).

IV. Homeostasis and Arousal

A. **Hypothalamus and limbic system**
  1. **The limbic system includes:** parahippocampal gyrus, cingulate gyrus, subcallosal gyrus, hippocampal formation (hippocampus, dentate gyrus, and subiculum), prefrontal cortex, and the amygdala.
     a. **The hippocampal formation** projects to the hippocampus through the subiculum. The subiculum is innervated by the hippocampus and the neocortex and innervates the hypothalamus via the fornix. This pathway is called the perforant pathway.
        i. The hippocampus is a three-layered cortex: molecular layer, granule cell layer, polymorphic cell layer
        ii. The hippocampus is covered by the white matter alveus
     b. **Amygdala** connected to hypothalamus, hippocampal formation, neocortex, thalamus reciprocally; afferents from olfactory; two major efferent projections
        i. Stria terminalis projects to nucleus of stria terminalis, nucleus accumbens, and hypothalamus.
        ii. The ventral amygdalofugal pathway projects to the hypothalamus, dorsal medial nucleus of the thalamus, and the rostral cingulate gyrus.
        iii. The amygdala functions primarily in learning the required coordination of different sensory modalities as well as emotional responses.
     c. The **parahippocampal gyrus** has a six-layered cortex.

d. **Circuit of Papez:** hippocampus ⇒ alveus ⇒ fimbriae ⇒ fornix ⇒ mammillary bodies of hypothalamus ⇒ anterior nucleus of thalamus ⇒ cingulate gyrus ⇒ amygdala ⇒ hippocampus
2. The **hypothalamus** has multiple **nuclei**.
   a. **Supraoptic** nucleus controls thirst and water balance.
   b. **Lateral** nucleus controls hunger.
   c. **Ventromedial** nucleus controls satiety.
   d. **Anterior** hypothalamus controls cooling and parasympathetics.
   e. **Posterior** hypothalamus controls heating.
   f. **Septate** nucleus controls emotions and sexual behavior.
   g. **Suprachiasmatic** nucleus controls circadian rhythms.
3. All connections in the hypothalamus are bidirectional except for hypothalamohypophysial tract, which contains efferents from paraventricular and supraoptic nuclei. Hypothalamus receives afferents from the retina.
4. The hypothalamus controls the **endocrine system**.
   a. **Neurohypophyseal system:** vasopressin and oxytocin transported down axons of magnocellular neurons to posterior pituitary where released into general circulation.
   b. **Adenohypophyseal system:** releasing or inhibiting factors are released by parvocellular neurons into the hypophyseal-portal circulation to control the synthesis and release of hormones from anterior pituitary into general circulation.
   c. **Hormone pairs** (releasing unless stated otherwise)
      i. Thyrotropin releasing hormone ⇒ thyrotropin, prolactin
      ii. Prolactin releasing factor ⇒ prolactin
      iii. Dopamine ⇒ inhibits release of prolactin
      iv. Corticotropin releasing hormone ⇒ adrenocorticotropin, β-lipotropin
      v. Gonadotropin-releasing hormone ⇒ luteinizing hormone (LH), follicle-stimulating hormone (FSH)
      vi. Growth hormone ⇒ GH
      vii. Somatostatin ⇒ inhibits release of GH, thyrotropin
      viii. Melanocyte stimulating factor ⇒ MSH, β-endorphin
      ix. Melanocyte stimulating hormone release inhibiting factor ⇒ MSH
   d. **Hormonal reflexes**
      i. Vasopressin is released at a rate dependent on serum sodium, blood osmolarity, and blood volume to maintain appropriate hydration. Skin temperature may also affect vasopressin release. Vomiting causes a large release of vasopressin.
      ii. Milk ejection from breasts: afferent pathway-suckling, efferent pathway-oxytocin

B. **Autonomic nervous system** (ANS)
   1. **Three divisions:** sympathetic, parasympathetic, and enteric
   2. **The ANS differs from somatic nervous system in three ways:** It is involuntary, it has synapses from the CNS and outside the CNS, thus is di-synaptic, and muscles are directly inhibited. For example, somatic system, muscles inhibited by inhibiting neurons that innervate them.
   3. The **sympathetic division** is located in spinal cord from T1–L3
      a. **Cell bodies** are located in the intermediolateral gray of the spinal cord (lamina VII).
      b. **Axons** travel in the ventral root of the spinal cord and then the white communicating ramus, where they synapse at the paravertebral chain ganglia with many postganglionic neurons. The ganglia where they synapse are usually at several levels, which can be up/down, or the same vertebral level. (A few do not synapse at the paravertebral chain ganglia; they synapse in prevertebral ganglia: celiac, superior, and inferior mesenteric ganglia.) They then project via gray communicating rami to structures they innervate. In the head, they travel with carotid arteries. In the rest of body, they travel with spinal nerves.
   4. The **parasympathetic division** is located in brainstem and spinal cord levels S2–S4.
      a. **Neurons** project to ganglia close to their ultimate targets of innervation.

b. It includes portions of many **cranial nerves**.
    i. Edinger-Westphal nucleus with CN III to the ciliary ganglion
    ii. Superior salivary nucleus with CN VII to pterygopalatine and submandibular ganglia
    iii. Inferior salivary nucleus with CN IX to the otic ganglion
    iv. Dorsal vagal nucleus and nucleus ambiguus with CN X. The ventrolateral nucleus ambiguus projects to cardiac ganglion, which innervates heart. The dorsal vagal nucleus projects to esophagus, lungs, stomach, liver, gallbladder, pancreas, and intestinal tract.
  c. The **sacral cell bodies** reside in the interomediolateral position but do not form an organized column. They project to the plexuses of pelvic ganglia and innervate the descending colon, bladder, and external genitalia.
5. The **enteric division** can function autonomously from the CNS; its neurons located in Auerbach and Meissner plexuses. It innervates the pancreas, gallbladder, and gastrointestinal tract. It has extrinsic innervation by both the sympathetic and parasympathetic nervous system to override normal function during stress.
6. The **hypothalamus** controls the autonomic nervous system. The major control of the autonomic nervous system is the nucleus tractus solitarius. It receives afferent information from throughout the body. It responds by control of the autonomic system by a system of reflexes as well as coordinating homeostasis with higher centers of control.
7. **Preganglionic synapses** are predominantly acetylcholine (ACh). Postganglionic sympathetics release norepinephrine. Postganglionic autonomics release ACh. Both also release peptides. Most targets are innervated reciprocally by both sympathetic and parasympathetic systems. One ANS division innervates sweat glands, liver, and spleen.

V.   Localization of Higher Functions

A. While localization of function may point to certain areas of the brain being more focused on one particular function, most functions require integrated actions of neurons of several different areas.

B. The association cortices are the areas of higher function in humans.
  1. They are the limbic, prefrontal, and parietal-temporal-occipital systems
  2. The limbic association cortex is located on the temporal pole, medial and ventral surface of frontal lobe (orbitofrontal cortex), and medial surface of the parietal lobe and includes the cingulate and parahippocampal areas. This allows emotion to affect motor planning.
  3. The prefrontal association cortex located anterior to the premotor area is important in the planning of responses. It projects to the premotor cortex.
  4. The parietal-temporal-occipital association cortex links sensory information from several different modalities.

C. The prefrontal areas are divided into two areas: the prefrontal cortex and the orbitofrontal cortex.
  1. **The prefrontal cortex has three divisions,** the principal sulcus, the superior prefrontal convexity, and the inferior prefrontal convexity.
    a. The principal sulcus mediates delayed responses to tasks through associated memory.
    b. Inferior prefrontal convexity mediates any type of delayed response. Lesions produce perseverance of previously learned behavior and inappropriate behavioral responses.
    c. Arcuate sulcus (not truly contained in anatomic prefrontal cortex, but adjacent to it, and shows a related function). Appears to mediate choice of motor response to a sensory cue.
  2. **The orbitofrontal cortex** is part of the limbic system.
  3. Both regions receive input from the **medial dorsal thalamic nucleus**. They both also contain granule cells, so that this region of the brain is sometimes referred to as the frontal granular cortex, as the motor and premotor areas do not have granule cells.

D. **Limbic system**
   1. **Orbitofrontal cortex** is involved in generalized arousal. Lesions in this area produce a decrease in aggressiveness and emotional responsiveness.
   2. **Temporal portion** of limbic system is reserved for emotional responses and memory.

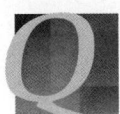

STUDY QUESTIONS FOR CHAPTER 2

Directions: Each of the numbered items or incomplete statements in this section is followed by answers or by completions of the statement. Select the ONE lettered answer or completion that is BEST in each case.

1. What are the projections to the globus pallidus?
   (A) Subthalamic nucleus
   (B) Neostriatum
   (C) Neostriatum and subthalamic nucleus
   (D) None of the above

2. What is the first layer in the retina to receive light?
   (A) Rods and cones
   (B) Inner plexiform
   (C) Outer plexiform
   (D) Ganglion cell

3. Hemiballismus is associated with a lesion in which area?
   (A) Subthalamic nucleus
   (B) GPi
   (C) GPe
   (D) Caudate

4. Which of the following is NOT correct of the infraspinatus muscle?
   (A) Nerve supply is the suprascapular nerve.
   (B) Nerve roots include C4, C5, C6.
   (C) It medially rotates the arm.
   (D) It stabilizes the shoulder joint.

5. What primary sensation bypasses the thalamus?
   (A) Hearing
   (B) Smell
   (C) Sight
   (D) Taste

6. What is the primary receptor for detecting an edge?
   (A) Merkel disk
   (B) Meissner corpuscle
   (C) Pacinian corpuscle
   (D) Ruffini ending

7. A 73-year-old man is found unresponsive by his family. After calling an ambulance, and arriving in the emergency department, you examine him. A full neurologic examination reveals only that he has difficulty with saccades. If this difficulty were to be caused by a stroke, what would be its localization?
   (A) Inferior colliculus
   (B) Superior colliculus
   (C) Fastigial nucleus
   (D) Interposited nuclei

8. A lesion in the ventroposterolateral thalamus would affect which sensation?
   (A) Ipsilateral proprioception and ipsilateral temperature sensation
   (B) Contralateral proprioception and ipsilateral temperature sensation
   (C) Ipsilateral proprioception and contralateral temperature sensation
   (D) Contralateral temperature sensation and contralateral proprioception

9. What cell group in the primary motor cortex will react to points of light?
   (A) Simple cells
   (B) Complex cells
   (C) Blob cells
   (D) None of the above

10. What is the function and projection of the dentate nucleus?
    (A) It integrates sensory and motor information and projects to the thalamus.
    (B) It functions in initiation of movement and projects to the motor cortex.
    (C) It functions in planning movement and projects to the premotor cortex.
    (D) It functions in preventing overshoot and projects to the interposited nuclei.

11. In women, the amygdala is larger than men. Which of the following stereotypes might be explained by this anatomic difference?
    (A) Women live longer than men.
    (B) Women are more thoughtful about emotions than men.
    (C) Women worry more than men.
    (D) Women seek more college degrees than men.

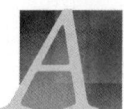# ANSWERS AND EXPLANATIONS

1. C. Neostriatum and STN. Likely you could have answered correctly by looking at the answers, even if you didn't know the answer. Occasionally, there are some questions for which you can deduce the answer from the answers offered. A and B are incomplete; D is a distracter.

2. D. Ganglion cell layer is the eighth layer. A. Inner plexiform is the seventh layer. B. outer plexiform is the fifth layer. C. Rods and cones are the second layer. The trick is that the ordering is from cornea outward.

3. A. Substantia nigra lesions cause hemiballismus. B. Lesions to the GPi have been helpful in treating medically intractable torticollis and the tremor of Parkinson disease. C. is a distractor. D. Caudate degeneration is seen in Huntington disease.

4. C. The infraspinatus muscle is innervated by the supraspinatus nerve with nerve roots C4, C5, C6, and laterally rotates arm and stabilizes the shoulder joint. Thus, A, B, and D are all incorrect answers.

5. B. Smell synapses in the MDN but also have direct connections to the limbic cortex that bypass the thalamus. A. Hearing synapses in MGN. C. Sight synapses in LGN. D. Taste synapses in VPN.

6. B. Meissner corpuscles detect edges. A. Merkel disk detects light touch. C. Pacinian corpuscle for pressure/vibration. D. Ruffini endings for pressure/stretch

7. B. Superior colliculus functions in saccades. A. Inferior colliculus is a distracter. C. Fastigial nucleus functions for antigravity. D. Interposited nuclei function in ongoing movement making movements smooth.

8. D. Pain and temperature as well as proprioceptive sensation ultimately project to the contralateral ventroposterolateral thalamus. Thus A, B, and C do not have the correct localizations.

9. C. Blob cells react to points of light and are important for color vision. A. Simple cells have oriented rectangular areas of activation surrounded by an area of inhibition. B. Complex cells have larger oriented rectangular areas than simple cells, but no area of inactivation. D. Distracter.

10. B. The primary function of the dentate nucleus is to initiate movement. It projects both to the thalamus and the motor cortex. C and D have the wrong projections. A. Tells what the dentate does, but not the function.

11. B. The function of the amygdala is in emotional processing, so this is likely. A. This may, in a small part, be due to the smaller average weight of women with increasing age. C. Although the amygdala functions in fear, it is not clear how closely fear is linked to worrying, so B is a better answer. D. This is likely due to the ability of women to obtain education more than any physical difference.

Anatomy II: Vascular Anatomy

I. Vascular Anatomy

We have provided angiograms and magnetic resonance angiography (MRA) and magnetic resonance venography (MRV) for review (Figures 3-1–3-4). Paired internal carotids (left from brachiocephalic trunk, right from innominate) splits into external and internal carotids at level of C4.

A. **Internal carotid segments**
   1. **C1** begins at carotid bifurcation and ends at the carotid canal of the petrous bone.
   2. **C2** ends at posterior edge of foramen lacerum.
   3. **C3** passes over the foramen lacerum and pierces dura; two small, inconsistent branches
   4. **C4** cavernous segment
      a. Meningohypophyseal trunk
         i. Inferior hypophyseal artery supplies posterior pituitary, occlusion implicated in Sheehan syndrome—postpartum pituitary failure
   5. **C5** ends at distal dural ring.
   6. **C6** ophthalmic segment ends just proximal to posterior communicating artery
      a. **Superior hypophyseal artery** supplies anterior pituitary and pituitary stalk.
      b. **Ophthalmic artery** supplies optic nerve; usually kinked on angiogram; a branch called the central retinal artery supplies the retina.
      c. **Posterior communicating artery**
         i. Thalamoperforators supply parts of optic tract, chiasm, and posterior hypothalamus
      d. **Anterior choroidal** supplies part of optic tract, globus pallidus internus, genu, part of posterior internal capsule (contralateral hemiplegia and hemianesthesia), optic radiation (homonymous hemianopia). These symptoms comprise Foix syndrome.

B. **Carotid artery dissection** usually occurs in patients with neck trauma who have congenital abnormality of arterial wall, e.g., fibromuscular dysplasia.
   1. Hemorrhage into medial layer of artery, spontaneous or posttraumatic.
   2. Presents with ipsilateral headache (H/A), incomplete or complete Horner (common carotid for complete, internal carotid artery [ICA] for incomplete or oculosympathetic palsy, i.e., ptosis and miosis), face, or hand pain; transient ischemic attack/cerebral vascular accident (TIA/CVA), especially with posttraumatic
   3. **Definitive diagnosis:** angiography—look for string sign or double lumen sign
   4. **Treatment:** Dissection may cause vessel occlusion. No bleeding, no emboli: intravenous (IV) heparin for 1 to 2 weeks, then warfarin for 6 to 12 weeks. Should do repeat angiogram to confirm canalization before discontinuing warfarin. Follow-up with antiplatelet medications.

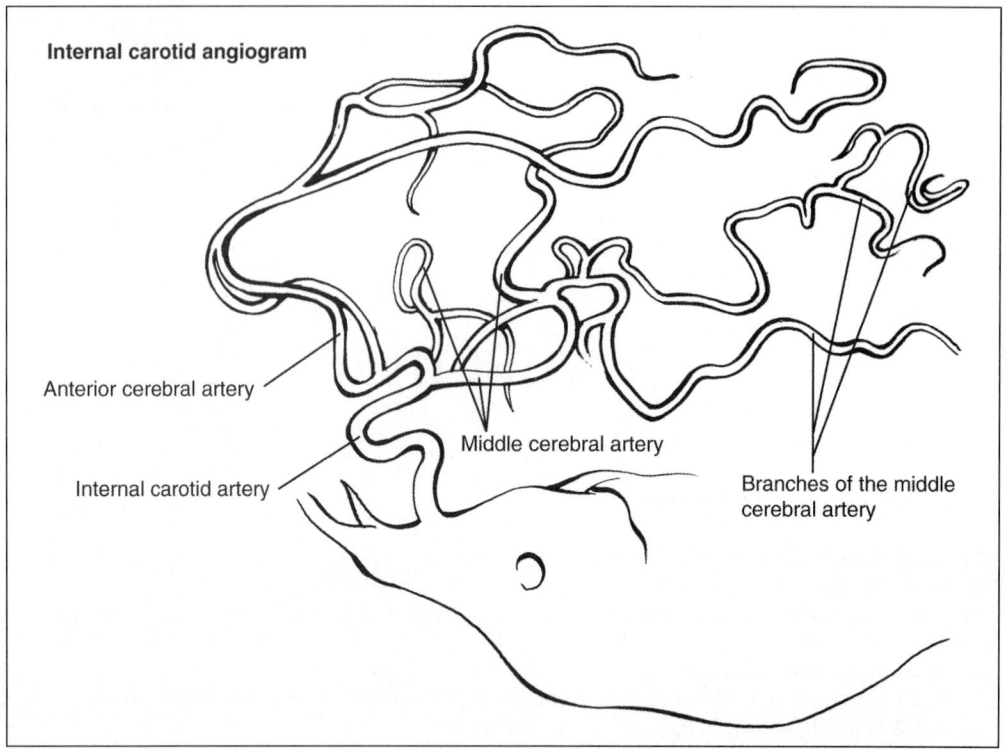

Figure 3-1 Angiogram of the internal carotid.

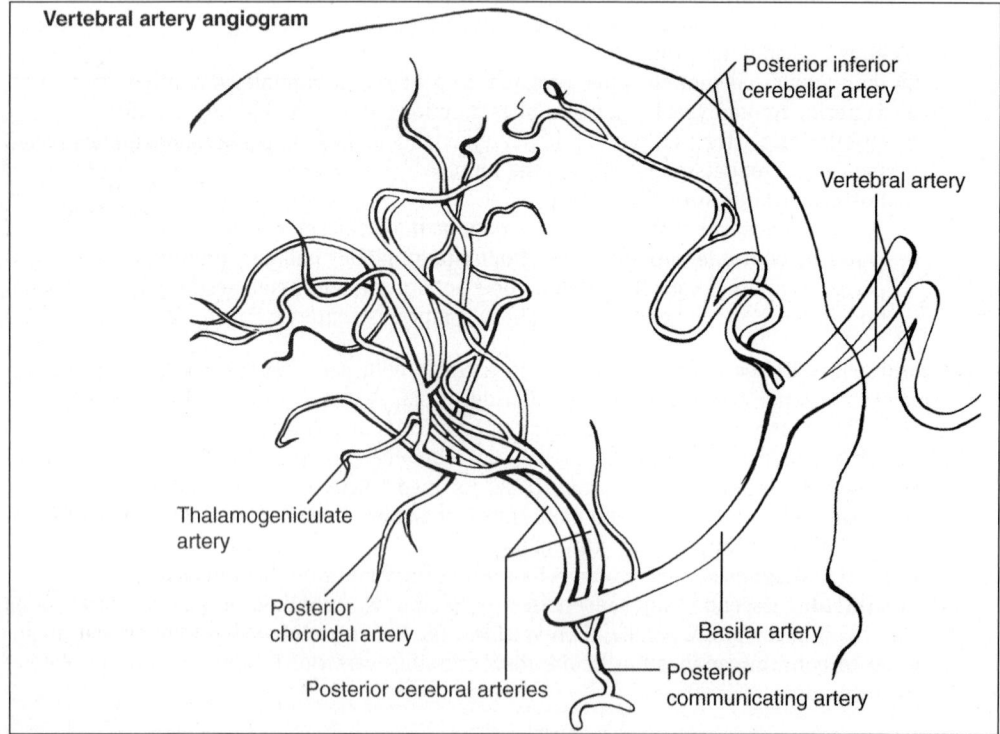

Figure 3-2 Angiogram of the vertebral artery.

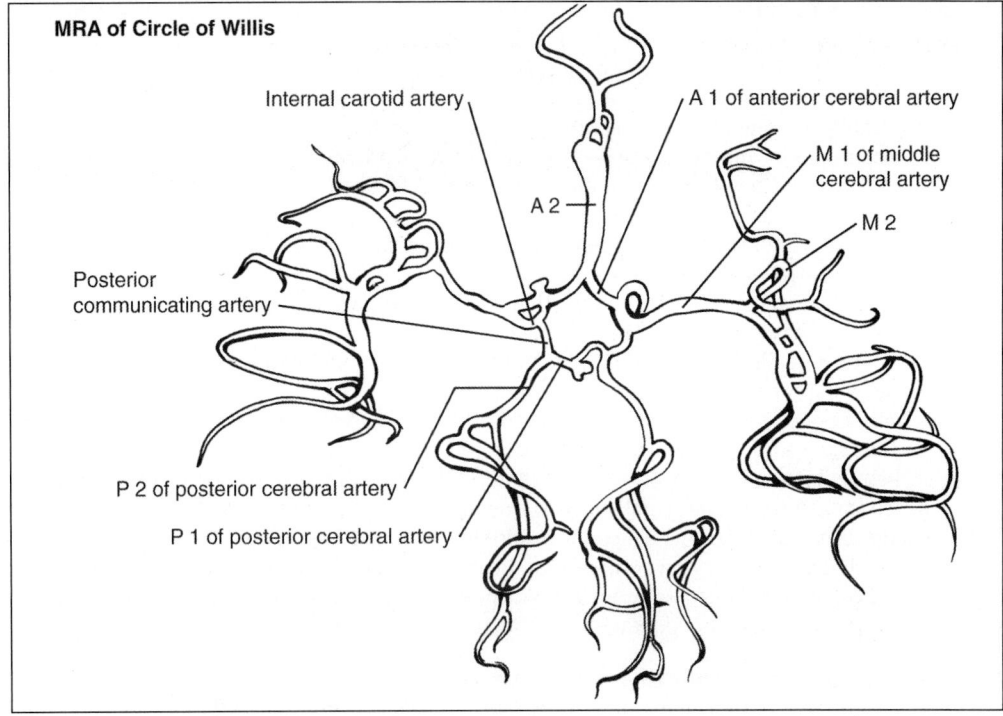

Figure 3-3 Magnetic resonance angiography (MRA) of the circle of Willis.

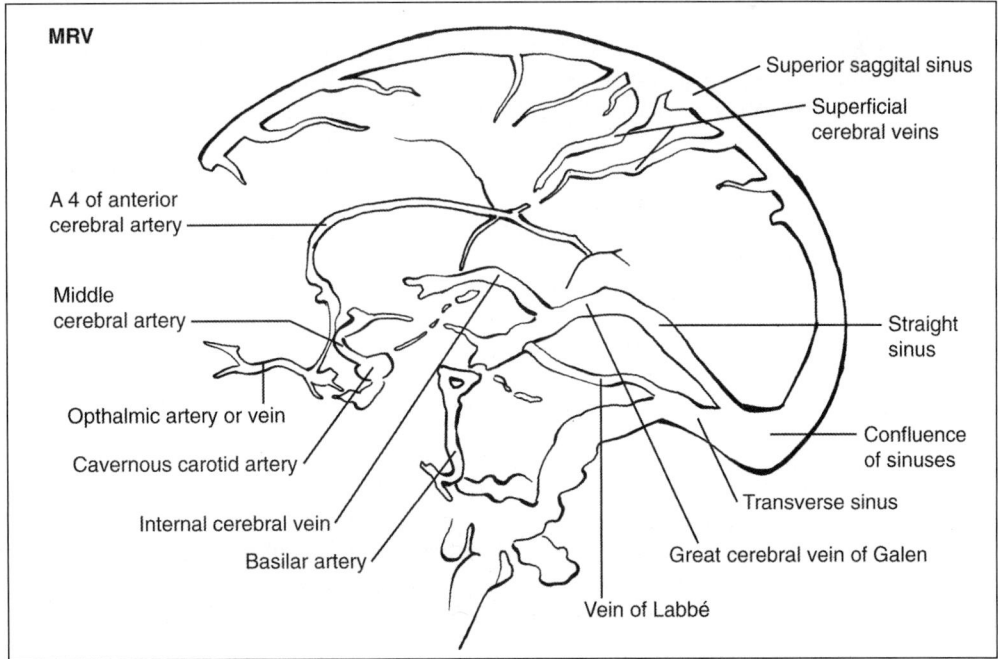

Figure 3-4 Magnetic resonance venography (MRV).

C. **Anterior cerebral artery**
   1. **A1** from end of C7 to anterior communicating artery
      a. Medial lenticulostriate arteries supply motor to hands, arms; lesion induces paresis.
      b. Orbital branches
      c. Usually present from A1-recurrent artery of Huebner supplies head of caudate and anteroinferior internal capsule. Occlusion of ACA proximal will produce facial weakness and arm spasticity. Nearby motor cortex for arm is left intact; good potential for recovery.
   2. **A2** to frontopolar artery
      a. Medial orbitofrontal artery supplies the inferomedial frontal region and damage to this region causes gait apraxia.
   3. **A3** until the callosal marginal artery (has middle and posterior internal frontal branches)
      a. Anterior internal frontal artery
   4. **A4** is the pericallosal artery; this splits into the superior and inferior internal parietal. There is also the artery of splenium of the corpus callosum.
      a. A4 supplies motor for the arm, leg, and bladder as well as sensation to foot and leg. Damage causes leg weakness with both brisk reflexes and extensor plantar response.
   5. If there is bilateral occlusion of ACA, there is weakness of both legs and urinary incontinence (bilateral posteromedial superior frontal gyrus). A2, A3, A4 run along the corpus callosum. Damage to corpus callosum results in dyspraxia and tactile aphasia of left limbs, and includes alien hand syndrome (hand can not be controlled by patient and carries out activities). ACA occlusion also results: grasp reflex, sucking reflex, paratonia (probably post frontal); abulia, lack of spontaneity, distraction, and perseveration.

D. **Middle cerebral arterycontralateral leg weakness**
   1. **M1** horizontal portion ends at trifurcation into anterior division, posterior division, and inferior division (anterior temporal artery).
      a. Lateral lenticulostriate arteries to globus pallidus externus, caudate and putamen, posterior internal capsule, and corona radiata. Damage to internal capsule causes contralateral motor weakness and anesthesia. Speech and vision may be affected (optic radiation). Within hours, areflexia and lack of plantar responses will change to hyperreflexia and extensor plantar response. With time, expect arm flexors and leg extensors to recover and patient shows arm flexed in front of the chest and walking with circumduction of affected leg.
      b. Infarctions affecting MCA are usually artery to artery or cardioembolic. M1 infarctions cause face, arm, contralateral leg weakness; hemianesthesia; homonymous hemianopia (lateral geniculate nucleus [LGN]). Head and eye deviation ipsilaterally is often seen. With normal dominance, left-sided lesions give global aphasia and right-sided lesions give anosognosia. These are devastating, with high risk of death from edema; poor potential for recovery.
   2. **M2** until emergence in the sylvian fissure
   3. Splits into anterior and inferior divisions
      a. The **anterior (or superior) division** supplies rolandic and prerolandic areas. Infarction causes the expected sensory and motor deficits: contralateral motor and sensory involving face, arm, and, to a lesser extent, leg. There will be ipsilateral deviation of head and eyes (motor areas 4+6—lateral gaze). If sensory deficit is particularly dense it is called the pseudothalamic infarct of Foix. If sensory deficit is ulnar or radial in distribution, it is called pseudoradiculopathy of Dejerine.
      b. **Inferior division** supplies lateral temporal and inferior parietal lobes. This is usually cardioembolic in origin. Infarction causes Wernicke aphasia, either superior quadrantopia or homonymous hemianopsia. There are four significant terminal branches.
         i. Precentral artery supplies motor to face and arm as well as Broca area. Infarction causes flaccid paralysis of the face and arm with total inability to speak and comprehension spared. Nondominant lesions replace dysphagia with dyspraxia.
         ii. Central artery supplies same and infarction causes arm and face paresis with mild-to-moderate dysphagia with same changes with nondominant hemispherical infarction.

iii. Posterior parietal artery supplies posterior parietal cortex. Dominant infarctions cause complete aphasia, with some creating neologisms, word salads. Some mild hemiparesis is possible. Nondominant causes geographical disorientation and dressing apraxia.
iv. Superior temporal artery supplies region of same name causing receptive aphasia.

E. **Vertebrobasilar and posterior cerebral arteries.** Many named syndromes (over 30).
  1. **Vertebral artery** (VA)
     a. **V1** first branch of subclavian artery
        i. Subclavian steal. Blockage of the subclavian proximal to V1 can cause ipsilateral arm weakness with exercise with or without headache when blood is drawn from the contralateral side
     b. **V2** begins at C6 transverse foramen
     c. **V3** begins at the exit of the C1 transverse foramen. Blockage of the VA may be asymptomatic.
     d. **V4 intradural segment**
        i. Medial medullary syndrome. V4 occlusion/basilar occlusion: CN 12 tract (ipsilateral paresis of tongue), pyramidal tract (contralateral arm, leg paresis), and medial lemniscus (contralateral decreased tactile and proprioception on that side of body)
        ii. Lateral medulla syndrome often called Wallenberg syndrome
           (a) Any of V4, posterior inferior cerebellar artery (PICA), or medullary artery occlusion
           (b) Tract, nucleus of CN 5 (pain or burning and impaired sensation of ipsilateral face), tract of CN 9+10 (dysphagia hoarseness and impaired gag), vestibular nuclei (nausea and vomiting [N/V], vertigo, nystagmus), descending sympathetic tract (ipsilateral Horner), nucleus gracilis/cuneatus (ipsilateral arm+leg impaired sensation), spinothalamic tract (contralateral impaired temperature and pain); some fall to side of lesion due to ataxia
        iii. Lateral pontomedullary syndrome; medial and lateral medulla always V occlusion
     e. **V4 has several branches,** the significant ones are the
        i. Posterior spinal (see spinal cord chapter)
        ii. PICA
           (a) Anterior medullary segment
           (b) Lateral medullary segment hence can be involved in Wallenberg
           (c) Supratonsillar segment; has one branch—the choroidal artery to the choroid plexus
           (d) Splits into two terminal branches: tonsillohemipheric (causing vertigo, limb dysmetria, N/V, gaze palsy, dysarthria, and ataxia) and inferior vermian (causing vertigo, ataxia, and nystagmus), although there is great variability in the arterial supply
        iii. Anterior spinal (see spinal cord chapter)

F. **Basilar artery** formed by the junction of the paired vertebrals
  1. **Anterior inferior cerebellar artery**
     a. Occlusion causes lateral inferior pontine syndrome; CN V tract and sensory nucleus (ipsilateral loss of facial sensation), CN VII nucleus/tract (ipsilateral facial paresis), CN VIII nucleus/tract (N/V, nystagmus, vertigo), paramedian pontine reticular formation (PPRF) (loss of conjugate gaze toward lesion), dorsal cochlear nucleus (ipsilateral deafness, tinnitus), middle cerebellar peduncle (ataxia), spinothalamic tract (contralateral loss of pain and proprioception)
     b. Inferior pontine syndrome—lateral and medial inferior pontine syndromes
  2. **Labyrinthine**
  3. **"Paramedian"** branches to the pons—syndrome depends on location
     a. **Medial inferior pontine syndrome**—several names; CN VI tract (ipsilateral lateral gaze diplopia), CN VII tract (facial weakness), CN VIII nuclei (nystagmus), PPRF (loss of conjugate gaze toward lesion), corticospinal/corticobulbar tract (contralateral face,

arm, leg paralysis), medial lemniscus (loss of tactile and proprioception of contralateral body)
  i. CN VI + hemiplegia = Raymond syndrome
  ii. CN VI, VII, hemiplegia = Millard-Gubler
  iii. Gaze palsy, facial weakness, facial numbness = Foville
b. **Medial midpontine syndrome**—middle/superior cerebellar peduncle (ipsilateral limb/gait ataxia), corticobulbar/corticospinal tract (contralateral face, arm, leg paresis); can occasionally affect the medial lemniscus (contralateral impairment of touch and proprioception)
c. **Medial superior pontine syndrome**—middle and superior cerebellar peduncle (ipsilateral cerebellar ataxia), medial longitudinal fasciculus (ipsilateral internuclear opthalmoplegia [INO]), central tegmentum (ipsilateral myoclonus anywhere in neck upward), corticobulbar/corticospinal tract (contralateral paresis of face, arm, leg), can rarely affect the medial lemniscus (contralateral impairment of touch and proprioception)
d. **Paramedian midbrain (Benedikt)**—CN III nucleus and tract (ipsilateral third palsy) and red nucleus (this is part of tract from opposite cerebellum so contralateral ataxia)
4. **Superior cerebellar artery**
  a. **Lateral superior pontine syndrome**—CN VIII nuclei (N/V, dizziness, horizontal nystagmus), middle/superior cerebellar peduncle (ipsilateral ataxia with falling to side of lesion), descending sympathetics (ipsilateral Horner), medial lateral lemniscus (contralateral impairment of touch and position leg > arm), spinothalamic (contralateral impairment of pain and heat), slurred speech

G. **Posterior cerebral:** Usually formed from basilar bifurcation, but in 20% one arises from basilar and the other from the internal carotid
  1. P1 until posterior communicating
    a. Mesencephalic perforators
    b. Interpeduncular thalamoperforators; Weber syndrome (see subsequent text), subthalamic nucleus (ipsilateral ballismus or choreoathetosis), mediodorsal (MD) nucleus (vascular Korsakoff)
    c. Medial posterior choroidal
  2. P2 until the posterolateral choroidal (we list only important branches)
    a. P2 occlusion results in basilar midbrain syndrome or Weber syndrome; CN III tract (ipsilateral third palsy), cerebral peduncle (contralateral face, hand, arm plegia)
    b. Lateral posterior choroidal
    c. Thalamogeniculate thalamoperforators supply the lateral geniculate and central and posterior thalamus
      i. Thalamic syndrome of Dejerine and Roussy; Complete sensory deficit, sometimes pain/temp > touch/proprioception, severe amnesia, taste alterations, and mood alteration possible; when sensation returns it can be accompanied by debilitating pain that can be unrelenting and excruciating.
  3. P3 occlusion results in dorsolateral midbrain infarction aka Nothnagel syndrome; CN III nucleus (ipsilateral third palsy), superior cerebellar peduncle (ipsilateral ataxia), mediolongitudinal (mlf), Horner.
    a. Quadrigeminal branches
    b. Geniculate branches to medial geniculate
    c. Posterior pericallosal—anastomoses with A4

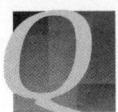 # STUDY QUESTIONS FOR CHAPTER 3

Directions: *Each of the numbered items or incomplete statements in this section is followed by answers or by completions of the statement. Select the ONE lettered answer or completion that is BEST in each case.*

1. Which stroke symptom is unlikely to be related to the others?
   (A) Dressing apraxia
   (B) Mild sensory difficulty in face
   (C) Flaccid plegia of arm and face
   (D) Geographical disorientation

2. For a brainstem stroke in single vascular territory, a patient has vertigo. Which of the following is likely to be an additional feature of the stroke?
   (A) Skew ocular deviation
   (B) Locked-in syndrome
   (C) Facial paresis
   (D) Facial anesthesia

3. A 68-year-old man has had painful paresthesias in the left side of his body for 3 years following a stroke. His primary care physician thinks that there must be another explanation, as a stroke cannot produce pain. Infarction in what vascular territory will most likely produce a stroke?
   (A) Quadrigeminal branches of the posterior cerebral artery
   (B) Mesencephalic perforators of the posterior cerebral artery
   (C) Interpeduncular thalamoperforators of the posterior cerebral artery
   (D) Thalamogeniculate thalamoperforators of the posterior cerebral artery
   (E) His primary care physician is correct—stroke cannot cause pain

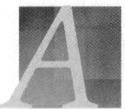

ANSWERS AND EXPLANATIONS

1. C. This question is about the four terminal branches of the MCA on the nondominant side. Three of the four symptoms A, B, and D all are consistent with posterior parietal or superior temporal artery occlusion. C is consistent with precentral or central branch occlusions.

2. D. Vertigo is most commonly associated with a lateral medulla stroke (PICA territory). Facial anesthesia is most consistent with lateral medulla, lateral caudal pontine, or lateral rostral pontine stroke. A. Skew deviation is seen with lateral rostral pons with superior cerebellar artery occlusion. B. Locked-in syndrome is a pontine stroke in the vascular territory of the basilar artery. C. Facial paresis is consistent with lateral caudal pons or inferior medial pons.

3. D. The thalamogeniculate thalamoperforators supply the lateral geniculate, central, and posterior thalamus and may produce the thalamic syndrome of Dejerine and Roussy. During recovery from this syndrome, sensation may be accompanied by debilitating painful paresthesias. The other territories noted would not be expected to produce pain.

CHAPTER 4

Physiology and Neurophysiologic Testing

I. Histology and Cytology

The nervous system is composed of two major types of cells: neurons and glial cells.

A. Nerve cell divisions
  1. **Nerves** have four components:
     a. **Cell body**—the metabolic center, consists of nucleus and perikaryon
     b. **Dendrites**—usually arborize, serve to receive inputs
        i. Pyramidal-shaped cell bodies have one group of long, thin apical dendrites and two or more groups of thicker, shorter basal dendrites.
     c. **Axon**—originates from axon hillock on cell body where action potential is generated.
        i. Axon does not have ribosomes so cannot synthesize proteins.
        ii. Specialized proteins are encased in organelles and transported to the axon terminal by axoplasmic transport.
        iii. Axons arborize: special swellings at nerve terminal called presynaptic terminals
        iv. Some nerves lack axons or have very short ones—these are interneurons, which directly affect secretion by passive spread of signals.
        v. Initial, unmyelinated portion of axon, which arises from axon hillock (initial segment). Both it and axon hillock integrate incoming signals and function as trigger zone.
     d. **Presynaptic terminals**—this is where one neuron communicates with another at the synapse.
  2. **Types of neurons**
     a. **Unipolar cells** have a single process from which arise the axon and dendrites. It is the primary type of neuron in invertebrates as well as vertebrate autonomic ganglia.
     b. **Pseudounipolar cells** develop as bipolar cells and fuse to form a single process that connects to the cell body. They are located in the dorsal root ganglia.
     c. **Bipolar cells** have two arborizing processes that leave the cell body: One ends in dendrites and the other is the axon.
     d. **There are three types of multipolar cells.** Each has one axon.
        i. **Spinal motor neurons** have several dendrites connected to cell body. Most excitatory synapses are close to cell body; inhibitory synapses farther away. Each motor neuron has few collateral branches of its axon (called recurrent), which synapse on Renshaw cells, a type of inhibitory interneurons that projects back to motor cells.
        ii. **Pyramidal cells**—apical dendrite and basal dendrites—are found in the hippocampus and the cerebral cortex. Easily destroyed from ischemia.
        iii. **Purkinje cells** of the cerebellum have extremely dense arborization of dendrites receiving over a 100,000 contacts per neuron.

35

e. **Interneurons** are two types: Golgi type I cells have long axons and convey information from one Brodmann area to another; Golgi type II cells have short axons and tend to stay in one Brodmann area.
      i. Inhibitory interneurons use glycine and γ-aminobutyric acid (GABA) as their neurotransmitters.
3. **Nerve cytology**
   a. Nerve cells do not, in general, regenerate after birth. Their nuclei exist in a relatively uncoiled state. Information to code proteins is contained in nucleus. A small portion is contained in circular DNA found in mitochondria.
      i. Mitochondrial DNA codes for ribosomal and transfer RNA (tRNA) (that is different from the nucleus), cytochrome oxidase, cytochrome b, an ATPase, and parts of ATP synthetase and NADH-Q reductase.

B. **Glial cells**—roughly 25 times more glial cells than nerve cells in vertebrates
   1. **Macroglia**
      a. **Oligodendrocyte** (central nervous system [CNS]) enwrap many (usually >10) axons in myelin
      b. **Schwann cells** (peripheral nervous system [PNS]) enwrap a single axon
      c. **Astrocytes** have many function: help endothelial cells form tight junctions, forming the blood–brain barrier; take up excess neurotransmitter at synaptic junctions; buffer high K during times of high activity; remove debris from dead neurons
   2. **Macroglial development**
      a. During development, Schwann cells arrange themselves at regular intervals along peripheral nerves. Each cell invaginates its external cell membrane (plasmalemma) to surround axon forming mesaxon. Mesaxon spirals in itself to form concentric layers and eventually condense to form mature myelin. The inner place of membrane invagination is called inner mesaxon. Last layer of myelin another invagination called outer mesaxon.
      b. Myelin coding genes activated by axons for Schwann cells and astrocytes for oligodendrocytes.
   3. **Myelin**—The major constituent of mature peripheral myelin is called P_0, myelin protein 0, sometimes also called myelin peripheral protein; it spans plasmalemma. It has glycosylated extracellular portion that interacts with other similar domains on other layers of the plasmalemma to help with compaction process.
      a. **Central myelin** is mainly composed of proteolipid protein. It lacks P_0. Proteolipids are soluble in organic solvents, their lipid moieties are covalently bonded to protein portion.
      b. **Central and peripheral myelin** contain myelin basic protein: seven related proteins.
         i. Experimental model of multiple sclerosis injects myelin basic proteins into animals causing focal inflammation and demyelination in CNS, like the disease.
         ii. Early example of successful gene therapy with mouse shiverer mutation: one exon coding for myelin basic protein not deleted. When mutation is homozygous, mouse has little to no myelin, shivers with a coarse tremor and convulsions, and dies young. When the normal gene is injected into homozygous shiverer fertilized eggs, mouse has a small amount of normal myelin but has normal lifespan and does not shiver.
   4. **Microglia derived from macrophage lineage**, which function in phagocytosis.

C. **Proteins**
   1. **Major membrane system** consists of the nuclear membrane, the endoplasmic reticulum, Golgi apparatus, secretory granules/lysosomes/endosomes, and the plasmalemma.
      a. All macromolecules made in neuron, except as detailed previously, made in this system. There are three classes of proteins made in neuronal cell: proteins made in gel-filled cytoskeleton (cytosol) and remain there; others later incorporated into nucleus, mitochondria, or peroxisomes; and proteins made in association with cell membrane system.

  i. Proteins that remain attached to membrane: They can be membrane-spanning, anchored (by covalent bonds), and associated (with weak bonds).
  ii. Proteins that remain inside the membrane
  iii. Both membrane attached proteins and proteins that remain inside the membrane are encoded by free ribosomes, called polysomes. After creation, these proteins are modified little.
  iv. Proteins in vesicles trans face of Golgi (the trans face of Golgi is where the secretary granules are produced; the cis face of Golgi receives transitional vesicles from the endoplasmic reticulum) are encoded by ribosomes rough endoplasmic reticulum and modified during creation (cotranslational) or after (posttranslational).
  v. A common cotranslational change is *N*-acetylation with acetyl group or myristoyl group (initiator methionine is enzymatically exchanged for the acetyl group). GTP-binding protein, cAMP dependent protein kinase, and calcineurin affected.
  vi. Common posttranslational changes are phosphorylation of serine, threonine, or tyrosine and the addition of ubiquitin.
  vii. The final destination of the protein depends on these changes.
 b. **Mitochondria and peroxisomes** are the other membrane systems. They are both thought to have been symbiotic organisms that were engulfed by our ancestors.
 c. **The two most abundant types of proteins** in the cytosol are enzymes for metabolic reactions and the cytoskeletal fibrillar elements.
2. **Axonal transport** is very different in the neuronal cell because of the length of transport that takes place. There are three types of transport:
 a. **Fast anterograde transport** as fast as 400 mm per day.
  i. Kinesins (structurally similar to myosins) are ATPases that form cross-bridges between organelles and microtubules. They appear to act like legs that walk down stationary tracts of microtubules.
 b. **Slow axoplasmic** flow faster component travels at about 0.4 to 5 mm per day
  i. Cytoskeletal elements and soluble proteins are moved by slow axoplasmic flow. It has two components: Slower component travels up to 2mm/day, contains neurofilament subunits, and α and β-tubulin all as polymers. Faster heterogenous composition
 c. **Fast retrograde axonal** transport is half the speed of fast anterograde transport.
Return of materials takes place in lysosomes propelled by dynein moving along microtubule tracts. This means that viruses like herpes, polio, rabies travel to nerve bodies.
 d. **Microtubules** are cylinders of 13 linearly arranged alternating α and β-tubulin dimers. Each monomer binds 2 GTP or one GTP and one GDP. There are more than 20 isoforms of tubulin.
 e. **Microtubule associated proteins** (MAPs) regulate stability of microtubules. MAP-1, MAP-2, and tau promote assembly. When tau and MAP-2 are phosphorylated, they minimally promote assembly. Both microtubules and microfilaments can rapidly alter their length (called dynamic instability).
 f. **Neurofilaments** are the most abundant fibrillar proteins in axons and are always polymerized. Bundles of filaments are called neurofibrils. They are oriented lengthwise along the axon. In Alzheimer disease can become modified forming neurofibrillary tangles. They are formed from 8 monomers ⇒ 4 coiled dimers ⇒ 1 tetrameric complex, which when linked linearly form a protofilament; 8 protofilaments ⇒ 4 protofibrils ⇒ 1 filament.
 g. **Microfilaments** are polymers of β and γ-actin wound in two filament helices. With hydrolysis of ATP to ADP, they can polymerize in one end and depolymerize in the other, called treadmilling. This is thought to be important for cell division and during growth and extension of axons and dendrites.

II. Ion Channels and Membrane Potential

A. **Cations** are surrounded by waters of hydration due to polarity of water. For an ion to move into lipid bilayer of cell membrane, must overcome electrostatic forces of attraction waters of hydration, making the lipid bilayer essentially impermeable to ions.

B. **Ion channels** allow the transport of ions across the lipid bilayer. They work at phenomenally fast rates—orders of magnitude faster than the fastest enzymes. Ion channels can either be selective for one of Na^+, K^+, Ca^{++}, Cl^- or nonselective. Current flows at low concentration are linear, although channels can fairly rapidly saturate.

C. **Ion channels** are allosteric proteins. Each has at least one open state, a closed state, and an in-between state called gating. There are more than a dozen types in neurons, each with multiple isoforms. Some, called nongated, are always open and maintain resting membrane potential.
   1. **Voltage-gated channels** have opening rates dependent on membrane potential; most enter a closed state due to a conformational change after activation (inactivation).
      a. Na^+ and K^+ voltage-gated channel inactivation is due to a conformational change in a region separate from the active channel.
      b. Na^+ voltage-gated channels have three conformations: resting, activated, and inactivated. K^+ channels have only resting and activated.
      c. Ca^{++} inactivation is due to Ca^{++} influx.
   2. **Ligand-gated channels** are dependent on ligands. Ligand-gated channels enter closed, or refractory, state when in the presence of a ligand, in a process called desensitization.
   3. Most **exogenous modifiers** to ion channels change conformation to the closed state.
   4. The **resting state** of most gated channels is closed.
   5. There are **four types of K^+ channels**, each with subtypes:
      a. Slowly activating K^+ channel of the action potential called the delayed rectifier
      b. Ca^{++} activated K^+ channel, activated by depolarization with voltage sensitivity dependent on Ca^{++}
      c. A type K^+ channel activates as fast as the Na^+ channel, but it also rapidly deactivates.
      d. M type K^+ channel activated by depolarization, inactivated by acetylcholine
   6. **Ca^{++} channels**
      a. Small concentration of Ca^{++} in normal cell $10^{-7}M$. With depolarization, voltage-gated Ca^{++} channels open, enough Ca^{++} enters cell to change Ca^{++} concentration near membrane, increasing activation rate of Ca^{++} sensitive K^+ channels. Net effect on the cell is increased sensitivity to a train of action potentials.
   7. **Voltage-gated channels** span cell membrane 6 times. The fourth segment (S4) is homologous between Na^+, K^+, and Ca^{++} voltage channels and likely represents gate. S4 of Na^+ channel highly conserved between species. Likely these channels are coded from same gene family.
   8. **Na^+ voltage-gated channels** are inhibited by tetrodotoxin.

D. **Membrane potential**
   1. **Neuronal cells** have membrane charge separation with excess positive charge outside and excess negative charge inside. Resting membrane potential in mammalian cells is -60 to -70 mV (this value is derived from convention of assigning potential outside the cell as 0).
      a. The Nernst equation: at equilibrium for K^+, -75 mV, due to the other ions.
   2. **Membrane potential** generated by ion concentrations. Na^+, Cl^- concentrated outside cell and K^+, organic ions concentrated inside. Increased permeability to K^+ would lead to more positive charge outside cell, hyperpolarizing membrane, and causing an inhibitory effect.
   3. **Glial cells** have open K^+ channels at resting membrane potential.
   4. **Na^+/K^+ ATPase** membrane protein with subunits: a transmembrane catalytic subunit, a glycoprotein regulatory subunit. Former has sites for K^+, irreversible inhibitor ouabain extracellularly, Na^+, ATP intracellularly. ATP brings 2 K^+ ions in, 3 Na^+ ions out.
      a. This pump maintains membrane potential even while nongated Na^+ and K^+ channels allow Na^+ and K^+ to fall down their concentration gradients.
   5. **Cl^- ions** usually passively distributed. If pump, Cl^- is actively pumped out of the cell.

E. Action potentials
  1. When an **excitatory synaptic potential** is great enough to cause some voltage gated Na^+ to open, Na^+ floods into the cell. This causes a net positive charge to develop in the cell, which increases depolarization, or a reduction in charge separation. Depolarization causes more voltage gated Na^+ channels to open in a positive feedback cycle.
     a. Rush of Na^+ into cell drives membrane potential toward Nernst equation's Na^+ equilibrium potential of +55 mV. It never reaches that value, in part due to counteracting effect of Cl^-.
     b. The membrane potential is returned to resting conditions due to:
        i. Inactivation of voltage-gated Na^+ channels if the channels are open long enough.
        ii. Voltage-gated K^+ channels take longer to open than Na^+ channels at all levels of depolarization. When the K^+ channels open, they counteract the effect of the Na^+, by having K^+ rush out of the cell. Note that the K^+ channels do not inactivate; they remain open as long as there is depolarization of the membrane.
     c. For most nerve cells, membrane potential has momentary hyperpolarization (afterpotential): Na^+ channels closed, more K^+ channels open than resting conditions.
     d. Net effect of all Na^+ channels inactivated is an absolute refractory period in which the neuron can not generate another action potential. After a period, some of the Na^+ channels have reverted to their resting state. At this point, the neuron has entered its relative refractory period when a large enough excitation could cause an action potential.
  2. **Larger diameter axons** are more easily stimulated because they have more ions per unit length, allowing a smaller current to stimulate them.
  3. The **speed of action potentials** in nerves is dependent on two variables:
     a. Diameter of axon, which increases speed. Briefly, for resistance r, diameter d, and capacitance c of the axon per unit length: $r \sim -d^2$, $c \sim d$. Ohm's law: $V = IR$. By definition, $v = q$ (charge)$/c$. Taking it all together, $d \sim -rc \sim I$.
        i. Extreme example is giant squid with neuronal axons up to 1 mm in diameter.
     b. More common mechanism is myelination. Myelination equals 100 times diameter. Myelination is interrupted by nodes of Ranvier every 1 to 2 mm; these are areas of very high density voltage-gated Na^+ channels. Interruptions reinforce passive depolarizing current so that it doesn't die out. Demyelination can block the axonal depolarization by allowing the passive currents to die out.
        i. Depolarization moves by saltatory conduction, leaping from one node to another. The reality is that its speed just slows down a lot because conductance is much higher in nodes.
        ii. The nodes of Ranvier metabolically favorable as less need for Na^+/K^+ ATPase.

III. Synaptic Transmission

A. **Synapses** are of two major types:
  1. **Chemical synapses** are a 30- to 50-nm gap between presynaptic active zones, postsynaptic receptors. Mediated by chemical transmitters with a synaptic delay of usually 1 to 5 msec
  2. **Electrical synapses** are gap junctions (1.5 nm); mediate transmission with a bidirectional ionic current that takes place virtually instantaneously. The ionic current causes positive charge to be deposited on the inside of the membrane of the postsynaptic cell depolarizing it. The excess current then leaves the cell through nongated conductance channels.
     a. Electrical synapses are unidirectional (rectifying) or bidirectional (nonrectifying). In nonrectifying electrical synapses, if presynaptic cell has significant afterpotential, postsynaptic cell will experience biphasic current (electrotonic transmission).
     b. Electrical synapses between cells act as resistors in series. Resistors in series are additive. Group of cells connected by electronic synapses act like one "large cell." This "large cell" will have a decreased depolarization to excitatory synaptic currents. In addition, they will all fire at virtually the same time if an action potential is generated. Electrical synapses are present when important for neurons to fire in a coordinated way.

3. **Gap junctions**
   a. Gap junctions are made up of two cylinders called connexons. One connexon is in the presynaptic cell and the other in the postsynaptic. Connexons made up of six connexins that assemble hexagonally to form cylinder, which attaches to sister connexon on other cell. Connexons closed when six connexins touch each other in center, open when connexins rotate slightly and form an opening in center. Many different types of connexins. Electrical synapses in neurons uses connexin 36 to form the gap junctions.
   b. Nonrectifying electrical synapses close with decreased pH or increased Ca^{++} concentration. Some can close with voltage. In addition, neurotransmitters act through signal transduction pathways to alter electrical synaptic transmission.
   c. In mammalian brain, good evidence for electrical synapses in mesencephalic nucleus of cranial nerve (CN) V; vestibular nucleus; inferior olivary nucleus; retina; and inhibitory interneurons of neocortex, hippocampus, and thalamus. Inferior olivary neurons can generate spontaneous, synchronous, subthreshold fluctuations of membrane voltage at 28 Hz due to electrical synapses. In hippocampus, CA1, 3 and dentate nucleus; function unknown. Connexin 36 knockout mice: scotopic vision (vision in dark) strongly impaired.
4. **Chemical synapses**
   a. **Presynaptic transmission** involves release of a chemical messenger. Most neurons have active zones, a specialized zone for focused release of neurotransmitters. Some do not, like the autonomic neurons innervating smooth muscles.
      i. Neurotransmitters can have multiple functions. It depends on the setting.
   b. **Postsynaptic transmission** involves receptors interacting with released neurotransmitters.
   c. **Receptors** are of two major types:
      i. Acetylcholine (ACh), glutamate, glycine, and GABA: upon recognizing a specific neurotransmitter undergoes a conformational change to open an ion channel.
      ii. Norepinephrine and serotonin: neurotransmitter recognition causes G protein to produce a second messenger. The second messengers can either act on the ion channels directly or activate a protein kinase, which interacts with the ion channels by phosphorylating them. In a few cases, the G proteins directly interact with ion channel.

IV. Motor Neurons

A. **The motor neuron axon** innervates muscle cells. When close to muscle cells, it loses its myelination and splits into several branches. At end of each branch are several spherical projections called synaptic boutons. Synaptic boutons lie on top of muscle and underneath them are several pits into the muscle called junctional folds lined with a basement membrane. Within the basement membrane is acetylcholinesterase, which hydrolyzes ACh into choline and acetate. ACh, which is released, is also rapidly diffused, causing a rapid decline in concentration.

B. **Synaptic bouton** have three components: synaptic vesicles containing ACh; specialized membrane for transmitter release (active zone), and voltage gated Ca^{++} channels.
   1. **With ACh release,** ACh receptors cause an excitatory postsynaptic potential called the endplate potential. The resting potential of muscle is −90 mV.
   2. **Curare and alpha-bungatoxin** (snake venom neurotoxin) are nicotinic ACh receptors are antagonists. Gallamine is a channel blocker. It is important to note that these work on neuromuscular junctions but not in autonomic ganglia nicotinic ACh receptors.
   3. **In the transmitter-gated channel,** when it activates, Na^+ rushes into cell and K^+ rushes out. This is in distinction from the action potential, where there are two separate channels for Na^+ and K^+ and they activate at different times. In addition, with Na^+ influx, more Na^+ channels are not recruited because this is dependent on ACh concentration.
   4. **A single channel** causes a 0.3 mV depolarization. Muscle needs about a 70 mV depolarization to fire.

5. **Acetylcholine receptors** are broadly muscarinic or nicotinic; there are five kinds of muscarinic receptors and four different classes of nicotinic receptors. Muscle has nicotinic receptor.
   a. These receptors are built of five subunits. 2 alpha1, beta1, epsilon, delta
   Two alpha1—each binds ACh with high affinity; both must be bound for the channel to be sufficiently open. Alpha-bungatoxin binds to this subunit. Typical location of myasthenia gravis antibodies
   b. There are no inhibitory synapses in the motor unit.

V. Neural Synaptic Transmission

A. **Most common types of synaptic connections** in the brain are called Gray connections.
   1. **Gray type I** usually glutamine, cleft sizes 30 nm, active zone 1 to 2 nm, and the synaptic vesicles are round after electron micrograph preparation.
   2. **Gray type II** usually GABA, cleft sizes 20 nm, active zone < 1 nm, the synaptic vesicles are oval, and there is little to no basement membrane.

B. **Glutamine receptor**
   1. Na^+ and K^+ are conducted equally.
   2. **Two major types**
      a. **Ionotropic** directly gate channels. Three major types of glutaminergic ionotropics, each named for their agonist; always excitatory activation
         i. *N*-methyl-D-aspartate (NMDA) blocked by APV
         ii. AMPA blocked by CNQX
         iii. Kainate blocked by CNQX
         iv. AMPA and kainate are together called non-NMDA.
      b. **Metabotropic** activate second messengers; excitatory or inhibitory
         i. Activated by APV
   3. In the motor neuron, non-NMDA generates large early EPSP (excitatory postsynaptic potential) with relatively low conductances and permeable to Na^+ and K^+. The NMDA receptor generates the late EPSP, with high conductance, is permeable to Na^+, K^+, and Ca^{++}, requires extracellular glycine to function, and its opening also depends on membrane voltage.
      a. In the NMDA receptor, Mg^{++} binds to the pore at rest. After depolarization of the membrane by non-NMDA receptors, the Mg^{++} is unbound and the receptor opens.
      b. PCP blocks the NMDA receptor producing hallucinations.
      c. In general, unless there is summation producing large depolarization of the postsynaptic cell, NMDA receptors contribute only a small current. When they contribute a large current, Ca^{++} activates Ca^{++}-dependent enzymes.
      d. Long-term synaptic modification due to NMDA receptors is called activity-dependent synaptic modification because of the activity required for NMDA to function.
      e. Excessive glutamate is toxic to most neurons, called glutamate excitotoxicity. This is thought to be mediated by excessive Ca^{++} inflow causing, perhaps, free radical creation.
   4. Glutamate receptors are composed of four subunits with pore similar to K^+ channels. AMPA receptors identical to NMDA receptors except for a single amino acid residue.

C. **Other excitatory receptors**
   1. Serotonin (5-HT) has several receptors, of which 5-HT 3 receptors are present in the CNS. These receptors are ionotropic.
   2. ATP is also a synaptic transmitter for smooth muscle cells, and a few CNS and PNS neurons. It is ionotropic.

D. **Inhibitory receptors:** GABA and glycine
   1. **Two types of GABA receptors:**
      a. GABA A, ionotropic receptor that gates Cl^-
      b. GABA B, metabotropic activates second messenger and usually activates a K^+ channel.

c. GABA receptors are composed of two α, two β, and one γ subunit. GABA can bind to any of receptor's subunits. It requires two molecules of GABA to activate the receptor.
      i. A missense mutation of the α subunit causes startle disease where the individual has hypertonic muscles and heightened responses to being startled.
   d. GABA also has separate binding sites for benzodiazepines, barbiturates, and alcohol. Binding of one will enhance the binding of any of the others. This is why alcohol and diazepam have additional effects when used together.
2. **Glycine** released by spinal cord interneurons to inhibit antagonist muscles. It gates Cl⁻ channels.
   a. Glycine receptors are composed of three α and two β subunits with glycine binding to the α subunit. Two or three glycine molecules are required to activate the receptor.
3. Inhibitory postsynaptic potentials (IPSPs) generated from increases in Cl⁻ conductance. With resting potential of resting neuron (−65 mV), Nernst potential of Cl⁻ is −70 mV, explaining why influx of Cl⁻ creates inhibition. During periods of very high excitation, intracellular concentration of Cl⁻ can double, causing a reversal of the Nernst potential to a level higher than −65 mV. In these conditions, Cl⁻ activation causes cell depolarization. This takes place during seizures and in newborns.

VI. Second Messengers

A. All G-protein receptors have single subunit; spans membrane seven times. Binding of transmitter activates G protein, which binds to enzyme. Specific enzyme depends on the pathway. These enzymes phosphorylate protein kinases, leading to signal amplification.
  1. The G protein itself is composed of three subunits α, β, and γ, which all exist on the intracellular aspect of the cell membrane. The α subunit is associated loosely with the cell membrane and it activates the associated effector enzyme. The β and γ subunits are more closely bound to the membrane.
  2. Each receptor that is bound activates many G proteins.

B. Nongaseous
  1. **cAMP**
     The binding of the receptor leads to activation of the stimulatory G protein called Gs, by the exchange of a GDP for a GTP. The Gs activates another integral membrane protein, adenylyl cyclase, which catalyzes the conversion of ATP to cAMP. In addition, the Gs acts as a GTPase, converting the GTP back into GDP, thereby inactivating itself and the adenylate cyclase.
     a. cAMP activates cAMP-dependent protein kinase, or protein kinase A (PKA); cAMP composed of two subunits: two catalytic and two regulatory. In the presence of cAMP, two molecules bind to two regulatory subunits revealing other two subunits for catalytic action. Catalytic units phosphorylate serine and threonine residues in specific phosphorylation sequence of amino acids. For PKA, this sequence is Lys/Arg, Lys/Arg, any, Ser/Thr.
  2. **Phospholipase C**
     This breaks PIP$_2$ (phosphatidylinositol 4,5-bisphosphate) into DAG (diacylglycerol) and IP$_3$ (inositol 1,4,5-triphosphate). DAG is hydrophobic and remains near the cell membrane where it activates protein kinase C, if the Ca^{++} levels are high enough. IP$_3$ activates a specific IP$_3$ receptor in the endoplasmic reticulum to release Ca^{++} stores into the cytoplasm.
     a. One of the ways that Ca^{++} acts is by the formation of a calmodulin Ca^{++} complex, which binds to the Ca^{++}/calmodulin-dependent protein kinase. This activated enzyme functions even in the absence of Ca^{++}.
  3. **Phospholipase A2** causes the formation of arachidonic acid from the cell membrane. Arachidonic acid is rapidly converted to any of active metabolites called eicosanoids. Cyclooxygenases produce prostaglandins and thromboxanes. Lipoxygenases form hydroperoxyeicosatetraenoic acid (HPETE), which becomes leukotrienes or other metabolites.

4. **Tyrosine kinase** receptor binds a specific peptide ligand. On binding, it associates with another tyrosine kinase forming a dimer that phosphorylates proteins in the cytoplasm. These proteins are believed to produce long-term functional changes.

C. **Gaseous**
   1. They have some special properties: they diffuse through cell membranes readily, they do not act on a cell membrane receptor, and they are short lived.
   2. They stimulate the synthesis of cGMP through guanylyl cyclase located in the cytoplasm. cGMP is important in retinal rod cell regulation. The greatest amount of cGMP-mediated phosphorylation occurs in cerebellar Purkinje cells contributing to long-term depression of synaptic transmission, probably part of motor learning.
   3. NO is produced when glutamate activates an NMDA receptor causing Ca^{++} influx and activation of a Ca^{++} calmodulin-dependent enzyme in neurons called NO synthase. CO is produced by heme oxygenase.

VII. Transmitter Release

A. Ca^{++} **channels**
   1. A large number of Ca^{++} channels are located on the active zones. Here Ca^{++} concentration can rise 1,000-fold on activation.
   2. Ca^{++} channels activate slower than Na^+ channels, allowing their activation during Na^+ channel repolarization.
   3. The types of Ca^{++} channels are L, N, P/Q, R, and T. They are composed of $\alpha 1$, $\alpha 2$, β, γ, and δ subunits. The $\alpha 1$ subunits determine the type of Ca^{++} channel.
      a. L-type channels are important for slow transmission neuropeptide release. L-type channels are blocked by dihydropyridines.
      b. N, R, P/Q are important for fast synaptic transmission. N is blocked by ω-agatoxin IVA (a neuropeptide from funnel web spider venom). P/Q is blocked by ω-conotoxin GVIA. Conotoxins are neuropeptides from marine snails of genus conus; ω-conotoxins affect Ca channels.
      c. The T type channels open in response to small depolarizations. Cardiac pacemaker cells.

B. **Neurotransmitter** is released in packages called quanta. In the motor neuron, about 5,000 ACh molecules are release, causing opening of 2,000 channels and a 0.5-mV depolarization. An action potential causes the release of about 150 quanta.
   1. Each quanta is, of course, a vesicle of neurotransmitter.
      a. Fusion pores allow release of a vesicle of neurotransmitter. They act like gap junctions, which have two states: open and closed. When in the presence of Ca^{++}, they become open, allowing a docked vesicle to release its contents. Fusion pores are basically the mechanism of exocytosis.
      b. The vesicle membrane is recycled through endocytosis into an endosome.
   2. Quanta of neurotransmitter released slow, constant rate in absence of action potential.

C. **Postsynaptic responses**
   1. The release of one quanta causes a 1-mV depolarization of the postsynaptic membrane. This is called a miniature end-plate potential, or MEPP. Frequency increased by increasing temperature and nerve depolarization. Frequency decreased with calcium deficiency and botulism. Amplitude increased by neostigmine. Amplitude decreased by myasthenia gravis and curare.
   2. End-plate potential, or EPP, is the summation of enough MEPPs to produce an action potential. A motor unit potential, or MUP, is an action potential at a motor unit.

D. **Proteins involved in neurotransmitter release**
   1. **Synapsins** are four proteins: Ia, Ib, IIa, and IIb that form a network of cytoskeleton that anchors the vesicles. With Ca^{++} influx, Ca^{++} calmodulin-dependent kinase is activated,

which phosphorylates synapsin I. The synapsin then undergoes a conformational change freeing the vesicles.
   2. **Rab3A and Rab3C** bind to synaptic vesicles allowing for efficient trafficking of vesicles.
   3. **Synaptobrevin** located on the vesicle, syntaxin located on the membrane, and SNAP-25, a peripheral membrane protein, work together to allow for vesicles to dock.
      a. Synaptobrevin is cleaved by tetanus toxin and botulinum toxin B. Syntaxin is cleaved by botulinum toxin C. SNAP-25 is cleaved by botulinum toxin A.
      b. Synaptogamin (or p65) is likely related to exocytosis, role has not been fully elucidated.
E. **Plasticity**
   1. **Synaptic effectiveness** can be changed by altering amount of steady state Ca^{++} influx.
   2. **Tetanic stimulation** has two effects:
      a. First, it increases the size of postsynaptic potentials called potentiation.
      b. Secondly, this increase persists for minutes or even an hour after stimulation ceases, called posttetanic potentiation. This occurs when amount of Ca^{++} influxed is too great for the cell's buffering systems and excess Ca^{++} remains in the cell. This keeps Ca^{++} enzymatic pathways activated, including the phosphorylation of synapsin. Therefore, further action potentials will cause even greater quanta of neurotransmitter to be released.

VIII. Neurotransmitters

A. **ACh**—all vertebrate neuromuscular junctions, all preganglionics in the autonomic nervous system (ANS), all parasympathetic postganglionics, nucleus basalis in the brain.

B. **Norepinephrine**—source of neurotransmitter is locus ceruleus, postganglionic sympathetics

C. **Dopamine**—nigrostriatal pathway, mesolimbic tract, mesocortical tract, hypothalamic arcuate nucleus

D. **Serotonin**—midline raphe nuclei of the brainstem

E. **Histamine**—hypothalamus

F. **Glutamate**—generally excitatory

G. **Glycine**—inhibitory spinal interneurons

H. **GABA**—throughout

I. **ATP and substance P**—pain C fibers and dorsal root ganglion (also use glutamete and glycine)

J. **Peptides**—there are more than 30. Most important may be substance P released by unmyelinated afferent pain fibers.

IX. Electroencephalogram (EEG)

A. **EEG basics**
   1. EEG is the cortical surface sum of EPSPs and IPSPs.
   2. To actually read an EEG you have to understand the different montages. For the boards, it is probably sufficient to know the abbreviations: ears are called A, the occiput O, frontal F, temporal T, parietal P. Odd numbers are left and even numbers are right.
   3. Activation procedures
      a. Hyperventilation causes slowing for 3 to 5 minutes. May provoke localized slowing in area of lesion or cortical dysfunction. About three fourths of absence seizures will be uncovered following this procedure.

b. Photic stimulation: expect no response or occipital driving at same frequency as driving. Can see complex waveforms with mixture of fundamental frequency and harmonics that mimic spikes/spike waves.

B. **Normal EEG** (Figure 4-1)
   1. **Alpha activity** 8–13 Hz. Alpha rhythm is alpha activity in the posterior regions while the subject is awake, relaxed, with eyes closed. Attenuates with eye opening (Figure 4-1A).
      a. Slow alpha variant notching due to 4–5 Hz component of the EEG
      b. Fast alpha variant is twice the normal alpha frequency
   2. **Beta activity** 13–40 Hz. Precentral increases with drowsiness, posterior dominant can be seen until 2 years, and frontocentral can be seen while under the influence of benzodiazepines or barbiturates (see Figure 4-1B)
   3. **Theta** 4–7 Hz, prevalent during drowsiness. In children, part of normal background.
      a. Subclinical rhythmic electrographic discharge of adults is seen with older adults, theta or mixed theta+delta, looks like seizures but is never accompanied by symptoms, background is often visible during discharge, and is of no significance.
   4. **Delta** 1–4 Hz, predominant activity seen in infants. It is not normal in adults. If present in asymptomatic teenagers, it is called posterior slow waves of youth.
   5. **Mu rhythm** 7–11 Hz, arch waveform does not attenuate with eye opening, but does attenuate with moving thumbs. Enhanced by hyperventilation. This is not an alpha variant, as it does not attenuate with eye opening.
   6. **Lambda waves** small spike-like waves in occipital region when subject scans a picture.

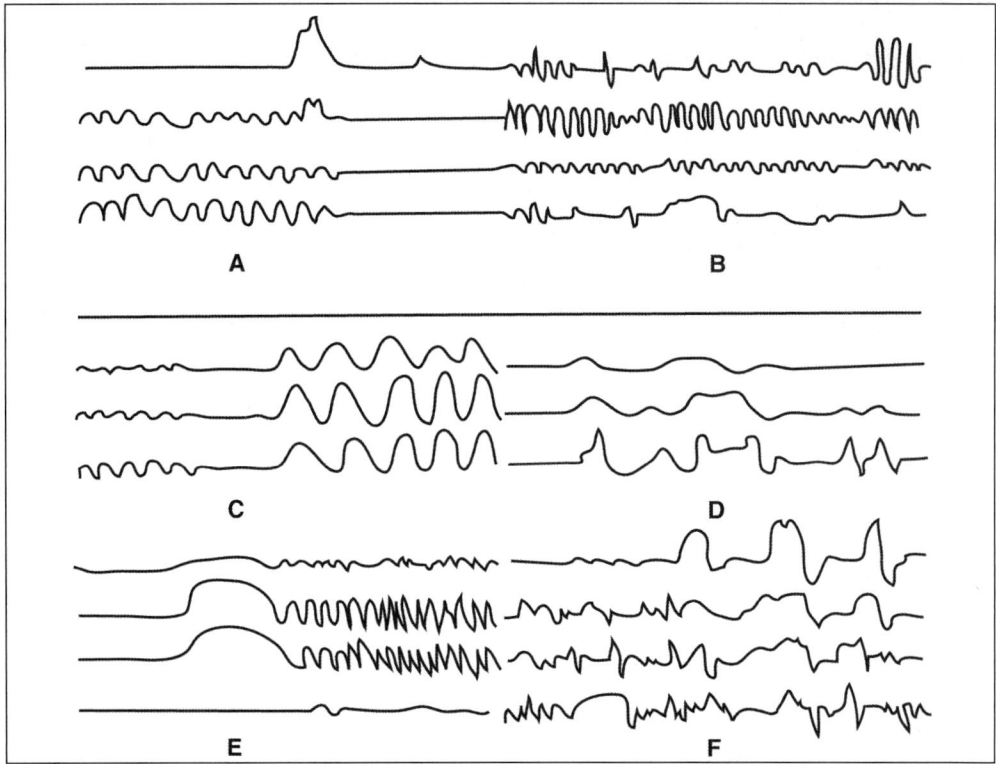

Figure 4-1 Normal electroencephalogram (EEG). Each 2-second segment of EEG uses a left parasagittal chain: Fp1-F3, F3-C3, C3-P3, P3-O1. **A:** Alpha rhythm showing eye opening and attenuation with eye opening. **B:** Diffuse beta maximal frontotemporally seen with benzodiazepines or barbiturates. **C:** Alpha intermixed with theta seen in drowsiness. **D:** Positive occipital sleep transients (POSTs) seen in sleep. **E:** K complex with normal 14-Hz spindle seen in stage 2 sleep. **F:** Low-amplitude, mixed frequencies, with rapid eye movements (REMs) seen in REM sleep.

7. **Drowsiness**—decreased alpha, increased theta, mu possible, sharp spikes in temporal region called wicket spikes are normal (Figure 4-1C).
8. **Vertex sharp transients** called V waves are sharp waves in the central vertex during sleep. f waves are similar but occur in the frontal region.
9. **Breech rhythm**—focal increase in waves over skull defect appears as epileptiform spikes.
10. **Rhythmic temporal theta bursts** of drowsiness are flat topped or notched and do not evolve into other waveforms or frequencies, enabling to discern the difference between this and epileptiform discharges.
11. **6-Hz spike and wave** occur during drowsiness or light sleep of (young) adults. They last up to 2 seconds; not associated with seizures of symptoms, and for that reason it is sometimes called phantom spike and wave.
12. **6-Hz and 14-Hz positive bursts** occur in the posterior temporal during light sleep. They last for about a second and occur in teens.
13. **Wicket spikes** are 6 to 11 Hz; they appear in temporal lobe during drowsiness and light sleep. No slowing after them, either locally or in the background.
14. **Mitten pattern** is fast wave–slow wave; looks like a mitten; seen during sleep.

C. **Sleep**
1. **Sleeping**—slow waves, 12 to 14 Hz activity in the central regions symmetrically lasting 0.5 to 1.5 seconds called sleep spindles = stage 2 sleep, vertex sharp transients or V waves occur maximally over the vertex, polyphasic wave maximal at vertex called a K complex, and sharp positive deflection over the occipital region called POSTs or positive occipital sleep transient of sleep (Figures 4-1D–E).
2. Can identify level of sleep based on **morphologic features**.
   a. **Stage W** (awake) = alpha or low-voltage mixed frequencies, vertical deflections from blinking
   b. **Stage I** = V waves, POSTs, slow waves 3 to 7 Hz, spindles <0.5 seconds possible
   c. **Stage II** = like stage I but also has regular sleep spindles and K complexes
   d. **Stage III** = like stage II but no V waves, <1/2 large amplitude (<75 V or >50 V in elderly) slow waves 0.5 to 2 Hz. Not delta waves; delta waves are NOT normal in adults.
   e. **Stage IV** = like stage III but >1/2 large amplitude slow waves
   f. **Rapid eye movement (REM)** sleep = low-voltage mixed frequency similar to stage I with episodes of REMs and, in some, sharp theta frequency waves that look like saw teeth and are called saw tooth waves (Figure 4-1F).

D. **Pathologic EEG** (Figure 4-2)
1. **Focal intracranial lesions** can produce focal EEG abnormalities.
   a. Temporal intermittent rhythmic delta activity = partial seizures with focal lesion
   b. Periodic lateralized epileptiform discharges = anatomic lesion/trauma. Can show an ischemic lesion before can be seen on computed tomography (CT).
   c. Intermittent rhythmic delta activity = distant effect of focal intracranial lesion, systemic metabolic, or electrolyte disorder; usually seen occipitally in children and frontally in adults and represents a distant effect. Usually increases with hyperventilation and disappears with sleep.
   d. If near convexity of hemispheres, likely to see focal decreased voltage of background. Can see increased voltage. A difference in alpha activity between sides of more than 1 Hz is likely a lesion on the side of the lower frequency
   e. Polymorphic focal delta = focal hemispheric lesion, usually a tumor and usually seen best during alert wakefulness (Figure 4-2A). If don't see attenuation of alpha with eye opening on one side, this can indicate a parietal or temporal lesion; this is called Bancaud phenomena (Figure 4-2B).
   f. Seizures controlled by medications and still delta waves—likely a tumor focus
2. **Ictal events** can take any form, which is why it is important to know the normal variants. They consist of repetitive morphology that has an abrupt onset and termination.
   a. Tonic-clonic ictus: tonic with fast spikes, clonic spikes, and slow waves gradually become more separated, postictal diffuse low amplitude and then diffuse slow waves.

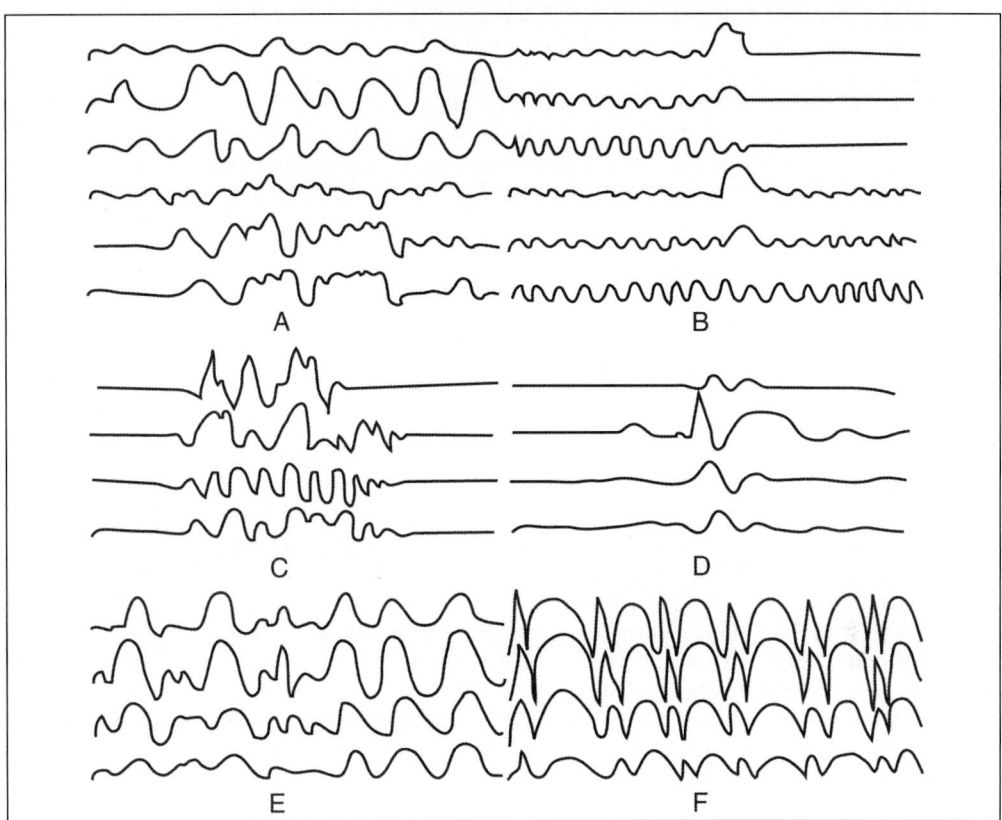

Figure 4-2 Abnormal EEG. Each 2-second segment of EEG uses a left parasagittal chain: Fp1-F3, F3-C3, C3-P3, P3-O1, except for **(A)** and **(B)**, which use F3-C3, C3-P3, P3-O1, F4-C4, C4-P4, P4-O2. **A:** Polymorphic rhythmic delta activity seen in focal abnormalities including tumor and stroke, diffuse atrophy, and cerebral edema. **B:** Unilateral attenuation of alpha can occur with parietal or temporal lesion called Bancaud phenomenon. **C:** Burst suppression. **D:** Frontal spike is a frequent discharge seen in adults. **E:** Nonconvulsive status. **F:** Absence seizure.

    b. Surface attenuation or an abrupt decrease in voltage is sometimes seen immediately before focal seizure activity, especially if the seizure is temporal.
    c. The slowing that is seen after a seizure is usually focal if the seizure was focal.
    d. Sometimes burst suppression can be seen postictally in patients who are comatose (Figure 4-2C), although it is more often associated with overdosage, anesthesia, or severe hypoxia.
3. **Focal spikes**
    a. Anterior temporal spike or sharp wave is >90% correlated with partial seizures; 30% to 50% with temporal lobe epilepsy will show spikes or spike-waves during wakefulness, 80% to 90% while sleeping. Anyone suspected of complex partial seizures gets sleep EEG.
    b. Frontal spikes are correlated with seizures in about 3/4, and are often correlated with an underlying pathologic condition (Figure 4-2D).
    c. Central temporal spike typically large amplitude, diphasic, followed by a slow wave seen in Rolandic epilepsy; normal background; seen during age 4 to 12 years and about 70% have seizures.
    d. Occipital spikes in children younger than 6: 40% have visual problem, 40% have seizures
4. **Status is an interictal pattern that does not abate.** They may be convulsive with physical movements or nonconvulsive without (Figure 4-2E).

5. **3-Hz spike and slow wave,** bilaterally synchronous, maximal superior frontal, no interictal changes. Absence seizures will appear if they last longer than 3 to 4 seconds. Discharge enhanced by hypoglycemia, hyperventilation (see Figure 4-2F)
6. **Sharp and slow wave** at 1.5 to 2.5 Hz, usually organic pathology, age 2 to 6 most common, can be any seizure type except typical absence; if more than one type of seizure consider Lennox-Gastaut; often subtle impairment even if no obvious seizure
7. **Atypical spike and wave** refers to a generalized spike and wave that is not at the standard 3 Hz with frequency between 2 and 5 Hz and admixed spikes. Can be multispike and slow waves and it lasts 1 to 3 seconds. Suggests that seizures are often myoclonic or tonic-clonic.
8. **Paroxysmal rhythmic fast activity** 12 to 20 Hz parasagittal. Tonic or tonic-clonic. Usually occur during sleep.
9. **Hypsarrhythmia large-voltage continuous multifocal spikes/sharp waves** with slow waves mixed in. Occurs age 4 months to 4 years. Associated with infantile spasms. Consider this when see large spike/slow wave followed by generalized decrease in amplitude of high frequency activity. This is called electrodecremental pattern.
10. **Nonfocal intracranial lesions** = encephalopathies; often appear as focal or generalized slowing. This is a nonspecific change.
11. **Periodic short-interval, diffuse discharges** are generalized synchronous sharp waves that recur at 1 to 2 Hz; they signify degenerative or toxic. If myoclonic jerks and progressive cognitive decline = Creutzfeldt-Jacob disease.
12. **Periodic long-interval diffuse discharges** are high-voltage sharp and slow waves that recur every 4 to 15 seconds = subacute sclerosing panencephalitis.
13. **Periodic lateralized epileptiform discharges** are focal, periodic sharp waves. They indicate a viral encephalitis, especially herpes simplex.
14. **Triphasic waves** are low-voltage negative deflection, followed by a prominent positive sharp wave and then a negative slow wave. They occur in metabolic and electrolyte disorders, toxins, hypoxia, degenerative disorders, or most commonly with hepatic encephalopathy.

E. Coma patterns
   1. **Alpha coma** pattern is a diffuse, unvarying alpha activity seen with hypoxic insult or brainstem lesions; prognosis is poor if seen with hypoxic insult.
   2. **Beta coma** pattern is generalized beta activity with delta slowing; occurs with drug toxicity or anesthesia.
   3. **Spindle coma** is unreactive spindles and some V waves. Sleep spindles during coma likely unrelated to prognosis.
   4. **Burst suppression** is episodic sharp waves and/or spikes on an attenuation pattern, which can be due anesthesia, drug intoxication, hypothermia, or hypoxia; if hypoxia, prognosis is poor.
   5. **Electrocerebral inactivity** is ≥30 minutes with no greater than 2μV deflection unreactive to afferent stimulation. Needs specific settings (≥8 scalp electrodes, 100 to 10,000 Ω interelectrode impedances, ≥10-cm interelectrode distance, sensitivity ≥2μV/mm) and qualified tech. It indicates drug overdose, hypothermia, or death. If the subject is age 7 days to 2 months, need two EEG separated by ≥48 hours. If age 2 months to 1 year, need two EEGs separated by ≥24 hours.

X. Nerve Conduction Velocity (NCV)

A. **Sensory nerve action potentials (NAPs)** are sensitive and specific measure of function of peripheral sensory nerve function. May specifically localize, classify peripheral neuropathy, can see effect on a large myelinated axon; technically difficult.
   1. **Two major strategies** for studying the sensory portion:
      a. Stimulate NAPs in mixed motor and sensory nerves or pure sensory, and record distal to where nerve splits into motor and sensory components. This makes an action potential travel opposite the normal direction (antidromic technique). Stimulate NAPs in sensory component record over mixed component (orthodromic technique).

b. Best sensitivity for diffuse problems over long nerve segments, for focal problems, over short nerve segments.
2. **Sensory NAPs** are frequently first sign of pathology, great to document neuropathy.
3. Measurements include **three values for each nerve**:
    a. First, the negative direction is oriented as an upward deflection
    b. Amplitude: deflection recorded from baseline to peak of maximum negative deflection
    c. Conduction velocity is distance divided by latencies.
    d. Latency is the time from stimulus artifact to initial baseline deflection (true latency) or peak of sensory NAP (peak latency).

B. Utility of NCV
   1. **In acute nerve injury**, initially NAPs will be normal. But when Wallerian degeneration takes place, NAP amplitude decreases to a nadir at 1 to 2 weeks.
   2. **Focal demyelination** causes normal NAPs distal to lesion and either increased latency or substantially decreased conduction velocity across lesion. True conduction block cannot be reliably determined by NAPs. If focal demyelination at terminus of the neuron, there will be increased distal latency.
   3. **Diffuse demyelination** shows prolonged distal latencies, decreased conduction velocities, and decreased amplitudes.
   4. **Neuropathy** decreased amplitudes, can have decreased conduction (but >70% lower limit of normal).
   5. **Normal NAPs** in the face of objective severe sensory loss is radiculopathy preganglionic (to dorsal root ganglion).
   6. **Superficial peroneal sensory** nerve for L5, sural sensory nerve for S1, and saphenous sensory nerve for L3 and L4.
   7. **To assess S1 radiculopathy**, test the Hoffman, or H, reflex.
       a. The H reflex is stimulation of tibial nerve in popliteal fossa at intensities less than needed for M wave (see subsequent text). The H reflex is a monosynaptic reflex similar to ankle jerk, except it bypasses muscle spindles that initiate reflex. Many factors affecting the reflex: increasing—passive stretch, mild contraction of agonists; decreasing—sleep, nicotine, diazepam, contraction of antagonists, or strong contraction of agonist.
       b. A difference of 1.2 msec in the latency between sides indicates S1 radiculopathy. Prolonged latency also: alcoholic, diabetic, nutritional, uremic, paraneoplastic, and cisplatin-induced neuropathies; Guillain-Barré syndrome; inflammatory polyneuropathies.
       c. The H reflex may not be present in healthy individuals older than 60 years.
       d. Can evaluate a C7 radiculopathy by testing the flexor carpi radialis.
       e. The radiculopathy needs corroboration from other data for a diagnosis.

XI. Compound Muscle Action Potentials (CMAPs)

CMAP = motor NCV

A. **Definition:** Action potential recorded from the muscle when stimulation of the motor nerve sufficient to activate some or all of the muscle fibers. Thus, it provides a way to measure descending motor axons, neuromuscular junction, and muscle fibers.

B. The waves
   1. **M wave** is CMAP recorded over a muscle from muscle's peripheral nerve. Most useful measurement is amplitude of the CMAP. Latency is time from stimulus artifact to first negative deflection. Latencies at two different points helps measure conduction velocity.
   2. **F wave** is CMAP from a single motor unit, which travels antidromically to anterior horn cells and then orthodromically back to motor cells without synapsing. F waves travel large nerve segments so are good for diffuse disease, proximal nerve disease.

C. **Findings associated with CMAPs**

1. **Conduction slowing**—increased distal latencies, decreased conduction velocity, and increased F wave latencies caused by segmental demyelination or axonal narrowing
2. **Conduction block**—no response proximal to the block, full response distal to the block caused by local anesthetics or myelin structural changes
3. **Reduced or absent CMAPs**—Wallerian or axonal degeneration, total conduction block
4. **Decreased amplitude** just proximal to a block is likely a localized mononeuropathy.

D. NCV/CMAP findings in various disease (amp = amplitude, cv = conduction velocity)
   1. **Myopathy**—neuromuscular transmission defect possible decreases CMAP amplitude.
   2. **Motor neuron disease**—large decrease in CMAP amplitude, mild increase in F wave latency, mild decrease (>70% LLN; LLN is short for lower limit of normal) CMAP conduction velocity (does not effect sensory NCV)
   3. **Axonal neuropathy**—decreased CMAP amp, large decrease sensory NCV amplitude, mild increases F wave latency, decreases in NCV/CMAP cv (>70% LLN)
   4. **Mononeuropathy**—similar to axonal neuropathy or demyelination but some differences: key is increased sensory NCV duration; also has large decrease in sensory NCV amplitude and decreases in NCV/CMPA conduction velocity (<70% LLN)
   5. **Demyelinating neuropathy**—slowed conduction velocity (<70% normal), temporal dispersion of CMAP, conduction block over a short segment or can be diffusely slowed
   6. **Regenerated conduction velocity** can still be slowed with low amplitude CMAP

XII. A Whirlwind Tour of Other Modalities

You should probably know something about these tests. The basics are covered here.

A. **Somatosensory evoked potentials** (SEPs or sometimes SSEPs)
   1. The basics
      a. SEPs are similar to sensory NCV, but can measure sensory conduction in proximal nerves, the spinal cord, and the brain.
      b. Most frequently used in evaluation of multiple sclerosis (MS) to produce objective evidence of a second lesion needed for diagnosis, as well as in spine surgery to monitor spinal cord functional status during anesthesia
      c. These tests are also frequently ordered when there is no neurologic deficit and sensory symptoms are vague. This test is something of a divining rod in these circumstances, showing where to go next by localizing a lesion to the brain, spinal cord, or PNS.
      d. They can also be helpful in conversion or malingering because they should be normal.
   2. The peaks
      a. SEPs are recorded as a series of peaks with (negative) upward deflections as N, (positive) downward deflections as P. Number after peak refers to average of normal latencies.
      b. No one is sure what the peaks indicate, but clear higher numbers represent sequentially higher levels. For specific nerves, the numbers can localize, but that localization is beyond what a general neurologist is expected know. As there is a large normal variation in range of amplitudes, slowed latencies are more helpful in making a diagnosis.

B. **Brainstem auditory evoked potentials** (BAERs or BAEPs)
   1. The basics
      a. This test uses sound clicks to test the responses of CN VIII and the brainstem auditory pathway. It does not require a participating patient.
      b. All activations are ipsilateral. Neurophysiologists may argue, but you may be asked (Figure 4-3A).
         i. Wave I is distal CN VIII action potential
         ii. Wave II is proximal CN VIII action potential or cochlear nucleus
         iii. Wave III is likely superior olivary nucleus
         iv. Wave IV is likely lateral lemniscus
         v. Wave V is likely inferior colliculus

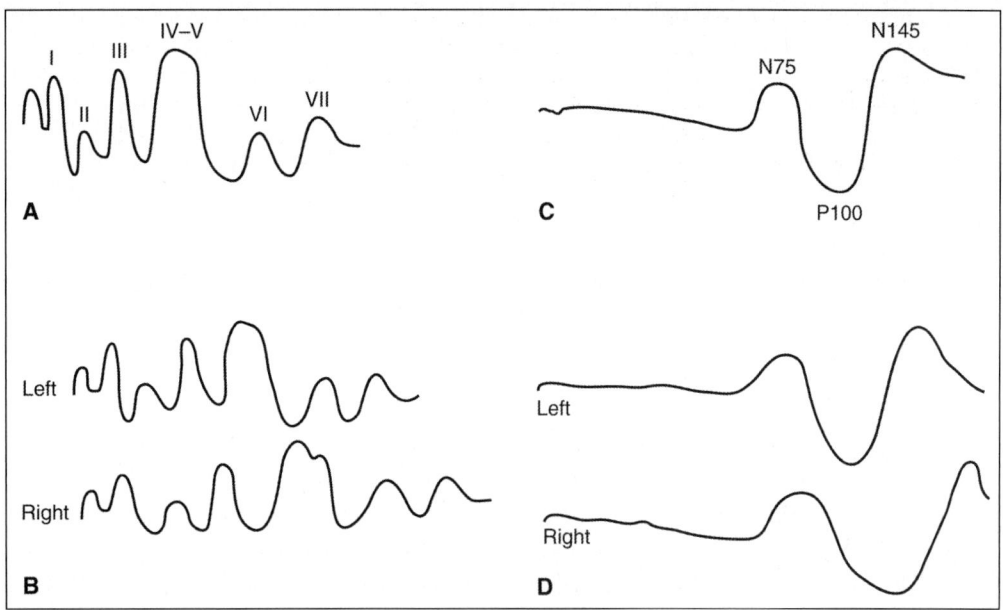

Figure 4-3 Evoked potentials. **A:** Brainstem auditory evoked potential (BAER) waves: I, distal action potential of cranial nerve (CN) VIII; II, proximal CN VIII; III, ipsilateral superior olivary nucleus; IV, lateral lemniscus; V, inferior colliculus; VI, medial geniculate body; VII, thalamocortical pathway. **B:** BAER showing prolonged I–V and I–III interpeak latencies seen on the right, which is typically seen in acoustic neuroma. **C:** Visual evoked potential (VEP) can be described in terms of either deflections N1P1N2—1st negative, 1st positive, 2nd negative deflection; or N75P100N145—negative deflection at 75 msec, positive at 100, negative at 145. **D:** VEP of multiple sclerosis with delayed P1.

vi. **Waves VI and VII** are not always present, so are not clinically useful.
c. The clinical data provided by the waves include waveform latencies, interpeak latencies between odd waves, and V/I amplitude ratio. If the I–III interpeak latency is prolonged but III–V is normal, the lesion is between distal CN VIII and superior olivary nucleus; whereas, I–III normal and III–V prolonged means the lesion is between the superior olivary nucleus and the inferior colliculus.
2. **Clinical utility**
    a. Hearing loss will show missing wave I, prolonged latencies of all the waves, or, in extreme cases, all the waves will be missing.
    b. In MS, more than 50% have abnormal BAER with prolonged I–V and decreased I/V amplitude. The abnormality can be unilateral or bilateral. It is even possible to monitor response to treatment for MS with serial BAERs (Figure 4-3B).
    c. In acoustic neuroma, both I–V and I–III are prolonged. BAERs are probably the most sensitive screening test for acoustic neuroma.

C. **Acoustic reflexes and evoked otoacoustic emissions**
1. **Acoustic reflexes** measure the contraction of the stapedius muscle in response to intense sound. It is involuntary so does not require a participating patient. Two measurements are produced: the sound needed to produce acoustic reflexes and acoustic reflex decay. The sensitivity and specificity for sensori-neural CN VIII lesions is 85%.
2. **Evoked otoacoustic emissions** (sometimes called just otoacoustic emissions) measure the cochlear response to sound. Most important frequencies are 1 to 4 kHz, the range for speech. Normal test results suggest normal middle ear and cochlea. This test is most often used for hearing screening of neonates. Can be used for young children as part of audiologic testing. For patients faking hearing loss, can be used to diagnose pseudohypacusis.

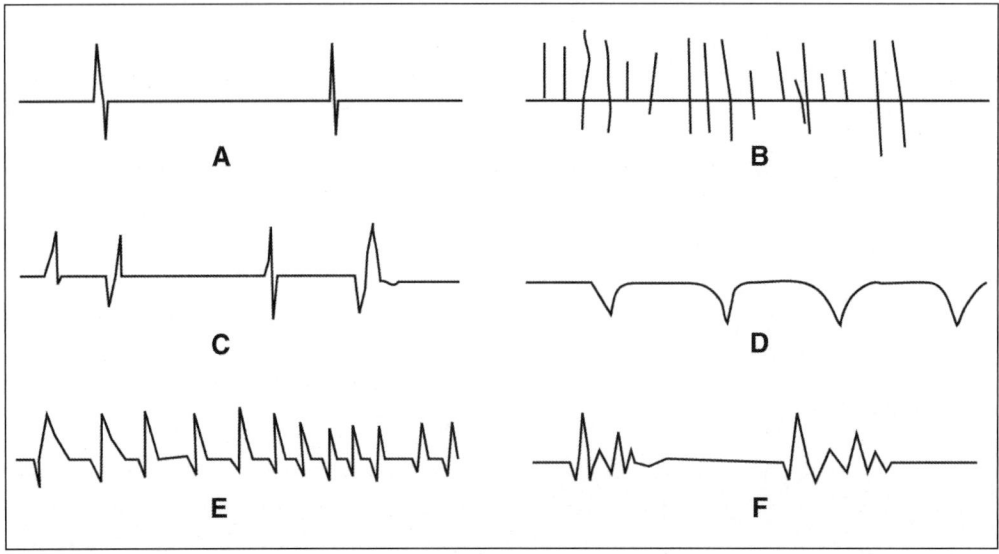

Figure 4-4 Electromyogram (EMG) in exaggeration. **A:** Normal motor unit action potentials. **B:** Motor units during recruitment. **C:** Fibrillations. **D:** Positive sharp waves. **E:** Myotonic discharge—high frequency trains of action potentials with varying frequency. **F:** Myokymic discharge complex grouped after potentials that repeat.

Table 4-1 Electromyographic patterns

Motor units	Recruitment	Variation	Differential diagnosis
Normal	Normal	Absent (−)	Normal or possibly systemic myopathy, polio
		Present (+) Decline in amplitude	Myasthenia
	Abnormal	−	Acute lesions, poor cooperation
Short-duration, polyphasics	Normal	−	Myopathy
		+	Botulism, re-innervation
	Abnormal	−	Severe myopathy, critical illness, muscular dystrophy
		+	
Long-duration, polyphasics	Usually abnormal	−	Chronic atrophy
		+	Progressive atrophy
Mixed-duration, polyphasics	Usually normal	−/+ (+ usually means active disease)	Myositis, ALS, SMA, Cori disease (a glycogen storage disease)

ALS, amyotrophic lateral sclerosis; SMA, spinal muscular atrophy

D. **Visual evoked potentials/responses**
   1. Studies the optic nerve and pathways; very useful in MS
   2. Normal response to pattern reversal checkerboard is a three-phase waveform: negative deflection at 75 msec (N1), positive at 100 msec (P1), and final negative at 145 msec (N2) in the midocciput (Figure 4-3C).
   3. Can help determine etiology of pathology: demyelination with P1 delayed latency, ischemia P1 amplitude loss, degeneration small losses in both (Figure 4-3D)

XIII. Electromyogram (EMG)

A. **EMG**
   1. EMG is used to assess the integrity of motor unit (Figure 4-4A,B for motor units)
   2. **Spontaneous activity at rest**
      a. **Insertional activity**—occurs when muscle is pierced by the needle. Prolonged insertional activity is seen in denervation, inflammatory myopathy, e.g., polymyositis. It can be reported as increased insertional activity, and you are expected to understand that they mean increased duration of insertional activity. Similarly decreased or no insertional activity is seen in neuromuscular disorders as muscle tissue is replaced with fat or scar. After insertional activity recedes, other activity can be seen.
         i. Myotonic discharges—trains of high frequency potentials that change in both amplitude and frequency during the train of impulses. Initiated by electrode movement or muscle contraction. Seen in an extremity in early chronic entrapment or postradiation; seen in the face with MS, polyradiculopathy, facial palsy. (Figure 4-4E.)
      b. **End-plate activity** corresponds to multiple monophasic negative (positive deflections)
         i. To qualify must have amplitude <10 mV and duration <3 msec
         ii. unless using single fiber electrodes, cannot usually distinguish individual end-plate potentials; so there is irregularity in the baseline called end-plate noise
      c. **Fibrillation potentials**
         i. Duration <5 msec, firing rate between 2 and 20 Hz, usually regular, with two or three phases, the first phase is always positive unless being recorded at the endplate
         ii. Occur in partially denervated muscle 3 to 5 weeks after acute insult, trauma, muscular dystrophy, poly or inclusion body myositis. In myopathy there is functional denervation with separation of muscle fibers from their end-plates (see Figure 4-4C).
      d. **Positive sharp wave**—initial positive deflection followed by an overshoot and slow return to baseline; seen in injured muscle, same meaning as fibrillations (Figure 4-4D)
      e. **Fasciculations** look like motor unit action potential that occur at rest. They can be normal, chronic partial denervation, or spinal cord pathology, amyotrophic lateral sclerosis (ALS).
      f. **Complex repetitive discharges**—trains of high frequency potentials, often polyphasic that have identical amplitude and frequency (thus can be easily distinguished from myotonic discharges); seen in muscular dystrophy, polymyositis, or partial denervation
      g. **Myokymic discharges**—groups of identically appearing action potentials separated by periods of inactivity; seen most commonly postradiation, but can occur with MS, radiculopathy, syringomyelia, gold intoxication (Figure 4-4F)
   3. **Recruitment**
      a. **Definition**—as voluntary effort increases, the motor unit fires more frequently, and additional motor units fire; this is called recruitment. Visually, the motor units will fire more frequently, and there will be additional peaks, representing recruited motor units (Figure 4-2B).
      b. **Polyphasics** are potentials with more than four phases; a turn (where the direction changes, but it does not cross the zero line) counts as a phase.
         i. Low amplitude, short duration are seen in myopathy, myositis, neuromuscular junction (NMJ)

ii. Large amplitude, long duration are seen in partial denervation with re-innervation, polymyositis
c. **Abnormal recruitment**
  i. Incomplete activation—relatively few motor potentials firing, seen with poor cooperation, pain, weight lifters
  ii. Increased recruitment—minimal effort produces many motor potentials, gives evidence of disease affecting the muscle
  iii. Reduced recruitment—higher recruitment frequency or decreased recruitment pattern.
4. **Localizing value**
   a. Has diagnostic utility comparable to imaging studies
   b. Partial denervation—classically appears in order of paraspinals, proximal muscles, distal muscles, and reappears in the same order as reinnervation occurs.
   c. Radiculopathy is shown with 2+ muscles in same nerve root but not by the same peripheral nerve. (You have to know your anatomy for this to be useful.)
   d. EMG patterns (Table 4-1)

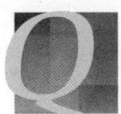 STUDY QUESTIONS FOR CHAPTER 4

Directions: *Each of the numbered items or incomplete statements in this section is followed by answers or by completions of the statement. Select the ONE lettered answer or completion that is BEST in each case.*

1. Among neurophysiologists, what is the importance of toxins?
   (A) Historical
   (B) They enable separation of actions and reactions
   (C) Basis for molecular understanding of neuronal action
   (D) Useful experimentally

2. A 76-year-old man falls and is brought in by family because of confusion. He is shown to have a subdural hematoma on CT, which is subsequently evacuated. He has a seizure after subdural hematoma evacuation. His EEG shows breech pattern. What do you do?
   (A) This is a medical emergency that needs to be treated with intravenous (IV) lorazepam
   (B) The patient has seizures on EEG, should be initially treated with phenytoin
   (C) EEG nondiagnostic; treat with phenytoin to prevent recurrence
   (D) EEG nondiagnostic; may treat with phenytoin

3. A man with objective sensory deficit in first two digits of right hand has sensory NCV with normal results. If this is first visit with you, what do you ask?
   (A) Ask if patient had a trauma to area of deficit
   (B) Test Tinel and Phalen
   (C) Ask about weakness
   (D) Do a routine history and physical

4. Colchicine is known to disrupt microtubules; this will seriously affect which component of axoplasmic flow:
   (A) Fast anterograde
   (B) Slow component of slow anterograde
   (C) Fast component of slow anterograde
   (D) None of the above

5. The resting membrane potential of the human neuron is
   (A) −50 to −60 mV
   (B) −60 to −70 mV
   (C) −70 to −80 mV
   (D) −80 to −90 mV

6. An EEG with large-voltage multifocal spikes and sharp waves with intermixed slow waves in a 1-year-old who is not developing as fast as he should is characteristic of what?
   (A) Infantile spasms
   (B) Temporal tumor
   (C) Anoxic brain injury
   (D) Epilepsia partial continuous

7. A 30-year-old man who has had his first seizure is having an EEG. He is supine with his eyes closed. His EEG shows repetitive central 12-Hz waves lasting for about a second. You deduce which of the following?
   (A) He is drowsy
   (B) He is in stage I sleep
   (C) He is in stage II sleep
   (D) He is in stage III sleep

8. A 67-year-old man with low back pain is referred to you for complaints of tingling in the fifth toe digit and difficulty everting his foot. You test
   (A) Peroneal sensory nerve
   (B) Saphenous sensory nerve
   (C) H reflex
   (D) M wave

9. A patient has I–III and I–V prolongation on both sides during a brainstem evoked potential test. The I/V amplitude is normal. What is the most likely diagnosis?
   (A) Hearing loss
   (B) Multiple sclerosis
   (C) Neurofibromatosis
   (D) Inferior colliculus tumors

10. An 88-year-old woman presents to the emergency room with difficulty opening her eyes, facial weakness, and slurred speech. She reports that she ate some canned food of indeterminate age the day prior to her visit. You make a clinical diagnosis of botulism. Which of the following is true about botulinum toxin?

(A) Synaptobrevin is cleaved by botulinum toxin A
(B) Synaptobrevin is cleaved by botulinum toxin B
(C) Synaptobrevin is cleaved by botulinum toxin C
(D) Syntaxin is cleaved by botulinum toxin A
(E) Syntaxin is cleaved by botulinum toxin B

11. A 67-year-old man with Parkinson disease is referred to you for management. He takes levodopa 100 mg, four times a day. Which of the following structures contains predominantly dopaminergic neurons?

(A) Nucleus basalis
(B) Locus ceruleus
(C) Mesocortical tract
(D) Midline raphe nuclei
(E) Postganglionic sympathetics

12. A 19-year-old college student had been taking herbal supplements as a study aid. Unfortunately, these supplements contained the glycine antagonist strychnine and he has now developed severe spasms and convulsions. What is the site of action of strychnine?

(A) Cerebral cortex
(B) Substantia nigra
(C) Hypothalamic arcuate nucleus
(D) Inhibitory spinal interneurons
(E) Neuromuscular junction

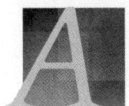

ANSWERS AND EXPLANATIONS

1. C. Here each answer is correct, so this is a tricky question. But the reason that toxins have historical importance, are useful experimentally, and enable separation of actions and reactions, is because they enable molecular understanding. Toxins are known to specifically activate a specific receptor that has a specific molecular action.

2. D. Breech pattern is expected after craniotomy due to the skull defect. Likely start on phenytoin to prevent further seizures, but starting treatment after first seizure is somewhat controversial. A, B. Breech pattern is nondiagnostic for anything other than a hole in the skull. C. Treating with phenytoin is a choice, not a guideline.

3. C. One should do a focused history and physical on every patient. This NCV suggests radiculopathy proximal to dorsal root ganglion. A. Trauma might be expected with decreased amplitude. B. Tinel or Phalen test for carpal tunnel syndrome, which would have prolonged latency. D. Not the best answer.

4. A. Fast anterograde flow uses microtubules as a road for the kinesins. B. Slow component of slow anterograde flow depends on many elements, so may or may not be affected. C. The fast component depends on neurofilament subunits and tubulins.

5. B. The resting membrane potential for all mammals is -60 to -70 mV. The rest of the answers are merely distracters.

6. A. The EEG shows hypsarrhythmia, which is infantile spasms until proven otherwise. B. Temporal tumor might show slowing in the temporal region. C. Anoxic brain injury might show periodic lateralized epileptic discharges. D. Epilepsia partial continuous would show continual partial epilepsy.

7. C. This is a sleep spindle. It lasts for 0.5 to 1.5 seconds during stage II sleep. A. No spindles are normally seen during drowsiness B. Sleep spindles last <0.5 seconds in stage I sleep. D. Would expect to see slow waves in addition to spindles in stage III.

8. D. The M wave is very helpful in testing neuropathy. A. Peroneal sensory nerve tests l5, but this is s1 distribution. B. Saphenous sensory nerve tests l4/l5. C. The H reflex is used for s1, but may not be present if >60, so D is the better answer.

9. C. Neurofibromatosis is associated with bilateral acoustic neuroma, which is the correct diagnosis. A. Hearing loss would expect missing wave I, prolonged latencies. B. MS would show decreased I/V amplitude. D. Inferior colliculus tumor would have I–III normal and I–C prolongation.

10. B. Synaptobrevin is cleaved by botulinum toxin B. SNAP-25 is cleaved by botulinum toxin A. Syntaxin is cleaved by botulinum toxin C.

11. C. The nigrostriatal pathway, mesocortical tract, mesolimbic tract, and hypothalamic arcuate nucleus contain predominantly dopaminergic neurons. The nucleus basalis contains mostly acetylcholine, the locus ceruleus and postganglionic sympathetics contain mostly norepinephrine, and the midline raphe nuclei release serotonin.

12. D. Glycine is the principal neurotransmitter of the inhibitory spinal interneurons. The cerebral cortex uses mostly glutamate and GABA, the substantia nigra and hypothalamic arcuate nucleus use dopamine, and the neuromuscular junction uses acetylcholine.

Pathology

I. Definition

A. **Study of morphologic changes** produced by diseases in the central nervous system (CNS) and peripheral nervous system (PNS). Diagnosis is predicated upon analysis of the gross and microscopic changes, location of lesion, and clinical-pathologic correlation.

II. Infectious Diseases—Generalities

A. **Brain constituents** are natural rich medium. Skull, dura matter, and blood–brain barrier (BBB) protect the brain and spinal cord from invasion by infectious agents.

B. **The infectious agents** reach the CNS via:
 1. The bloodstream: embolic source
 2. Direct invasion from adjacent bones (osteomyelitis), sinusitis, or mastoiditis; and trauma including surgical or septic spinal punctures
 3. Retrograde invasion via cranial and peripheral nerves such as in some viral infections (rabies)

C. **Infections** can be pathogenic in healthy hosts or opportunistic in immunocompromised hosts.

III. Bacterial Infections

A. Acute pyogenic infections
 1. **The bacterial pyogenic infections** can be described in relation to the dura mater
  a. **Epidural abscesses:** more frequent in thoracic spine in the region of true epidural space. Source of infection is adjacent skin: furunculosis, skin infections, or sepsis. Organisms: *Staphylococcus aureus* and *Streptococcus* species. Compression of spine is major complication.
  b. **Subdural empyema or abscess:** Frontal or ethmoidal sinusitis or mastoiditis is source. Extension from pyogenic meningitis usually in children and *Haemophilus influenzae*. Organisms: *Streptococcus*, anaerobic organisms, *Escherichia coli*, *Pseudomonas*.
  c. **Acute pyogenic leptomeningitis:** infiltration of the subarachnoid space by bacteria
  d. There are **age-related organisms:**
   i. **Newborns:** group B streptococci and *E. coli*.
   ii. **Infants:** *H. influenzae*.
   iii. **Children and college age students:** meningococci (*Neisseria meningitides*).

60 SECTION I   SCIENTIFIC UNDERPINNINGS

        iv. **Adults:** *Streptococcus pneumoniae.*
- e. *Klebsiella, Proteus,* and *Pseudomonas* after lumbar punctures, spinal anesthesia, or shunting procedures. Any organism can be seen in immunosuppressed patients. Lesions consist of presence of dense infiltrate by polymorphonuclear cells in subarachnoid space.
- f. **Complications:** cortical vein thrombophlebitis and hemorrhagic cerebral infarcts; thrombophlebitis of large dural sinuses; sensorineural deafness; hydrocephalus; subdural effusions, or hygromas
2. **Brain abscesses:** source of infection local contiguous infections such as sinuses, skin, penetrating head injuries. Hematogenous: frequently multiple, located at the junction of cortex with white matter; sources are infectious endocarditis, pulmonary infections (paradoxical septic emboli–foramen ovale). Children with cyanotic congenital heart diseases: tetralogy of Fallot are at high risk. (Figure 5-1.)
3. **Cerebritis:** starts with arrival of bacteria to brain, brain necrosis followed by purulent brain necrosis surrounded by granulation tissue; formation of an early capsule in 10 to 13 days, gets thicker with time; marked vasogenic edema around abscess; abscess layers include (i) necrotic purulent center, (ii) granulation tissue, (iii) dense fibrous capsule, (iv) marked edema and perivascular lymphocytic infiltrate
   - a. **Complications:** increased intracranial pressure, herniations, and intraventricular rupture–pyocephalus

B. **Subacute bacterial infections**
  1. **Tuberculous (Tb) infections:** epidural infections produce osteomyelitis and bone deformities such as Pott disease; meningitis characterized by dense basilar fibrinous exudate that

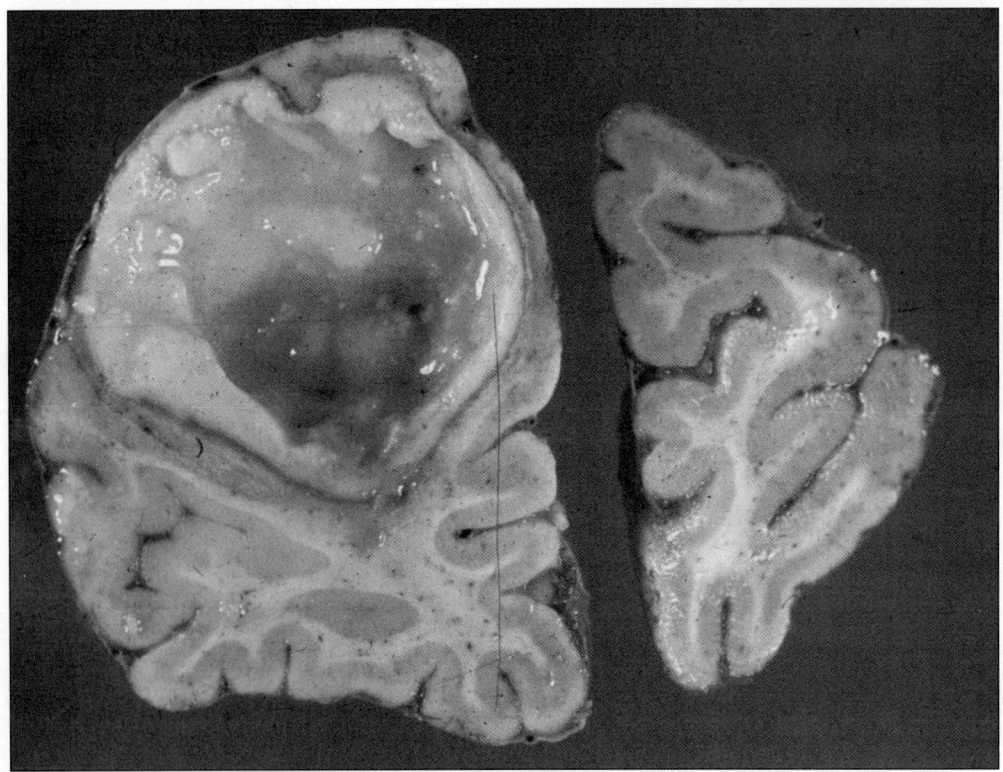

Figure 5-1   Frontal lobe abscess in a child with tetralogy of Fallot. Note the cyanotic brain and encapsulated abscess.

involves cranial nerves and obliterates basal cisternal spaces to produce hydrocephalus; Tb arteritis produces cerebral infarcts; tuberculomas can be found in the cerebellum, ponds, and insular area

2. **Whipple disease:** multisystem disease involves intestines and brain; produced by Gram-positive actinomycete (*Tropheryma whipplei*); produces lymphocytosis and gliosis with sickle-shape inclusion and bacteria in subcortical areas, hypothalamus, periaqueductal gray matter, and nuclei of brainstem and dentate nuclei of the cerebellum
3. **Lyme disease** or erythema chronicum migrans is produced by the spirochete *Borrelia burgdorferi* transmitted by the tick *Ixodes dammini*; produces aseptic meningitis or meningoencephalitis with cranial and peripheral nerve involvement

C. **Bacterial toxins** induce neurologic diseases including tetanus, diphtheria, and botulism

IV. Mycotic (Fungal) Infections

A. **Mycotic infections** are secondary to a focus elsewhere but the symptoms are primarily in the CNS and are seen in immunocompromised patients.
   1. Most frequent fungal infection is chronic meningitis produced by *Cryptococcus neoformans* that elicits minimal inflammatory reaction. The fungus can produce intraparenchymal gelatinous pseudocysts.
   2. Mucor infection (zygomycosis, phycomycosis) is seen predominantly in diabetics and drug addicts, where it produces nasal infection with spread to the cavernous sinus and orbit.
   3. Carotid artery vasculitis produces extensive hemorrhagic infarction. Basal ganglia necrosis may be seen in drug addicts.
   4. Aspergillosis can be seen in patients with lymphoma or leukemia who are immunocompromised.

V. Parasitic Infections

A. **Metazoal infections**
   1. **Cysticercosis** is produced by larval stage of *Taenia solium*. Embryonated eggs ingested in feces-contaminated food or regurgitation in intestines. Encysted larva produces meningeal, intraventricular or miliary parenchymal forms. Some brain cysts calcify.
   2. **Schistosoma mansoni** can produce a granulomatous thoracic myelopathy, a reflexive paraplegia, or cauda equina syndrome.

B. **Protozoal infections**
   1. **Amebiasis**
      a. *Acanthamoeba* is seen in immunocompromised patients, usually secondary to a silent pulmonary focus; it produces multiple granulomatous hemorrhagic brain lesions.
      b. *Naegleria fowleri* is acquired through the nose by healthy young swimmers in hot stationary waters and produces acute fatal amebic meningitis.
   2. **Toxoplasmosis:** congenital form acquired *in utero* from infected mother, produces hydrocephalus and granulomatous calcified cortical and basal ganglia lesions; acquired form in AIDS patients, produces single or multiple noncalcified granulomatous lesions.
   3. **Malaria** produced by *Plasmodium falciparum* acquired via mosquito bite.

VI. Viral Infections

A. **Acute viral infections** Virus can invade CNS and PNS and produces encephalomyelitis and neuritis. Pathologic features of CNS infections consist of perivascular lymphocytic cuffs, microglial nodules, predominantly gray matter shows satellitosis neuronophagia and microglial cells. The

CNS infections can be acute, predominantly in gray matter (neurotrophic viruses) and have a topographic predilection.
1. **Dorsal root ganglia** are infected by the varicella zoster virus producing a dermatomal nerve–skin lesion (shingles). Rarely the virus can invade the spinal cord and has been found in intracranial granulomatous arteritis.
2. **The leptomeninges** can be infected by enteroviruses (ECHO, coxsackie), mumps, herpes simplex virus type 2 (HSV-2), and others, and can produce an aseptic meningitis.
3. **Anterior horn cells** of spinal cord are affected by poliovirus (RNA enterovirus), which produces asymmetrical pure motor paralysis, poliomyelitis; same viruses can affect medulla producing bulbar form; coxsackie virus affects predominantly spinal cord of children and is associated with myocarditis; and rabies virus (rhabdovirus) can involve spinal cord and produce a paralytic form or "dumb" rabies. A distinctive histopathologic feature of rabies is presence of intracytoplasmic inclusions known as Negri bodies.
4. **Medulla and cerebellum** are affected by rabies virus and produce the agitated or "furious" form of rabies. Negri bodies are seen in Purkinje cells, hippocampal neurons.
5. **The midbrain** is affected in encephalitis lethargica or von Economo encephalitis. Pathologic and epidemiologic features suggest a virus (possibly influenza?), although no virus has been isolated at this time. The sequela of the encephalitis is postencephalitic Parkinson disease.
6. **Cortex** affected by arboviruses (arthropod-borne) transmitted by infected mosquitoes during hot summer period (seasonal); includes the St. Louis, western, eastern, Venezuelan equine encephalitis, West Nile, Japanese, Australian. Most frequent sporadic form of encephalitis is herpes simplex type 1, produced by a DNA virus, which produces a focal hemorrhagic necrosis of temporal or frontal lobes or insular areas. Intranuclear inclusions are seen predominantly in oligodendrocytes around hemorrhagic areas.

B. **Subacute viral infections** have a subacute course, affect the gray and white matter, are gliotic, and have viral inclusions. Slow progressive course takes weeks to months.
1. **Subacute sclerosing panencephalitis** (SSPE) is produced by the measles virus, a paramyxovirus, and occurs in children several years after a severe episode of measles. Intranuclear inclusions are see in oligodendrocytes.
2. **Cytomegalovirus infection** in congenital form produces necrotic granulomatous lesions in periventricular areas. Infection is acquired from infected mother. Acquired adult form predominantly in HIV-infected patients; can produce focal CNS infiltration, myelitis, and radiculitis. Cytomegalic intranuclear or cytoplasmic inclusions are diagnostic.
3. **Progressive multifocal leukoencephalopathy** (PML) is produced by a human polyoma virus (JC virus); affects immunocompromised patients, predominantly HIV infected; areas of demyelination with prominent gliosis, intranuclear oligodendrocyte inclusions
4. **HIV encephalitis** is produced by the retrovirus that invades the brain via macrophages that serve as reservoirs and agent for dissemination. Perivascular macrophages and diffuse demyelination are prominent features.
5. **HTLV-1**, or human T-cell leukemia/lymphoma virus 1, associated myelopathy (inflammatory gliotic myelopathy) produces the tropical spastic paraparesis seen in the Caribbean and South America.

VII. Prion Diseases

Produced by abnormal isoform of a normal prion brain protein. Agent is devoid of DNA and RNA. The Prion protein cellular (PrPc) is encoded in the short arm of chromosome 20. The diseases are characterized by spongiform (vacuolated) gliotic lesions in the gray and white matter, hence the name spongiform encephalopathy, with presence of amyloid plaques in most of these disorders. The diseases are inherited or acquired (sporadic) forms and include:

A. **Sporadic form of Creutzfeldt-Jakob disease and Kuru**

B. **Familial Creutzfeldt-Jakob disease**—cognitive decline, cerebellar dysfunction, visual changes, later seizures and cranial nerve involvement

C. **Gerstmann-Straussler-Scheinker**—ataxia, dysarthria, personality change

D. **Fatal familial insomnia**—insomnia with stuporous episodes that include hallucinations, autonomic dysfunction, myoclonus, and seizures

VIII. Demyelinating diseases

A. **The CNS myelin** can be secondarily affected as part of different processes including hypoxia, CO intoxication, viral infections (progressive multifocal leukoencephalopathy [PML], HIV), metabolic disorders causing osmotic demyelination (central pontine myelinolysis [CPM]). Most commonly there is primary demyelinating disease.

B. **Acute forms**
   1. **Acute disseminated encephalomyelitis (ADE):** monophasic disease usually immune-mediated complication of infections outside CNS
      a. Postinfections occur after viral infections (measles, chickenpox, other) or mycoplasma
      b. Postvaccinial: rabies, smallpox
      c. The pathology consists of perivenous mononuclear cell infiltrate surrounded by a halo of perivenous demyelination.
      d. A hemorrhagic severe variant of the disease is known as Hurst acute or subacute necrotizing hemorrhagic encephalomyelitis.
   2. **Devic neuromyelitis optica**: disease of children, young adults and consists of the simultaneous or successive involvement of the optic nerves and spinal cord. The eye involvement precedes or follows a transverse necrotizing myelitis. Pathologic features consist of marked inflammatory process; also destructive lesions in spinal cord and optic nerves. In most cases disseminated lesions seen on imaging or autopsy studies.
   3. **Optic neuritis:** an acute inflammatory demyelination of one optic nerve that can be isolated and monophasic but in 50% of the cases is part of MS

B. **Chronic forms** most commonly multiple sclerosis: most frequent form of demyelination that affects young adults. Lesions are disseminated throughout entire CNS with predilection for periventricular areas. Macroscopic lesions show gray irregular but well-demarcated plaques of demyelination randomly distributed in entire CNS. Microscopic findings: perivascular mononuclear inflammatory reaction more prominent in acute lesions, loss of myelin, oligodendroglial cells with proliferation of astrocytes. In chronic lesions, inflammation less prominent with more gliosis, axonal loss.

C. **Leukodystrophies** are heterogeneous group of disorders characterized by:
   1. **Bilateral symmetrical and widespread degeneration or failure** of myelin formation of the CNS and in some cases the peripheral nerve myelin.
   2. **Hereditary metabolic disorders** inherited as autosomal recessive or X-linked
   3. **Clinical manifestations** include progressive spasticity, ataxia, and optic atrophy.
   4. **Metachromatic leukodystrophy:** autosomal recessive (22q13.31) disorder due to lysosomal aryl sulfatase A deficiency. On macroscopic inspection, the brain shows diffuse loss of myelin. Microscopically there is loss of myelin with excessive accumulation of sulfatides in tissue that stain brown with acidic cresyl violet (metachromasia). Peripheral nerves are involved and diagnosis established by sural nerve biopsy. There are infantile, juvenile, and adult forms.
   5. **Krabbe disease or globoid cell leukodystrophy:** autosomal recessive (14q31) due to deficiency of galactocerebroside β-galactosidase deficiency. The brain shows atrophy and diffuse demyelination. Microscopically there is marked loss of myelin with perivascular

macrophages with abundant cytoplasm or "globoid" cells. Peripheral nerves are involved. Onset of the disease is before 6 months with rapid course and early death.
6. **Adrenoleukodystrophy and adrenomyeloneuropathy:** X-linked (xq28) peroxisomal recessive disorder with accumulation of very-long-chain fatty acids in adrenal gland and brain. Disease affects young boys with adrenal insufficiency and progressive spasticity, adult females (symptomatic carriers) with spastic ataxia. Peripheral nerves are involved.
7. Pelizaeus-Merzbacher disease: an X-linked recessive disease due to mutations involving proteolipid protein-1 (PLP-1) gene. Brain is atrophic with diffuse demyelination, with small areas of perivascular preserved myelin, thus termed "tigroid leukodystrophy." Peripheral nerves are spared. Young males present with nystagmus, ataxia, and spasticity.
8. Alexander disease: an autosomal recessive disorder due to mutations in the glial fibrillary acidic protein (GAFP) gene. There is megalencephaly, mental retardation, seizures, and spasticity. The brain shows diffuse loss of myelin, predominantly in the frontal lobes, with presence of Rosenthal fibers, which are elongated tapered rods found in astrocytes of cortex and white matter.

IX. Metabolic Disorders

A. Carbon monoxide Lesions are due to hypoxia and are variable. Acute phase—brain shows marked swelling and "cherry red color" produced by carboxyhemoglobin in blood. Lesions after CO exposure are variable, dependent on amount and time of exposure; consist of necrosis of globus pallidus, white matter demyelination, or laminar cortical necrosis.

B. Vitamin deficiency disorders
1. **Thiamine deficiency:** the acute deficiency as seen in food poisoning, hyperemesis graviderum, or in alcoholics produces swelling of the mamillary bodies and petechial hemorrhages of the periaqueductal and third ventricular areas and explain the ophthalmoplegia, delirium, and ataxia seen in the acute Wernicke encephalopathy. Chronic phase or Korsakoff confabulatory psychosis is produced by pigmentary atrophy of the mamillary bodies that are connected with the thalamus and the hippocampus.
2. **Vitamin B_{12} deficiency** produces pernicious anemia causes subacute combine degeneration in spinal cord. Spinal cord lesions consist of spongy changes in corticospinal tract and posterior columns. Optic atrophy may be seen and mental changes may be due to chromatolysis of cortical neurons. Vacuolar myelopathy seen in HIV patients and copper-deficient myelopathy have same pathologic changes.

C. Central pontine myelinolysis: originally described in alcoholic patients and is due to rapid correction of hyponatremia in patients with other metabolic problems including liver disease. Also may rarely occur in young women undergoing surgery with general anesthesia. The lesion is reversible and consists of loss of myelin in the central portion of the pons with preservation of the neurons of pontine nuclei and no inflammation.

D. Methanol intoxication: methanol is metabolized into formaldehyde and formic acid that produces marked systemic acidosis. The CNS lesions consist of massive brain swelling, edema, and necrosis of the optic nerves and necrosis of putamen and claustrum.

E. Ethylene glycol: used in antifreezes and coolants and produces severe metabolic acidosis with elevated serum oxalic acid. The brain shows mild inflammatory infiltrate in the meninges and birefringent perivascular calcium oxalate crystals.

X. Congenital Malformations

A. Deviations of normal development of the CNS that usually occur during the first trimester of gestational life and are due to hereditary genetic or chromosomal abnormalities. Genetic counseling is important to differentiate these lesions from destructive or encephaloclastic acquired disorders produced by infections, toxic substances including medications, radiation, and hypoxia.

B. Neural tube defects are the most frequent malformations and include most severe form (range from anencephaly–amyelia to spina bifida occulta). Recurrence of the defect can be prevented with prenatal folate supplement. Meningomyelocele is associated with small posterior fossa and the Chiari II malformation that includes a downward displacement of the lower brainstem and cerebellar tonsils.

C. Holoprosencephaly: due to trisomy in chromosome 13 or 18 or inherited as autosomal recessive or X-linked forms. There are different variants associated with midline facial abnormalities. The alobar type consists of an undivided cerebrum, and absent septum, corpus callosum, and third ventricle, and a holospheric cerebrum. Arrhinencephaly or absence of the olfactory bulbs and tracts is the least severe variant.

D. Agenesis of the corpus callosum may be total or partial and may be associated with lipoma. In the total variant, the cingulate gyrus is replaced by perpendicular gyri and the ventricles in coronal planes have the bat-wing appearance (Figure 5-2).

E. Cortical disorders range from minor cortical, focal dysplasias that cause seizures to focal absence of gyri (pachygyria) to diffuse form (agyria–lissencephaly) (Figure 5-3). Excessive and irregular folding of gyral pattern: microgyria or polymicrogyria. Some are hereditary.

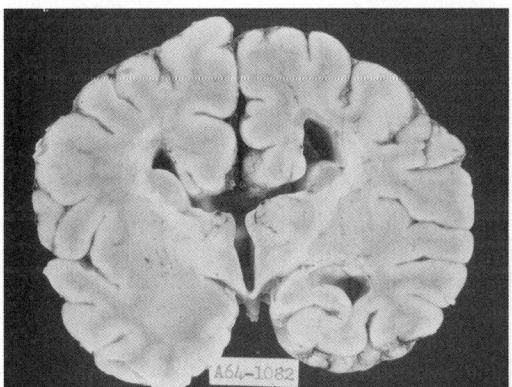

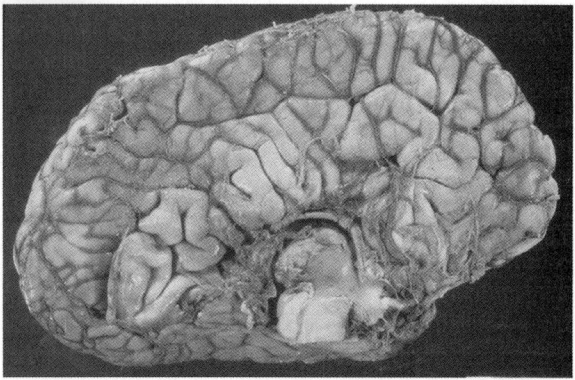

Figure 5-2 Agenesis of the corpus callosum. On the **left**, a coronal section showing the bat-wing shape of the ventricle. On the **right**, a midsagittal section showing the absence of the cingulated gyrus and the radiating pattern of the gyri.

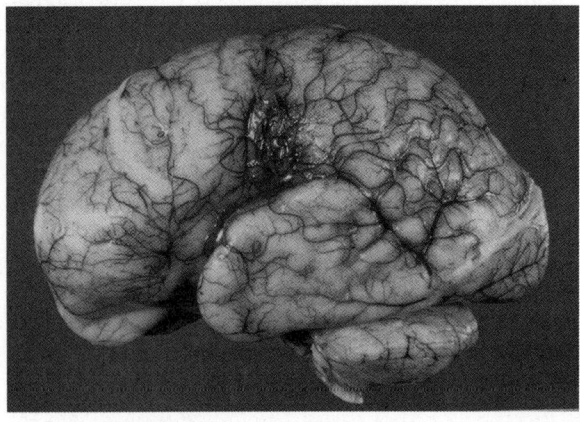
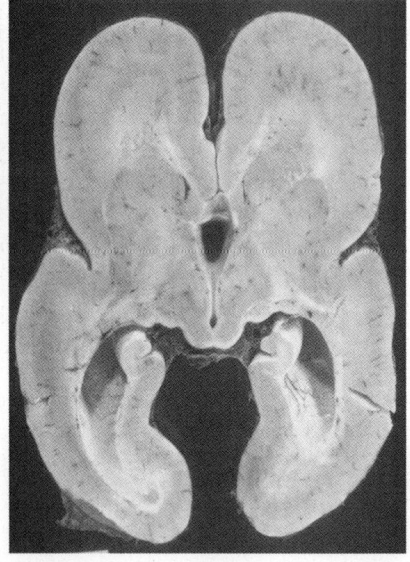

Figure 5-3 Agyria-lissencephaly; lateral view on the **left** and sagittal view on the **right**.

F. Aqueduct of Sylvius: isolated stenosis is rare and is the cause of hydrocephalus in an X-linked inherited form. It may be part of other malformations.

G. Dandy-Walker malformation: partial or total agenesis of the vermis produces an enlarged cystlike fourth ventricle and enlarged posterior fossa and hydrocephalus. It may be isolated or as part of other malformations. Acquired gestational lesions of the brain and range from massive hemispheric necrosis to minor lesions of the white matter.

H. Hydranencephaly: a multifactorial cause of massive necrosis of already formed brain producing a sac ("bubble brain") replacing portion of cerebral hemispheres irrigated by the carotid arteries. Viral infections, trauma, intoxication implicated as possible etiologic agents.

I. Multicystic encephalomalacia: multiple cysts are seen throughout the white and gray matter of both cerebral hemispheres separated by glial tissue. Hypoxia in late in pregnancy or early neonatal period has been implicated.

J. Germinal matrix lesions: periventricular germinal matrix composed of primitive dark blue neuroectodermal cells that migrate into mature neuronal and glial cells. Germinal matrix capillaries are thin and delicate and vulnerable to hypoxic and hemodynamic changes. Periventricular hemorrhages are frequent in immature infants with neonatal respiratory distress (Figure 5-4). Hemorrhages vary from small, localized lesions to massive hemorrhages that extend into the ventricles to produce massive hemicephalus and hydrocephalus.

K. Periventricular leukomalacia are white-matter hypoxic periventricular cystic lesions that contain reactive astrocytes, capillary proliferation, and perivascular "globules" that may calcify. Lesions are usually seen in premature infants that survive with cerebral palsy.

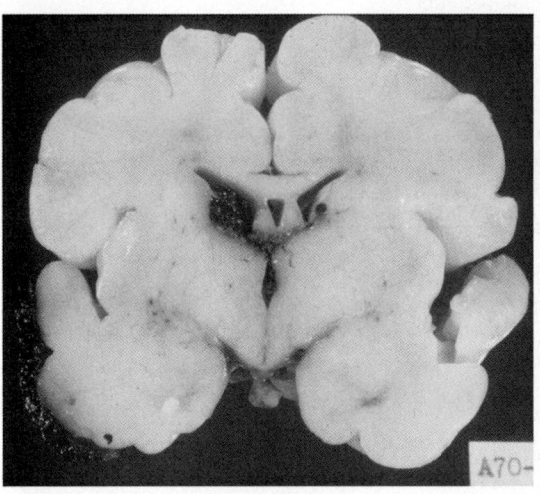
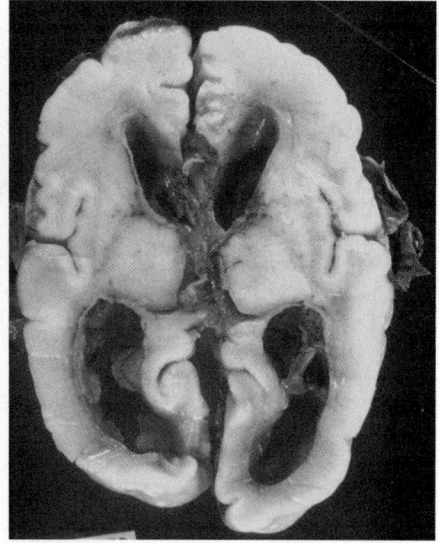

Figure 5-4 **A:** Small periventricular germinal matrix hemorrhage. **B:** Posthemorrhage hydrocephalus is evident.

XI. Pathology of Vascular Diseases

A. **Anatomic variations:** knowing anatomy of cerebral blood vessels and anatomic variations found in circle of Willis is important to understand ischemic events. Hypoplasia of segments or entire vessel is frequent and explains why occlusions of same vessel can produce infarcts of different sizes with different clinical manifestations. Size of ischemia depends on efficiency of collateral circulation in circle of Willis.

B. **Atherosclerosis:** most common cerebrovascular disease
  1. **The risk factors** for atherosclerosis include dyslipidemias, hypertension, diabetes mellitus, tobacco use (cigarette smoking), and aging.
  2. **Atherosclerosis** is an arterial systemic lipid disorder that begins early in life as a nonpathologic fatty streak. Over time, some of the fatty streaks develop into fibrous plaques located in the outer areas of bifurcation where the laminar flow is disturbed. The fibrous plaques contain connective tissue, smooth muscle cells, and lipid that continues to accumulate and eventually produce stenosis of the vessel wall, but without reducing significantly the blood flow to cause neurologic symptoms. This is a multifocal vascular disorder.
  3. **Complicated plaque:** Calcification inside plaque is frequent (Figure 5-5). Hemorrhage within plaque can accelerate arterial stenosis. Focal loss of endothelium of plaque or ulcerated plaque can be source of microemboli to retinal vessels (amaurosis fugax) or brain (some transient ischemic attacks [TIAs]). Microembolism may consist of platelets, fibrin, or calcium. Damage to endothelium of plaque can release tissue factors that activate coagulation and formation of thrombus. Thrombus can completely occlude lumen of the vessel or be source of emboli distally (artery to artery embolic phenomena). Anterograde extension of a thrombus or stagnation thrombus can also be source of emboli.
  4. **Cerebral infarction:** encephalomalacia or brain softening refers to necrotic brain tissue produced by ischemia in certain vascular territory.
      a. **Pale, anemic, or bland infarct:** macroscopic changes require at least 6 hours depending on the site and size of lesion for visible changes in cerebral infarcts. Swelling, congestion, and softening are earliest signs followed by fragmentation, and then clear liquefactive

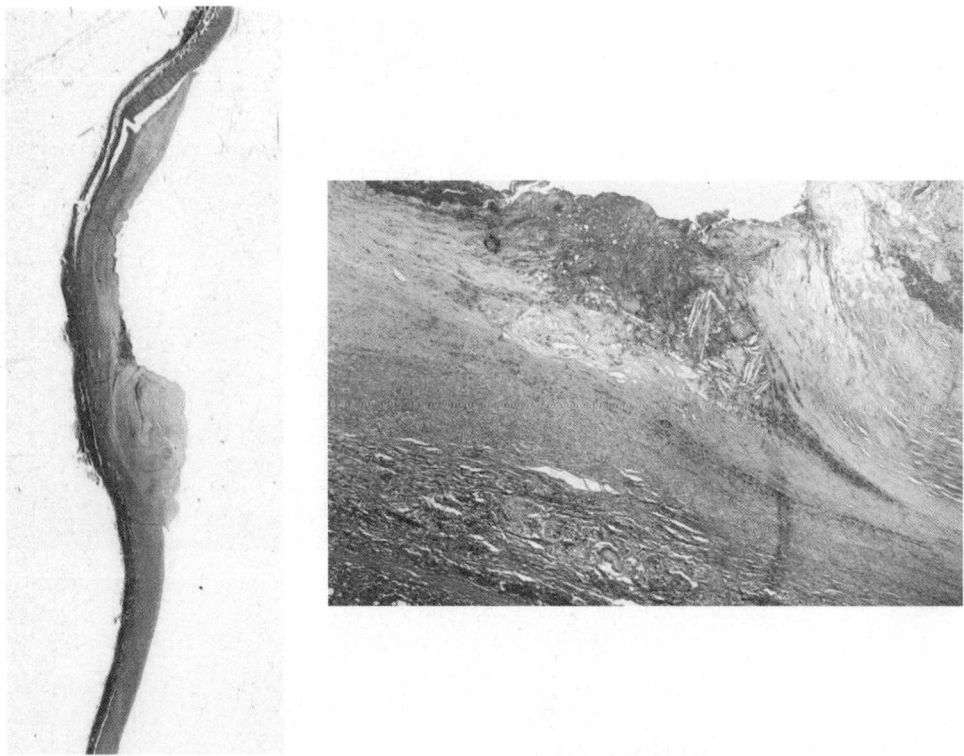

Figure 5-5 On the **left**, longitudinal section of carotid artery showing atherosclerotic ulcerated plaque. On the **right**, high power of the ulcer showing fibrin, cholesterol clefts, and platelets.

       necrosis. End-stage of infarct is a cystic space. Microscopic changes occur after 8 hours when neurons first show eosinophilia of cytoplasm and nuclear shrinkage with endothelial swelling of vessels and edema. After 24 hours neutrophils can be detected, and after 48 hours the macrophages begin to ingest and remove necrotic tissue. Astroglial reaction appears after 72 hours and persists for life (Figure 5-6A).
    b. **Hemorrhagic infarct:** areas of hemorrhage predominantly in infarcted cortex and basal ganglia, where capillaries are more numerous than in white matter (Figure 5-6B). Hemorrhage results from extravasation of red cells when reperfusion of blood reaches capillaries already damaged by ischemia (Figure 5-6C). Reperfusion occurs after thrombolysis or mobilization of a thrombus as may happen in cardiac embolic lesions or following venous sinus thrombosis.
    c. Embolic infarcts: can be cardioembolic or artery to artery. Fragmentation, migration of embolic material (thrombus) explains hemorrhagic nature of these lesions. Other sources of embolism include fat as seen in bone trauma and air as seen after chest trauma.
5. **Small vessel disease:** In hypertensive angiopathy hypertension accelerates atherosclerosis, produces small vessel disease and arteriolar sclerosis. Arterioles in chronic hypertension become thickened from proliferation of smooth muscle cells in response to intraluminal pressure. Arteriolar wall becomes hyalinized and may undergo fibrinoid change. Foamy macrophages in vessel wall are so-called lipohyalinosis. Arteriolar changes mainly in basal ganglia and pons where terminal arterioles are at a short distance from large mother vessel and where blood pressure is higher than in convexity of brain. Arteriolar changes can lead to occlusion of vessel lumen and produce lacunes or produce a diffuse form of disease known as arteriopathic leukoencephalopathy of Binswanger. Arterioles can rupture and produce intracerebral hemorrhages. Lacunes are small, less than 1.0 cm cystic lesions seen

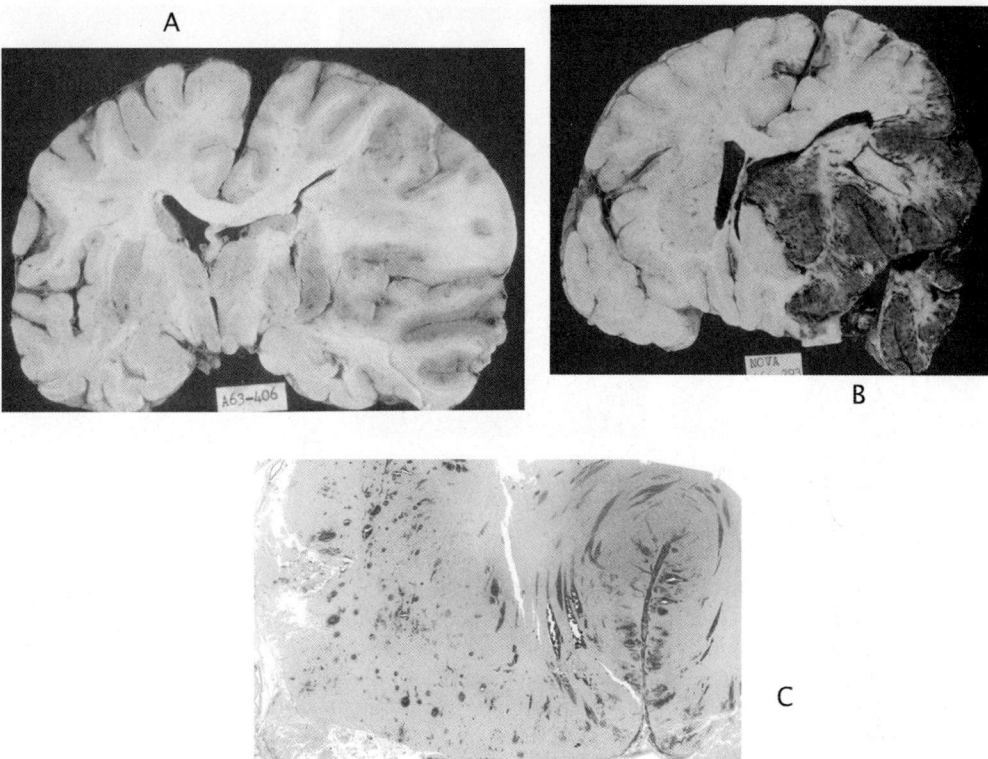

Figure 5-6 **A:** Recent ischemic "pale" infarct in the middle cerebral artery distribution. **B:** Hemorrhagic infarct of the middle cerebral artery distribution. Note the hemorrhagic component is mainly in the gray matter. **C:** Microscopic section of a hemorrhagic infarct. Note the predominant perivascular extravasation of blood.

usually in hypertensive elderly are due to arteriolar disease but may be due to other causes. Charcot-Bouchard micro- or miliary aneurysms can rupture and produce hematomas. Intracerebral hemorrhages: spontaneous hemorrhages may remain small and eventually may be reabsorbed, or may expand to rupture into the ventricle or produce mass effect with herniations and death. Most hemorrhages are found in the putamen followed by thalamus, pons, and cerebellum (Figure 5-7).

6. **Vasculopathies:**
   a. **Cerebral amyloid angiopathy:** produced by deposition of Aβ amyloid precursor protein (APP) in meningeal and cortical medium-sized arteries and arterioles of elderly patients. Amyloid is detected in tissue with Congo red stain that polarizes giving apple-green birefringence. "Lobar" hemorrhages occur in cortex and subcortical white matter of patients older than 60 years; may be multiple.
   b. **Moyamoya angiopathy:** obliterative, noninflammatory angiopathy seen in young stroke pateints. There is stenosis or occlusion of terminal portions of carotid arteries with externalization and duplication of the elastic layer. Ischemic and hemorrhagic events frequently occur.
7. **Vasculitis:**
   a. **Giant cell arteritis** patients older than 55 years, affects predominantly temporal artery, extends into ocular arteries producing monocular blindness. Microscopic findings include mononuclear inflammatory infiltration of vessel wall and giant cells next to elastic layer.

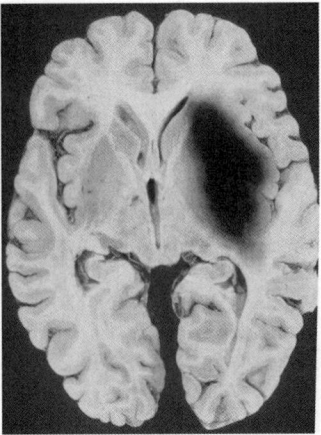 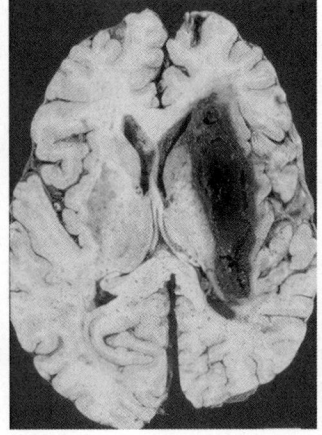 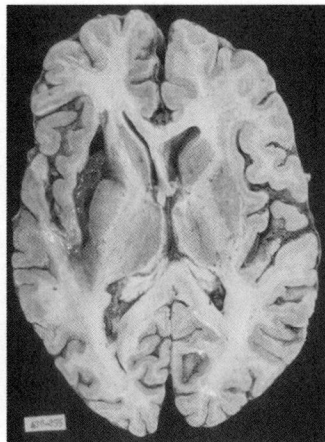

Figure 5-7 Hypertensive putaminal hemorrhage in different stages.

    b. **Primary angiitis** of CNS in adults and the histologic findings are variable, with mild mononuclear inflammatory infiltrate to granulomatous lesions.
    c. **In systemic lupus erythematosus** most common change in brain is multiple foci of infarction. Histologic findings in brain vessels similar to those in kidneys, including fibrinoid necrosis, mononuclear inflammatory infiltrate, and fibrosis of the vessel wall.
8. **Saccular (berry) intracranial aneurysms** are saclike dilations of arterial wall, usually seen at bifurcation of major branches of anterior portion of circle of Willis; 10% found in vertebrobasilar system. Most are found between the ages of 40 to 60 years; 50% of these patients are hypertensive. Most cases are sporadic and may be associated with polycystic kidney disease, Marfan syndrome, Ehlers-Danlos syndrome, fibromuscular dysplasia, coarctation of aorta, and sickle cell disease: 10% is familial, 20% with multiple aneurysms.
Clinical course:
    a. Some aneurysms never bleed and may be found in imaging studies or at autopsy.
    b. Others rupture into subarachnoid space, produce subarachnoid hemorrhage (SAH).
    c. The annual risk of bleeding for an unruptured intracranial saccular aneurysm found incidentally on imaging studies and confirmed by angiography is estimated to be approximately 1% for aneurysms 7 to 10 mm in diameter, and the risk of rupture increases with aneurysm size. Rebleeding is frequent in the first week.
    d. Some aneurysms rupture directly into brain parenchyma or ventricular system and a few may rupture directly into the subdural space and produce subdural hematomas.
    e. Aneurysms may grow and compress neighboring structures like temporal lobe (produce complex partial seizures) or third nerve (oculomotor palsy) or other cranial nerves.
    f. Distal ischemia due to vasospasm, or microembolism from the sac may occur.
    g. Hydrocephalus may occur in acute phase or chronic phase following bleeding after SAH.
9. **Dolichoectasia and fusiform aneurysms:** dilations on axis of large vessel possible in elderly hypertensive diabetic patients with advanced atherosclerosis. Intimal damage (endothelial and elastic layers) from atherosclerosis prevents normal elasticity of vessel wall; this with hypertension produces vessel dilation and uncoiling, which produce dolichoectasia of vessel (<4 mm in diameter). Basilar artery and supraclinoid portion of carotid arteries most frequently affected. Further dilation of dolicoectatic vessel produces fusiform aneurysm and can compress adjacent area, and cranial nerves and pons in basilar artery lesions. Fusiform aneurysms may thrombose but rarely rupture to produce SAH. Dolicoectatic and fusiform aneurysms seen in young patients with metabolic disorders, including Marfan syndrome, α-galactosidase deficiency, and arteritis.
10. **Infective or inflammatory aneurysms:** called mycotic if produced by infected emboli in patients with infective endocarditis. Aneurysms are small, usually fusiform in shape, and

seen in middle cerebral arteries branches. SAH and ICH is a frequent complication. Some resolve following antibiotic treatment, and others require surgical management.
11. **Dissecting aneurysms:** due to blood extravasation into arterial wall between intima and media and less frequently between media and adventitia. Lesions in young patients (25–40 years) associated with neck trauma including neck manipulations (neck dissections); may be spontaneous (intracranial vessels) in fibromuscular hyperplasia, Marfan syndrome, and connective tissue disorders. Dissections may be associated with lumen thrombus. Some vertebral dissections rarely rupture and produce SAH. Ischemia is the result of dissections.
12. **Miliary aneurysms** are arteriolar microdilations seen in hypertensive patients, described by Charcot and Bouchard as the cause of hypertensive intracerebral hemorrhages.
13. Veins and dural sinuses: no-infectious venous or sinus thrombosis is seen in children with diarrhea, dehydration or cyanotic congenital heart diseases. In young adult females, sinus thrombosis is found in pregnancy, the puerperium, or with the combined use of birth control pills and cigarette smoking. Venous thrombus impairs venous return, thereby producing swelling, congestion, and venous infarction, which may be hemorrhagic.

XII. Pathology of Brain Tumors

A. **The classification** based on the histologic features with the help of immunostains.
  1. The tumors are primary if they arise from structures in the brain, meninges, and calvaria
  2. Or secondary or metastatic if they originate outside the CNS
  3. Classification based on age, location, and clinicopathologic correlation; 70% of tumors in children infratentorial (posterior fossa) and 70% of tumors in adults supratentorial.

B. **Infratentorial tumors in children**
  1. **Circumscribed pilocytic cerebellar astrocytomas:** most frequent posterior fossa tumor in children; is slow growing, usually cystic, may be vermal or hemispheric. Histologic features are a compact astrocytic component with Rosenthal fibers and a loose or spongy component with microvascular proliferation. Surgical resection frequently cures this lesion.
  2. **Medulloblastoma:** malignant fast-growing embryonal, poorly differentiated, small blue cell tumor seen in early life with a second peak in adulthood (Figure 5-8). Tumor originates in posteromedullary velum of cerebellum, arises in roof of fourth ventricle, and grows rapidly to occupy fourth ventricle, with a tendency to meningeal spread. Cells form Homer-Wright rosettes and may show neuronal, glial, or even mesenchymal differentiation. Subtypes include desmoplastic medulloblastoma, medullomyoblastoma, and melanotic medulloblastoma. PNET or primitive neuroectodermal tumor (World Health Organization [WHO IV]) is a controversial term for small dark blue cell neoplasm, similar to the medulloblastoma but found in the cerebral hemispheres.
  3. **Pontine astrocytoma:** a diffuse fibrillary infiltrative astrocytoma of children and adolescents, produces a "hypertrophy" of pons with exophytic areas. The patients present with cranial nerve involvement and long tract signs. Radiation is a mainstay of therapy.
  4. **Ependymoma:** slow-growing tumor, originates in ependymal cells of ventricular system, in phylum terminalis of spinal cord. Usually originates in floor of fourth ventricle in children and adolescents and produces hydrocephalus. Cells are polygonal and form perivascular pseudorosettes: true ependymal rosettes resemble central canal of spinal cord.
  5. **Subependymoma:** is frequently asymptomatic tumor found on imaging studies or incidental autopsy material of adults. The tumor is found in the fourth ventricle attached to the dorsal medulla oblongata. The cells resemble the subependymal glial cells.

C. **Supratentorial tumors of children**
  1. **Pineal tumors:** pineal parenchymal tumors rare.
     a. Pineocytoma well-differentiated and slow growing; it enlarges pineal gland of young.
     b. Pineoblastoma embryonal, poorly differentiated, dark blue cell usually affects young males. Cells may form rosettes, pseudorosettes; they resemble other embryonal and

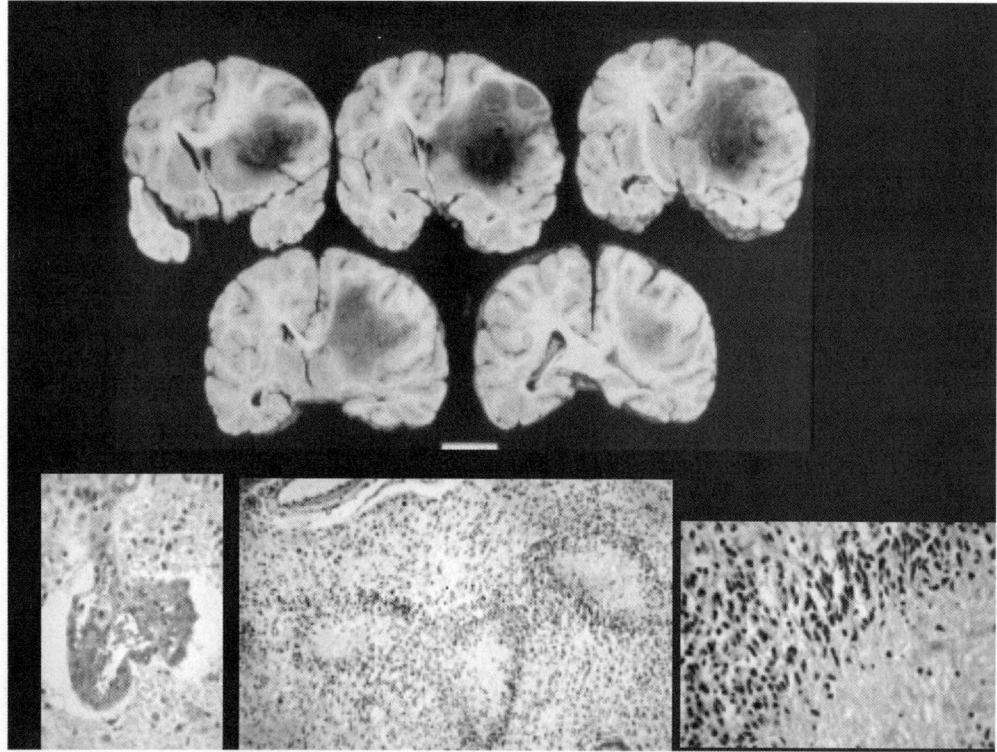

Figure 5-8 Glioblastoma multiforme. On **top**, gross sections showing a hemorrhagic, necrotic, infiltrating tumor. On the **bottom left**, endothelial hyperplasia; **bottom center**, areas of necrosis with palisading nuclei; on **bottom right**, nuclear palisades and pleomorphism of cells.

primitive neuroectodermal tumors such as the medulloblastoma. Meningeal spread may occur.
2. **Germ cell tumors:** arise from gonadal cells in midline structures of the body including third ventricle and pineal area, predominately in young Asian males. Germinoma, the most frequent type, often produces meningeal spread; highly radiosensitive. Other variants include embryonal carcinoma, choriocarcinoma, and teratomas. Serum and cerebrospinal fluid (CSF) can be assayed for oncoproteins such as α-fetoprotein, β-chorionic gonadotrophin, and carcinoembryonic antigen (CEA) for diagnostic confirmation and response to treatment.
3. **Craniopharyngioma:** most frequent benign epithelial suprasellar calcified neoplasm in children. Irregular cysts filled with dark material contain cholesterol and calcium. The childhood histologic variant resembles the adamantinoma of the jaw. The papillary non-calcified form is most frequently seen in adults. The tumor locally invades the adjacent hypothalamic region eliciting an exuberant gliotic reaction with Rosenthal fibers.
4. **Hemispheric astrocytomas in children:** Pleomorphic xanthoastrocytoma is a slow growing low-grade tumor that can be solid or cystic and found near the cortex of the temporal lobes. The cells have nuclear variations with a xanthomatous cytoplasm.
5. **Subependymal giant cell astrocytoma:** predominantly in tuberous sclerosis, grows from the wall of the lateral ventricles and obstructs the third ventricle producing hydrocephalus. The tumor grows slowly, is vascular, and can be calcified. The prognosis is usually good, seen in patients with tuberous sclerosis.

D. **Supratentorial tumors of adults**
1. **Metastatic tumors:** most frequent tumors in adults; may be found in any region of the CNS; hematogenous spread from primary including the lungs, breast, skin, gastrointestinal tract,

or kidneys. Well-circumscribed and usually multiple, necrosis or cystic degeneration. Bleeding can occur in any metastasis but most frequently occurs in metastatic melanomas, hypernephroma, and choriocarcinoma; also pituitary tumor. Meningeal carcinomatosis occurs independent of brain metastasis and is associated with adenocarcinomas of the stomach, breast, and lung.

2. **Glioblastoma:** most common primary tumor in adults; occurs most frequently in males and is supratentorial (Figure 5-9). Tumor may occur *de novo* and arise from low-grade diffuse astrocytoma. Highly malignant, infiltrative, grows fast, and shows areas of necrosis and hemorrhage. Vascular proliferation, cellular pleomorphism, areas of necrosis surrounded by rim of cells arranged in pseudopalisading pattern are diagnostic. Poor response to treatment.

3. **Pituitary tumors:** benign anterior lobe adenomas predominantly in women. Microadenomas are small lesions localized to gland, which cause endocrine symptoms: galactorrhea–amenorrhea, acromegaly, Cushing disease. Some enlarge, expand sella, and compress optic chiasm to produce visual field defects. Necrosis and bleeding (pituitary apoplexy) produces sudden expansion of tumor; this compresses chiasm to produce acute blindness and subarachnoid hemorrhage. Sensitive radioimmunoassays measure serum pituitary hormones; immunoperoxidase stains have made classification more accurate.

    a. Prolactinoma most frequent pituitary tumor in young females, usually microadenomas that produce amenorrhea and galactorrhea. Medical (dopaminergic medication) and surgical treatments are available.

    b. Growth hormone cell adenomas are associated with gigantism in young growing patients and acromegaly in adults.

4. **Meningiomas:** Benign slow-growing tumors, arise from meningothelial (arachnoidal) cells. Attached firmly to dura. Predominant in middle-aged females and occurs with increasing

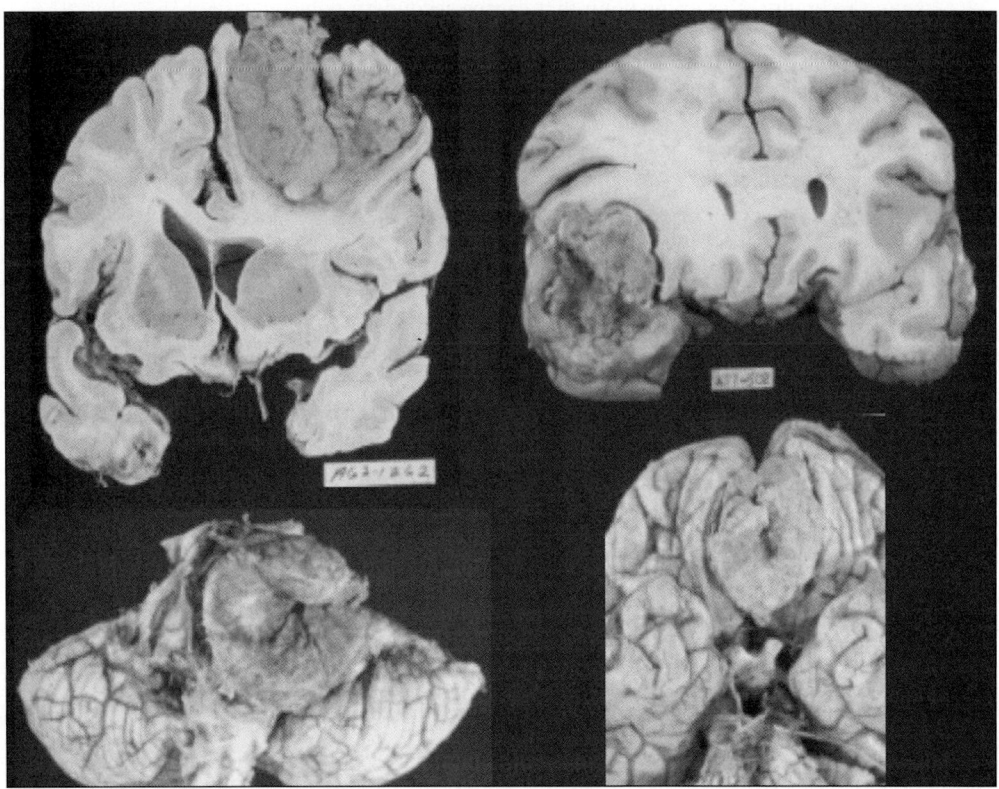

Figure 5-9 Meningiomas. **Upper left**, parasagittal, **upper right**, sphenoid wing area, **lower left**, clivus area, **lower right**, subfrontal.

frequency in association with breast cancer. Soft well-circumscribed lesions located over convexity around parasagittal region but may also occur in olfactory groove, parasellar area, sphenoid ridge, clivus, tentorium, and ventricles. Histologic features are variable; heterogeneous but presence of lobules, whorl formation, and psammoma bodies is distinctive. Histologic variants include meningotheliomatous, fibrous, and syncytial. Malignant meningiomas show anaplasia and brain invasion.
5. **Oligodendrogliomas:** infiltrating, well-differentiated, predominantly frontal lobes of adults. Regularity of tumor cell nuclei with clear cytoplasm or "fried egg" artifact in "honeycomb" pattern with mucoid areas; microcalcifications are distinctive diagnostic features. Malignant features include cellular pleomorphism and areas of necrosis.
6. **Diffuse infiltrating astrocytomas:** group of glial tumors of adults with malignant degeneration usually located in frontal or temporal lobes.
   a. Fibrillary astrocytoma most common type
   b. Gemistocytic astrocytoma abundant cytoplasm, peripherally displaced nucleus. Can progress to anaplastic astrocytoma or glioblastoma.
   c. Anaplastic astrocytoma—pleomorphic cellular features but without areas of necrosis. It may appear *de novo* or arise in a preexisting astrocytoma.

E. **Infratentorial tumors in adults**
1. **Schwannoma:** (neurilemoma, neurinoma) benign slow-growing tumor of peripheral nerves. Can be sporadic; usually single or associated with neurofibromatosis type 2 (NF2), multiple. Most frequent intracranial Schwannoma arises in the vestibular division of the CN VIII, the acoustic neuroma or the cerebellopontine angle tumor.
2. **Cerebellar hemangioblastoma:** solitary tumor or sporadic form most frequent. However, can be part of von Hippel-Lindau syndrome. Tumor usually cerebellar cystic lesion with mural nodule. Two cellular elements: stromal or large vacuolated cells and a rich capillary network. Produces erythropoietin that causes secondary polycythemia.

F. **Miscellaneous CNS tumors and cysts**
1. **Lymphomas:** most CNS lymphomas are primary, malignant B-cell type. Incidence has sharply increased since AIDS epidemic; more prevalent in males than females. Most tumors supratentorial, solitary or multiple, frontal, temporal periventricular regions. Lymphomas can originate in spinal cord in HIV patients. The prognosis is poor despite RT and CT.
2. **Lipomas:** fat tumors similar to lipomas elsewhere. Associated with partial, total agenesis of the corpus callosum; quadrigeminal areas, dysraphism of the spinal cord possible.
3. **Chordomas:** derived from remnants of the notochord and found in the sacrum and clivus areas. The tumor is benign but difficult to eradicate.
4. **Benign cystic lesions**
   a. **Colloid cyst:** epithelial-lined cyst with proteinaceous material found in anterosuperior third ventricle of young adults. Can produce acute hydrocephalus and sudden death.
   b. **Arachnoid cyst:** lined by meningothelial (arachnoidal) cell and contains normal CSF. The lesion is frequently found in the temporal fossa and is rarely symptomatic.
   c. **Epidermoid and dermoid cysts:** cysts lined by benign squamous epithelium. Dermoid cysts also contain cutaneous adnexa. The cysts can be found in the cerebellopontine angle, sellar area, and fourth ventricle.
   d. **Rathke cleft cyst:** intrasellar or suprasellar lined by columnar or cuboidal epithelium.

XIII. Neurodegenerative Diseases

A. **Neurodegenerative diseases** are a group of disorders.
1. Affect the aging population
2. Neuronal loss and variable astrocytic and microglial reaction
3. Presence of inclusions due to accumulation of abnormal proteins
4. Have a regional (topographic) predilection

B. **Etiologies implicated** include oxidative stress, genetic predisposition, and apoptosis.
   1. Apoptosis or programmed cell death is a genetically controlled process. The neurons show chromatic condensation and margination, nuclear condensation, and cytoplasmic blebbing. Caspases are proteases that regulate cell death and may be implicated in apoptosis.
   2. In this review a topographic and clinicopathologic correlation is used.

C. **Diseases that affect the cortex**
   1. **Alzheimer disease:** most common neurodegenerative disorder and most common cause of dementia. Risk factors include age, family history, low education, head injury, atherosclerosis, and elevated serum homocysteine. The familial cases affect younger patients. Genotype at the apolipoprotein E-4 (APOE) locus seems to increase risk.
      a. **Macroscopic changes** in the brain consist of:
         i. Cortical atrophy predominantly in hippocampus and midtemporal structures and amygdala, frontal lobes, and olfactory bulb
         ii. Enlargement of the lateral and third ventricles
      b. **Microscopic changes** consist of:
         i. Senile (neuritic) plaques with central core of amyloid deposits of Aβ-peptide derived from APP, surrounded by degenerating nerve cell processes: astroglial microglial reaction, predominantly hippocampus, entorhinal cortex, neocortex
         ii. Neurofibrillary tangles (neurofibrillary degeneration), intracellular inclusions made by abnormal tau proteins. When affected neurons die, insoluble tangles remain in neuropil as "ghost tangles." These elements are part of the peripheral elements of the plaques. Tangles are found in the amygdaloid, anterior thalamic nucleus, basal nucleus of Meynert, reticular and mesencephalic nucleus, and locus ceruleus.
         iii. Amyloid deposition in the cerebral blood vessel (amyloid angiopathy) may be seen in the posterior cortex of patients with AD.
   2. **Dementia with Lewy bodies:** typically affects patients older than 65 years and is associated with well-formed visual hallucinations and parkinsonism with episodes of loss of consciousness. The pathology consists of cerebral atrophy, predominantly in the limbic system, and pallor of the substantia nigra. Microscopic findings include presence of Lewy bodies in the locus ceruleus and substantia nigra. There are ubiquitin and α-synuclein–positive deep cortical Lewy bodies in hippocampus, singular and insular cortex.
   3. **Frontotemporal dementia:** patient characteristics include disinhibition, apathy, compulsive behavior, and alcoholism. The macroscopic lesion is severe atrophy of the frontal and temporal lobes and hydrocephalus. The microscopic features include presence of tau proteins in the neurons and glia of affected areas.
   4. **Pick disease:** associated with speech impairment, long survival.
      a. **Macroscopic findings:** cortical "knife edge" or "dry walnut" appearance. Frontotemporal atrophy spares precentral gyrus and two thirds of superior temporal gyrus. Marked atrophy of limbic structures, especially Ammon horn (Figure 5-10).
      b. **Microscopic findings:** cortical and subcortical gliosis with microvacuolation of the superficial layers and ballooned neurons or Pick cells; some contain spherical argentophilic (tauproteins) cytoplasmic inclusion (Pick bodies). The inclusions are predominantly in dentate gyrus of the hippocampus, amygdala, and septal nuclei.

D. **Diseases that affect the cortex and basal ganglia**
   1. **Corticobasal degeneration:** asymmetric atrophy of the cortex, basal ganglia and the substantia nigra with accumulation of tau protein in neurons and glia. The patients are rigid and clumsy with apraxia, the "alien limb" phenomenon. There is loss of neurons and glia and presence of large globose pale neurofibrillary tangles.
   2. **Huntington disease:** is an autosomal dominant trinucleotide expansion disorder manifested by dementia, behavioral disorders including psychoses, involuntary movements, and cachexia. Mean age of onset is 40 years with duration of approximately 17 years. Paternal inheritance increases length of expansions (anticipation) with an earlier age of onset and more severe disease.
      a. **Macroscopic findings:** moderate-to-severe cortical atrophy with some preservation of temporal lobes, predominant atrophy of caudate nucleus, and putamen (neostriatum)

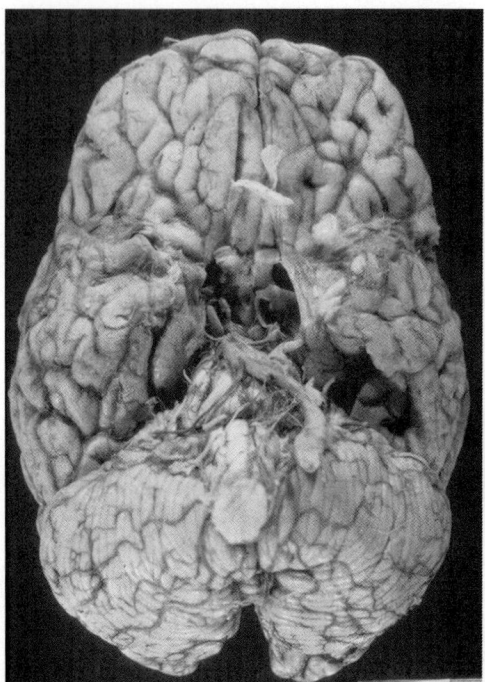 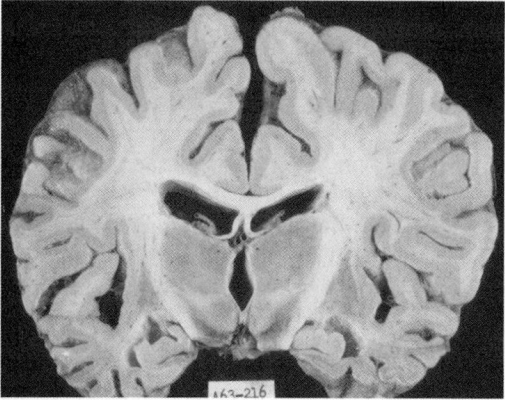

Figure 5-10 On the **left**, a basal view of a Pick dementia brain showing lobar atrophy of the left temporal lobe. On the **right**, a coronal section showing predominant left temporal atrophy.

with marked dilation of ventricular system. Normal bulging appearance of caudate nucleus; on coronal section becomes flat or concave.
  b. **Microscopic findings:** loss of medium spiny neurons in the striatum and reactive astrogliosis and microgliosis, the Huntington protein is encoded by the defective gene in chromosome 4 and can be detected in high quantities by immunostaining in the affected cortex.

E. **Diseases that affect predominantly the brainstem**
  1. **Parkinson disease:** frequent neurodegenerative movement disorder characterized by akinesia, rigidity, resting tremor, and postural instability.
      a. **Etiology:** progressive deterioration and loss of pigmented neurons in pars compacta of substantia nigra affects entire dopaminergic nigrostriatal system. The disease is associated with specific intracytoplasmic Lewy bodies and dystrophic Lewy neuritis.
      b. **Macroscopically:** mild atrophy and hydrocephalus but diagnostic feature is pallor of substantia nigra and locus ceruleus with normal appearance of striatum and globus pallidus (Figure 5-11).
      c. **Microscopic findings:** severe loss of melanized neurons and gliosis of substantia nigra and locus ceruleus with presence of classical Lewy bodies. These bodies are intraneuronal cytoplasmic, round eosinophilic structures. The cortical Lewy bodies are granular "pale bodies" better detected by immunohistochemical stains including ubiquitin and α-synuclein. Cortical Lewy bodies are ubiquitous in the dementia of Lewy body. In postencephalitic Parkinson disease the neurons of the substantia nigra and locus ceruleus contain predominantly neurofibrillary tangles rather than Lewy bodies.
  2. **Progressive supranuclear palsy** (PSP) or Steele-Richardson-Olszewski disorder of middle age characterized by severe axial rigidity without tremor, retrocollis, supranuclear ophthalmoplegia, pseudobulbar palsy, and dementia.

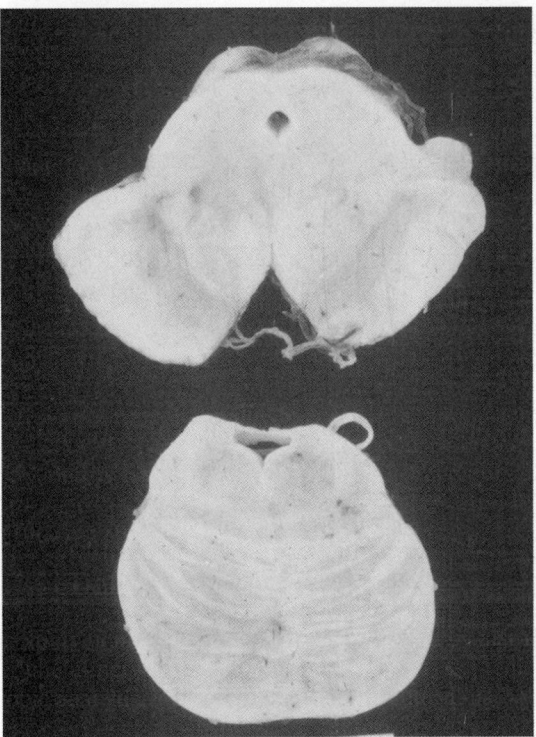 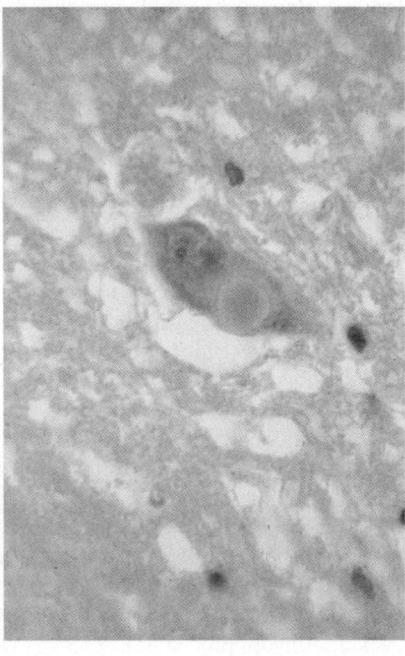

Figure 5-11 On the **left**, a midbrain of a patient with Parkinson disease. Depigmentation of the substantia nigra and locus ceruleus. On the **right**, pigmented neuron with Lewy body.

   a. **Macroscopic findings:** atrophy of midbrain, predominantly superior colliculi: dilation of aqueduct and paleness of the substantia nigra.
   b. **Microscopic changes:** loss of nerve cells, gliosis, accumulation of tau protein in neurons, glia. Neurons show globose neurofibrillary tangles strongly stain to tau protein.
3. **Multisystem atrophy** (MSA): adult-onset sporadic neurodegenerative disease characterized by α-synuclein glial cytoplasmic inclusions (Papp-Lantos inclusions). MSA includes three disorders that had been considered separate entities.
   a. **Sporadic form of ataxia** known as olivopontocerebellar atrophy, predominantly autonomic failure or Shy-Drager disease, parkinsonism form—striatonigral degeneration
   b. **Macroscopic findings:** variable, depend on clinical finding; may include mild brain atrophy, paleness of substantia nigra and locus ceruleus, atrophy of the striatum and atrophy of the brainstem and cerebellum.
   c. **Microscopic findings:** loss of nerve cells, astrocytosis, and myelin loss in affected areas. System related presence of inclusions in the cytoplasm of oligodendrocytes (Papp-Lantos inclusions) is the diagnostic hallmark. These inclusions may be seen less frequently in astrocytes and neurons and are not seen with hematoxylin and eosin, but are silver positive with Gallyas or Bodian stains and specifically stain with α-synuclein.

F. **Diseases that affect predominantly the spinal cord**
   1. **Spinocerebellar ataxias:** clinical and genetic heterogeneous group. Presentation includes truncal and limb ataxia, ataxic speech, nystagmus, associated with sensory impairment, weakness, parkinsonism, cognitive impairment, and autonomic dysfunction.
      a. Genetic abnormalities autosomal dominant with a few autosomal recessive and X-linked forms. Autosomal forms CAG triplet repeat that correlate with the age of onset, severity of the disease, and genetic anticipation. Macroscopic and histologic findings are

similar except for topography of lesions; ≥25 different genotypes with genes identified in at least 12 different phenotypes.
- b. **SCA3 Machado-Joseph disease** (14q24.33q31): pyramidal, extrapyramidal signs, nystagmus, lid retraction, decreased saccades, peripheral neuropathies, amyotrophy with fasciculations.
- c. Dentatorubral-pallidoluysian atrophy DRPLA (12p13.31): chores, seizures, dementia, and myoclonus. Most patients present with spastic ataxia and associated features.
2. **Friedreich ataxia** (FA): autosomal recessive due to homozygous intronic GAA repeat chromosome 9 (9q13–21.1), encodes frataxin, a mitochondrial protein reduced in FA.
   - a. **Clinical features:** preadolescent onset, truncal and limb ataxia, scanning speech, proprioception and vibratory sense impairment, areflexia, Babinski sign, peripheral neuropathy associated with cardiomyopathy and diabetes mellitus.
   - b. **Macroscopic findings:** demyelination and astrogliosis of posterior columns, corticospinal, spinocerebellar tracts, axonal neuropathy, and degeneration of some brainstem tracts. The cerebellar involvement is mild when compared with the spinal cord lesions.
3. **Hereditary spastic paraparesis:** Group of disorders manifested by progressive spastic weakness of the legs, urinary urgency late in the disease, and subtle dorsal column involvement. Most cases are transmitted as autosomal dominant, but autosomal recessive and X-linked inheritance can occur. There are pure forms of the disease and in some cases there may be deafness, optic nerve involvement, and other associated findings.
4. **Motor neuron diseases:** progressive disorder of motor neurons of cortex, brainstem, spinal cord to produce weakness and atrophy of affected muscles. There are different clinical patterns according to the neurons involved.
   - a. **Amyotrophic lateral sclerosis (ALS)** involves the upper motor neurons, producing spastic weakness with hyperreflexia and Babinski sign and also lower motor neurons producing early atrophy and fasciculations of affected muscles. ALS may begin with bulbar muscle involvement known as progressive bulbar palsy. A progressive lower motor neuron form of ALS affecting predominately the spinal cord is known as progressive spinal muscular atrophy.
   - b. Predominantly upper motor neuron with spasticity is primary lateral sclerosis.
   - c. Bulbar involvement and respiratory failure are the final stages.
   - d. Ten percent of the cases are hereditary in an autosomal dominant pattern and are due to mutations of the co-zinc superoxide dismutase gene (SOD1)
   - e. Macroscopic findings: atrophy of the precentral gyrus, thinning of spinal cord, and atrophy of anterior roots
   - f. Microscopic findings: atrophy and loss of motor neurons of cortex, motor brainstem nuclei, and anterior horn cells in spinal cord. Reactive astrogliosis is seen in the affected areas along with loss of myelin and gliosis in the corticospinal tracts of the spinal cord. Ubiquitin-stained inclusions have been seen in the cortex and hippocampal areas.
5. **Spinal muscular atrophy** (SMA): hereditary motor neuron disease predominately in infancy, childhood, and adolescence. Autosomal recessive with homozygous deletion of survival motor neuron (SMN1) gene in chromosome 5q13. Severe weakness, atrophy, and features of muscle denervation due to loss of anterior horn cells and gliosis of cord without involvement of corticospinal tracts. Spinal cord atrophy of anterior roots.
   - a. Three phenotypes according to age of presentation: type I or Werdnig-Hoffman disease, chronic infantile type II, childhood type, or Kugelberg-Welander disease.

XIV. Traumatic Brain Injury (TBI)

A. **Brain damage** from TBI is important cause of death and disability. It is complex, has different causes, mechanisms, different types of clinical manifestations, and prognosis. The severity and distribution of the trauma are very important and can be:
1. Focal or impact injuries to skull and brain; the lesions are immediate and include intracranial hematomas, contusions of the brain, and hemorrhages of brain or meninges

2. Diffuse or acceleration–deceleration injuries like brain contusions and axonal injuries
3. Hypoxia, brain swelling, and vascular damage can occur and produce delayed effects.

B. **Cerebral concussion** is a reversible traumatic paralysis of nervous function.
   1. Produced by blunt nonpenetrating head injury, either a severe blow to the static head (accelerative), or a moving head that is arrested by a hard unyielding surface (decelerative)
   2. Always immediate loss of consciousness; may last from seconds to hours or longer
   3. Mechanisms of concussion: the brain is subjected to sheering stresses produced by rotational acceleration of the head that affects
      a. The high midbrain and subthalamic area that contain the upper reticular formation to explain the immediate loss of consciousness
      b. The hemispheric white matter producing diffuse axonal shearing injury
         i. Is the cause of some of the early and late clinical effects
         ii. Produces microglial "clusters" or "stars" in 5 to 10 days, but can be detected in 3 hours after the trauma with staining for β-amyloid precursor protein.
   4. **Clinical features**
      a. Immediate loss of consciousness, suppression of all reflexes, bradycardia, hypotension, apnea
      b. Gradual recovery of consciousness with amnesia
         i. Retrograde amnesia or loss of memory of events preceding the trauma
         ii. Anterograde amnesia or loss of memory of events after trauma
         iii. Duration of anterograde amnesia most reliable predictor of severity of concussion

C. **Surface contusions and lacerations of the brain**
   1. Size, location, and extent of contusions depend on circumstances of injury. Lesions may be superficial, involve cortex and white matter, and can be associated with hematomas, edema, and subarachnoid hemorrhage; may be multiple, usually asymmetric

D. **Axonal injury**
   1. Axonal injury variably related to severity of the injury; can be mild and reversible in some brain concussions or severe and diffuse in severe head injuries.
      a. Axonal injury is produced by angular or rotational acceleration–deceleration forces in unconscious patients who have no imaging lesion to explain the neurologic status.
      b. Gross examination may not show clearly visible lesions; extensive sampling of white matter hemispheric areas and brainstem may be necessary to detect the lesions.
      c. Antibodies to β-amyloid precursor protein can be detected 2 hours after the injury; axonal swelling or bulbs are visible 12 hours after the injury and microglial "clusters" or "stars" are seen 5 to 10 days after the injury. Gliosis and wallerian degeneration can be detected in longstanding cases.

E. **Coup and contrecoup fractures**
   1. Coup fractures occur at the site of the impact.
   2. Contrecoup fractures at opposite side from impact not connected with impact fracture.
   3. Contrecoup fractures frequently occur at roof of orbit and ethmoidal plate in occipital injuries.

F. **Coup and contrecoup contusions**
   1. Coup contusions are usually produced by a blow to the stationary head; occur at the site of the impact and are not associated with impact fractures.
   2. Contrecoup contusions occur opposite to site of impact, are produced by deceleration of head, and can be seen in frontotemporal areas in backward falls that hit the occiput.
   3. Other features of brain trauma: hypoxia in acute injury can produce laminar cortical necrosis and infarcts in border zones. Dementia pugilistica or punch-drunk encephalopathy occurs due to repeated head trauma in boxers, soccer or football players, and jockeys. In these cases brain shows rupture of interventricular septum, pallor of substantia nigra, widespread cortical neurofibrillary tangles, amyloid plaques, and neuropil threads.

G. **Epidural (Extradural) Hemorrhage**
   1. Epidural hemorrhage is usually due to severe impact to the head with skull fracture and vascular damage. The impact produces loss of consciousness followed by a lucid interval and then a rapid, usually focal, deterioration of brain function.
   2. Arterial bleed. The meningeal arteries lie in the grooves of the skull outside the dura. Laceration of the middle meningeal artery produces immediate bleed under arterial pressure with acute compression of the adjacent brain.
   3. Venous bleed. Rarely the impact produces laceration of a venous sinus producing a slower accumulation of venous blood.

H. **Subdural hemorrhage**
   1. **Subdural hematomas** can be acute or chronic.
   2. **Acute subdural hematomas** usually associated with brain contusions due to severe head trauma are a mixture of arterial and venous blood. May be seen in abused children.
   3. **Chronic subdural hematomas** venous in nature, produced by minor head trauma in patients with atrophic brains. Atrophy of brain in elderly patients and alcoholics stretches the bridging veins that drain the circulation to the dural sinuses. Minor trauma produces tear in veins with slow bleeding. Chronic subdural hematomas are frequently encapsulated.
   4. **Subdural hygromas** collection of CSF or high protein fluid due to traumatic tear to arachnoid membrane. More frequently seen in children and the elderly.

I. **Whiplash or recoil injury of the neck**
   1. Produced by sudden and violent extension followed by flexion of the neck, frequently in rear-end collisions in motor vehicle accidents, or, when the accelerating person or vehicle is suddenly stopped the head moves forward (flexion) followed by violent backward displacement (extension). The injuries occur in the neck muscles, ligaments, and soft tissues of the neck, not spinal cord. Injures range from minor sprain of muscles and ligaments to severe damage of bone and soft tissues. Psychologic and compensation factors play an important role in the recovery of mild injuries.

XV. Cerebral Edema

A. **Cerebral edema** represents increased brain volume due to increased water volume. Different types affect different brain compartments and respond differently to treatment.

B. **Vasogenic edema**, the most common type of edema, is due to increased permeability of the BBB to macromolecules (proteins).
   1. Is seen around abscesses and brain tumors
   2. Responds to steroids
   3. Can be detected by imaging studies

C. **Cytotoxic edema** is caused by intracellular accumulation of water produced by injury that damages the capacity of the cells to maintain tonic homeostasis.
   1. Affects neurons, glial, endothelial cells, myelin: seen in ischemia, trauma, toxin exposure
   2. Does not respond to steroids
   3. Is not usually detected by imaging studies

D. **Interstitial, hydrocephalic, or "pressure" edema:**
   1. CSF accumulation in periventricular white matter in hydrocephalus
   2. Can be detected by imaging studies
   3. Does not respond to steroids
   4. Treat with shunt

E. **Some brain edemas are combination** of both vasogenic and cytotoxic types.

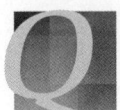 STUDY QUESTIONS FOR CHAPTER 5

Directions: *Each of the numbered items or incomplete statements in this section is followed by answers or by completions of the statement. Select the ONE lettered answer or completion that is BEST in each case.*

1. Perinatal hypoxia is thought to be the basis of the following lesions, EXCEPT

   (A) Hydranencephaly
   (B) Multicystic encephalopathy
   (C) Holoprosencephaly
   (D) Ulegyria (sclerotic microgyria)
   (E) Leukomalacia

2. The following changes are constantly found in Pick disease, EXCEPT

   (A) Loss of nerve cells
   (B) Amyloid deposits in blood vessels
   (C) Cortical and subcortical astrogliosis
   (D) Tau-positive antibodies in inclusions
   (E) Intraneuronal argentophilic inclusions

3. The neuropathologic lesion associated with (HbSS) sickle cell disease is

   (A) Venous thrombosis and hemorrhagic infarcts
   (B) Presence of miliary aneurysms in hematomas
   (C) Arterial occlusions associated with cerebral infarcts
   (D) Telangiectatic vascular malformations with hemorrhage
   (E) Sagittal sinus thrombosis

4. Neuropathologic changes in delayed death produced by methanol intoxication is

   (A) Necrosis of the lateral aspect of putamen and claustrum
   (B) Pigmentary atrophy of the mamillary bodies
   (C) Atrophy of the cerebellar vermis
   (D) Atrophy and gliosis of the hippocampus
   (E) Laminar cortical necrosis

5. Complications of fibrous atherosclerotic plaque in carotid artery include all the following, EXCEPT

   (A) Calcification and stenosis
   (B) Ulceration of the intima
   (C) Bleeding within the plaque
   (D) Resolution with diet in a few days
   (E) Formation of a thrombus

6. Subependymal giant cell astrocytoma is a tumor found in patient with

   (A) Down syndrome
   (B) Sturge-Weber syndrome
   (C) Neurofibromatosis
   (D) Tuberous sclerosis
   (E) von Hippel-Lindau syndrome

7. Primary noninfectious thrombosis of dural sinuses are seen in

   (A) Neonates in respiratory failure
   (B) School age children after head trauma
   (C) Dehydrated infants and postpartum young females
   (D) Heavy smokers (male) with cardiac disease
   (E) Sickle cell disease

8. Progressive supranuclear palsy is associated with which of the abnormal structures?

   (A) Lafora bodies
   (B) Lewy bodies
   (C) Globose neurofibrillary tangles
   (D) Buscaino bodies
   (E) Hirano bodies

9. A 41-year-old heroin addict is admitted to the neurosurgery service with fever, weakness of the lower extremities, and urinary incontinence. Strength in his upper extremities is normal. Magnetic resonance imaging of the brain and entire spine is performed and a diagnosis of epidural abscess is made. What is the most likely location of this patient's abscess?

   (A) Frontal convexities
   (B) Cervical spine
   (C) Thoracic spine
   (D) Conus medullaris
   (E) Cauda equina

10. A 3-year-old girl is brought to the emergency room with profound weakness of the left arm with absent reflexes. The remainder of her neurologic examination is normal. What is the most likely causative viral agent?

    (A) Herpesvirus
    (B) Enterovirus
    (C) Rabies
    (D) Measles
    (E) Arbovirus

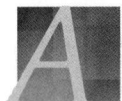 ANSWERS AND EXPLANATIONS

1. C. Holoprosencephaly is chromosomal disorder. A, B, D, E caused by perinatal hypoxia.

2. B. Amyloid angiopathy is not a feature of Pick disease; other answers are.

3. C. Large arterial disease associated with multiple infarcts is the usual finding.

4. A. Methanol intoxication produces optic nerve damage and necrosis of lateral aspect of putamen and claustrum. Others answers would not be expected.

5. D. Formation of atherosclerotic plaque takes years; does not clear in a few days. Each of the other answers is correct.

6. C. Subependymal giant cell astrocytoma originates in about the third ventricle and produces hydrocephalus in patients with tuberous sclerosis. No other answer is associated.

7. C. Spontaneous thrombosis of the longitudinal sinus is seen in infants with diarrhea and dehydration and postpartum females.

8. C. Globose neurofibrillary tangles are seen in the brainstem in the basal nucleus of Meynert and in the subthalamic nucleus. None of the other answers are associated with supranuclear palsy.

9. C. The thoracic spine is the most common location of an epidural abscess.

10. B. Although vaccinations have made it uncommon, poliovirus is an enterovirus that can affect the anterior horn cells of the spinal cord, producing asymmetrical weakness. The other viral agents listed are not as likely to produce this clinical picture.

CHAPTER 6

Pharmacology

Drugs every neurologist should know to pass the boards. Abbreviations—MOA, mechanism of action; C, cautions; CI, contraindications. Some drug descriptions include testable uses that have not received a US Food and Drug Administration (FDA) indication (the drug cannot be advertised as such by drug companies, but any qualified health care professional—MD or NP and PA under supervision—can use them with proper knowledge). The FDA pregnancy categories are A (safe, based on human studies), B (safe, based on animal studies), C (uncertain), D (evidence of risk), and X (highly unsafe, never use).

I. Alzheimer's

A. **donepezil (Aricept)** mild to moderate Alzheimer's
   1. **MOA:** Selective reversible cholinesterase inhibitor; does not affect butyrylcholinesterase
   2. **C:** increased risk of gastrointestinal (GI) bleeding, especially with history of ulcers or nonsteroidal anti-inflammatory drug (NSAID) use, frequent aggravation of asthma and benign prostatic hyperplasia (BPH)

B. **galantamine (Reminyl, Razadyne)** mild to moderate Alzheimer's, pregnancy category B; enhances cognitive function, but does not alter course of dementia
   1. **MOA:** Reversible competitive acetylcholinesterase inhibitor
   2. **C:** Vagal stimulator leading to bradycardia and atrioventricular (AV) block, nausea, vomiting, and increased gastric acid secretion

C. **memantine (Namenda)** moderate to severe Alzheimer's, pregnancy category B
   1. **MOA:** N-methyl-D-aspartate (NMDA) antagonist, 5-hydroxytryptamine-3 (5-HT3) antagonist
   2. **C:** Renally excreted—not recommended with severe renal dysfunction; most common side effects are dizziness, confusion, headache

D. **rivastigmine (Exelon)** mild to moderate Alzheimer's
   1. **MOA:** Selective irreversible cholinesterase inhibitor, affects butyrylcholinesterase
   2. **C:** Take with food; significant nausea, vomiting, anorexia, and weight loss frequent; β-blockers with intrinsic sympathomimetic activity and Ca channel blockers—increased bradycardia

II. Antibiotics/Antivirals

A. **acyclovir (Zovirax)** Herpes simplex virus (HSV) encephalitis, prevention of cytomegalovirus (CMV) infection after bone marrow transplantation; dose by ideal body weight; pregnancy category B
   1. **MOA:** Viral specific thymidine kinase activates; incorporated into viral DNA
   2. **C:** Increased side effects with zidovudine and probenecid, most important side effects—light headedness, anorexia, acute renal failure, Stevens-Johnson, thrombotic thrombocytopenic purpura/hemolytic-uremic syndrome (TTP/HUS)

B. **ampicillin (Principen)** empiric treatment of meningitis if 60 years of age for listeria
   1. **MOA:** Inhibits bacterial wall synthesis
   2. **C:** Renally excreted; rash with mononucleosis; effect of warfarin may be increased; can cause seizures, fever, anemia

C. **ceftazidime (Fortaz)** empiric treatment of meningitis, abscess after neurosurgical procedure, can be synergistic with aminoglycosides against pseudomonas
   1. **MOA:** Third-generation cephalosporin, inhibits cell wall synthesis
   2. **C:** If penicillin (pcn) allergy, especially immunoglobulin E (IgE); large amount of Na, adjust for renal impairment

D. **ceftriaxone (Rocephin)** empiric treatment of presumed bacterial meningitis, no adjustment necessary for with either renal or hepatic impairment, pregnancy category B
   1. **MOA:** Third-generation cephalosporin, inhibits cell wall synthesis
   2. **C:** If pcn allergy, especially IgE, discontinue if gallbladder disease, large amount of Na

E. **chloramphenicol (Chloromycetin)** used to treat infection due to *Streptococcus pneumoniae*, although in a patient allergic to penicillin or cephalosporins, probably use vancomycin; pregnancy category C
   1. **C:** Aplastic anemia, reversible bone marrow suppression (>25 mg/mL), gray man syndrome (>50 mg/mL), inhibits phenytoin metabolism, may decrease absorption of vitamin B_{12}
   2. **Gray man syndrome**—circulatory collapse, cyanosis, acidosis, coma/death

F. **foscarnet (Foscavir)** used for acyclovir resistant HSV, pregnancy category B
   1. **MOA:** Noncompetitive inhibitor of several viral enzymes, does not need activation by thymidine kinase
   2. **C:** Renally dose; monitor electrolytes including magnesium, calcium, and phosphate carefully; low ionized calcium at risk for paresthesias, tetany, and seizures; acute renal failure is the norm; avoid concurrent use of ciprofloxacin, which increases seizure risk

G. **gentamycin** empiric treatment of meningitis when Gram-negative rods are a concern
   1. **MOA:** Binds to 30S, 50S of bacterial ribosome interfering with protein synthesis
   2. **C:** Ototoxicity, nephrotoxicity, vertigo/ataxia common; renally dose; use ideal body weight; pcn/cephalosporins increase nephrotoxicity

H. **metronidazole (Flagyl)** for empiric treatment of brain abscess with antibacterial drug; not used alone
   1. **MOA:** DNA strand breakage
   2. **C:** Nausea very common, metallic taste very common, disulfiramlike reaction with alcohol, inhibits CYP 3A4, so can increase serum levels of benzodiazepines, Ca channel blockers, increases prothrombin time (PT) prolongation with warfarin, urine discoloration to red-brown
   3. **CI:** First trimester, concomitant statin use

I. **penicillin-G (Pfizerpen)** treatment of listeriosis, infection due to *Neisseria meningitides*, or neurosyphilis
   1. **MOA:** Inhibits cell wall synthesis, good cerebrospinal fluid (CSF) penetration with inflammation

2. **C:** Seizures, Jarisch-Herxheimer reaction, renally dose, may increase effects of warfarin

J. **vancomycin (Vancocin)** erratic CSF penetration but generally good with inflammation, for methicillin-resistant *Staphylococcus aureus* (MRSA), *S. pneumoniae*, pregnancy category C
   1. **MOA:** Blocks glycopeptide polymerization blocking cell wall synthesis
   2. **C:** Monitor drug levels, renally dose, red man syndrome, common taste change, nausea and vomiting

III. Anticholinergic and Myasthenia Gravis

A. **atropine,** pregnancy category C
   1. **MOA:** Muscarinic cholinergic blocker used in 2-pyridylethylamine (PEA), asystole, and to reverse Tensilon test
   2. **C:** Anticholinergic psychosis possible
   3. **CI:** Narrow-angle glaucoma, myocardial ischemia, GI obstruction, urinary obstruction

B. **edrophonium (Tensilon)** diagnosis of myasthenia gravis; pregnancy category C
   1. **Tensilon test:** 10 mg of edrophonium in 10 mL saline. Give 2 mL every 30 seconds. If muscarinic side effects noted, give atropine 0.5 mg IV and discontinue test.
   2. **CI:** Bronchial asthma, mechanical intestinal obstruction

C. **pyridostigmine (Mestinon)** Myasthenia gravis safe for use in children
   1. **MOA:** Acetylcholinesterase inhibitor of the myoneuronal junction
   2. **CI:** Bronchial asthma, mechanical intestinal obstruction

IV. Anti-Emetic and Motion Sickness

A. **meclizine (Antivert)** anti-emetic, motion sickness, antihistamine; pregnancy category B
   1. **CI:** Asthma, glaucoma, urinary problems

B. **metoclopramide (Reglan)** chemotherapy associated nausea and vomiting, anti-emetic
   1. **CI:** GI obstruction or hemorrhage, pheochromocytoma, receiving other medications that might cause extrapyramidal side effects
   2. **Side effects:** Mental depression, acute dystonic reaction can occur while in the first day or two, seizures, hallucinations, oculogyric crisis

C. **odansetron (Zofran)** chemotherapy associated nausea and vomiting
   1. **MOA:** Selective 5-HT3 blocker
   2. **C:** Extrapyramidal reactions, hypokalemia, seizures

D. **prochlorperazine (Compazine)** antinausea and antivertigo
   1. **MOA:** Dopamine antagonist that acts on the chemoreceptor trigger zone
   2. **C:** Pregnancy, sedation, children with acute illness have high risk of acute dystonias

E. **promethazine (Phenergan)** vertigo, anti-emetic, motion sickness; pregnancy category C
   1. **C:** Sleep apnea, narrow-angle glaucoma, asthma, urinary problems
   2. **CI:** Comatose patients, central nervous system (CNS) depressants

F. **scopolamine (Transderm-Scop)** motion sickness; pregnancy category C
   1. **C:** Glaucoma, use with ethyl alcohol (ETOH), CNS depressants, activity needing alertness
   2. **Side effects:** Orthostatic hypotension, acute narrow-angle glaucoma, disorientation

G. **trimethobenzamide (Tigan)** nausea and vomiting
   1. **C:** Extrapyramidal syndrome, ETOH, CNS active drugs, may contribute to Reye syndrome after a viral illness

V. Antiparkinsonian

A. **amantadine (Symmetrel)** antiparkinsonian used for Parkinson's, influenza A, spastic pseudosclerosis of Creutzfeldt-Jakob disease
   1. **MOA:** Unknown, evidence for several effects on dopamine, including blocking reuptake
   2. **C:** Seizures (in children with seizures increases seizure frequency), psychoses, eczematoid dermatides, hepatic dysfunction, congestive heart failure

B. **carbidopa-levodopa (Sinemet)** dopaminergic agent used for Parkinson's
   1. **MOA:** Carbidopa prevents peripheral conversion of levodopa, which is converted to dopamine in basal ganglia
   2. **C:** Asthma, peptic ulcer disease, psychiatric symptoms
   3. **CI:** Cardiac care unit (CCU) only to start med with h/o myocardial infarction and any residual arrthymia

C. **entacapone (Comtan; part of Stalevo with Sinemet)**
   1. **MOA:** Reversible catechol-O-methyltransferase (COMT) inhibitor allowing for more sustained levels of levodopa and thereby increased passage through the blood–brain barrier
   2. **C:** Do not treat with nonselective monoamine oxidase inhibitor (MOAI), increased risk of orthostatic hypotension with dopaminergic therapy, weak inhibitor of many CYP enzymes, possible decreased metabolism and increased side effects of COMT substrates like norepinephrine, dopamine, dobutamine, 10% will have brown-orange urine discoloration, rare pulmonary. fibrosis

D. **pergolide (Permax)**
   1. **MOA:** Ergot dopamine agonist D1, some D2
   2. **C:** Symptomatic hypotension in 10%, can cause fibrosis of heart valves, lungs, sleep attacks, pathologic gambling
   3. **CI:** CYP 3A4 substrate so macrolide antibiotics or azole antifungals can cause overdosage with vasospasm and ischemia

E. **ropinirole (Requip)** also used for moderate to severe restless legs syndrome
   1. **MOA:** Nonergot dopamine agonist D2, 3, 4. At doses >0.25 mg causes postural hypotension due to D2 mediated blunting of noradrenergic response
   2. **C:** CYP 1A2 substrate (inducers: carbamazepine, phenobarbital; inhibitors: amiodarone, ketoconazole), CYP 2D6 inhibitor (some β-blockers, fluoxetine, tricyclics; prodrug substrates include: codeine, oxycodone, hydrocodone; tramadol will decrease effects of these). Can cause rebound or augmentation in restless leg syndrome (RLS).

F. **selegiline (Eldepryl)** weak evidence for neuroprotection, modestly effective for PD
   1. **MOA:** Monoamine oxidase type B (MOAB) inhibitor, so only rare problems with tyramine-containing foods
   2. **C:** Avoid concomitant tricyclics or selective serotonin reuptake inhibitors (SSRIs), malignant hyperthermia with lithium, serotonin syndrome with meperidine, severe hypertensive reaction with pseudoephedrine

G. **pramipexole (Mirapex)**
   1. **MOA:** Nonergot dopamine agonist
   2. **C:** Can cause compulsive gambling, lower extremity edema, compulsive behaviors

VI. Antiplatelet

A. **aspirin** antiplatelet agent; pregnancy category C
   1. **MOA:** Irreversibly acetylates cyclooxygenase, thereby inhibiting platelet aggregation
   2. **CI:** Nasal polyps, severe asthma, relative for children <12 years as can cause Reye syndrome

B. **clopidogrel (Plavix)** antiplatelet
   1. **MOA:** Directly inhibition of ADP binding
   2. **C:** Monitor complete blood count (CBC) with differential every 2 weeks during first 3 months for risk of neutropenia/thrombocytopenia

C. **dipyridamole (Aggrenox)** antiplatelet used as a combination with aspirin
   1. **MOA:** Inhibits uptake of adenosine into platelets and endothelial cells inhibiting platelets
   2. **C:** Dose-dependent vasodilation careful: coronary artery disease (CAD), coagulation disorders, liver/kidney failure

D. **ticlopidine (Plavix)** antiplatelet second line for aspirin-allergic patients
   1. **C:** Do not give to children less than 18 years, CBC every week for 3 months, as can cause life-threatening agranulocytosis and neutropenia
   2. **CI:** Active bleeding

VII. Anti-Epileptic

A. **acetazolamide (Diamox)** antiepileptic used for clonic tonic seizures, absence seizures, benign intracranial hypertension
   1. **MOA:** Depresses neuronal excitability by inhibition of carbonic anhydrase in glial cells
   2. **C:** Concurrent aspirin use associated with anorexia, coma, death, aplastic anemia
   3. **CI:** Closed-angle glaucoma, hyponatremia, hypokalemia, adrenal failure

B. **carbamazepine (Tegretol, Carbatrol)** antiepileptic used for tonic clonic seizures, partial seizures, chronic pain, Bell's palsy; pregnancy category C
   1. **MOA:** Antagonism of voltage-dependent sodium channels
   2. **C:** Aplastic anemia (need frequent white blood cell (WBC) checks in the first 3 to 4 months of initiating therapy), agranulocytosis, Lennox-Gastaut absence seizures, syndrome of inappropriate antidiuretic hormone secretion (SIADH)
   3. **CI:** MAOI must be discontinued for 2 weeks before using carbamazepine

C. **clonazepam (Klonopin)** benzodiazepine used in akinetic seizures, myoclonic seizures, Lennox-Gastaut syndrome, absence seizures
   1. **C:** Operating a motor vehicle, ETOH/CNS depressants, can increase incidence of generalized tonic clonic seizures so should never be used for them, combined with valproic acid may induce absence seizures

D. **diazepam (Valium)** benzodiazepine used primarily during status epilepticus, night terrors, anxiolytic, rectal form available if do not have IV access

E. **ethosuximide (Zarontin)** antiseizure first line for absence seizures (as well as valproic acid and lamotrigine)
   1. **MOA:** Inhibits thalamic T type calcium channels
   2. **C:** Aplastic anemia, liver function test (LFT) values increase, drug-induced lupus, abrupt withdrawal can produce absence status, children <3 years

F. **felbamate (Felbatol)** antiepileptic used for partial seizures, Lennox-Gastaut generalized seizures; pregnancy category C
   1. **MOA:** Unknown, but known to affect glutamate receptors
   2. **C:** Aplastic anemia, hepatotoxicity; get CBC with differential, LFTs every 1 to 2 weeks
   3. **CI:** Hepatic dysfunction, blood dyscrasia

G. **lamotrigine (Lamictal)** anti-epileptic used adjunctively for partial seizures, Lennox-Gastaut generalized seizures; pregnancy category C
   1. **MOA:** Antagonism of voltage-gated sodium channels

2. **C:** Do not use if <16 years old, do not stop abruptly due to increase in seizure frequency

H. levetiracetam (Keppra) anti-epileptic used adjunctively for partial seizures; pregnancy category C
 1. **C:** Reduced dose in renal failure

I. lorazepam (Ativan) benzodiazepine sedative and anxiolytic; anti-emetic, especially in combination with other agents or for cisplatin, alcohol withdrawal
 1. **MOA:** Limbic, thalamic, hypothalamic γ-aminobutyric acid (GABA)–mediated effect
 2. **C:** Depression, psychosis, additive effect with ETOH or barbiturates, <18 years, use longer than 4 months has not been evaluated
 3. **CI:** narrow-angle glaucoma, arterial injection

J. oxcarbazepine (Trileptal) structurally similar to carbamazepine
 1. **C:** May cause hyponatremia diplopia, rare Stevens-Johnson syndrome usually at about 3 weeks after initiation; does not have aplastic anemia like carbamazepine

K. pentobarbital (Nembutal) barbiturate used for Wada testing, status epilepticus, barbiturate coma, and short term for insomnia
 1. **MOA:** Acts throughout CNS but especially on midbrain reticular formation
 2. **C:** Rapid IV use associated with respiratory depression and vasodilation, abrupt discontinuation can cause seizures
 3. **CI:** Porphyria, severe hepatic dysfunction

L. phenobarbital (Luminal) barbiturate in generalized tonic clonic seizures, partial seizures; pregnancy category D
 1. **C:** Do not discontinue abruptly, cognitive deficits in children
 2. **CI:** Porphyria, liver impairment

M. phenytoin (Dilantin) and phosphenytoin (Cerebyx) anti-epileptic used for generalized tonic clonic seizures, partial seizures, and status epilepticus (here use fosphenytoin, which can be used faster IV)
 1. **MOA:** Blocks voltage-dependent sodium and possibly calcium channels
 2. **C:** Do not use in absence seizures, may induce insulin resistance, ETOH
 3. **CI:** Sinus bradycardia, second- and third-degree AV block

N. primidone (Mysoline) anti-epileptic used for partial or tonic clonic seizures
 1. **C:** Risk of drowsiness, risk of suicidality with suicidal tendencies, avoid abrupt withdrawal as can lead to status epilepticus, avoid with ETOH/drug abuse

O. tiagabine (Gabitril) anti-epileptic used for partial seizures; pregnancy category C
 1. **MOA:** Possibly increases availability of GABA
 2. **C:** Periodically monitor eye due to melanin binding, generalized weakness that resolves with decreasing dose, do not discontinue abruptly

P. topiramate (Topamax) anti-epileptic used for partial and tonic clonic seizures, chronic pain, depression; pregnancy category C
 1. **MOA:** Multiple-antagonism of voltage-gated sodium channels and α-amino-3-hydroxy-5-methylisoxazole-4-proprionic acid (AMPA) glutamate receptor, enhances GABA-A effect
 2. **C:** Increased risk of developing renal stones, do not discontinue abruptly

Q. valproic acid (Depakene, Depakote) anti-epileptic used for complex partial seizures and absence seizures; pregnancy category D
 1. **MOA:** Increases GABA and frequency-dependent antagonism of voltage-dependent sodium channels
 2. **C:** Thrombocytopenia, hyperammonemia, monitor liver function (LFTs) as can cause hepatic failure

R. **zonisamide (Zonegran)** anti-epileptic for partial seizures, Lennox-Gastaut syndrome
   1. **MOA:** Several including enhanced GABA
   2. **C:** Aplastic anemia, hyperthermia, renal calculi, do not discontinue abruptly

VIII. Antithrombotics and Anticoagulants

A. **alteplase (t-PA)** fibrinolytic agent 0.9 mg/kg (max 90 mg) 10% bolus, give the remainder over 1 hour
   1. **MOA:** Converts plasminogen to plasmin, promoting fibrinolysis, use within 3 hours of acute ischemic stroke or 6 hours if endovascular intra-arterial
   2. **CI:** Acute or history of intracranial hemorrhage, recent intracranial surgery or stroke, blood pressure >185 mm Hg systolic or >100 mm Hg diastolic, seizure at onset of stroke, acute internal bleeding, anticoagulant use, platelets <100,000

B. **enoxaparin (Lovenox)** antithrombotic; pregnancy category B
   1. **MOA:** Low-molecular-weight heparin with higher affinity for factors Xa and IIa
   2. **C:** Recent/anticipated surgery have risk of spinal/epidural hematoma
   3. Should not significantly affect PT, partial thromboplastin time (PTT), bleeding time

C. **heparin** anticoagulant; pregnancy category C
   1. **MOA:** Promotes inhibitory action of antithrombin III, used in low doses to prevent recurrence of stroke or thromboembolism; measure by increased PTT
   2. **C:** Risk of spontaneous fracture with at least 15,000 U for 6 months or more

D. **warfarin (Coumadin)** anticoagulant; pregnancy category X
   1. **MOA:** Interferes with vitamin K synthesis causing depletion of factors II, VII, IX, X, C, S monitor PT-INR (international normalized ratio)
   2. **CI:** Pregnancy, alcoholism, psychosis, noncompliant patient

IX. Migraine

A. **almotriptan (Axert)** except as indicated in the preceding text, identical to sumatriptan
   1. **MOA:** 5-HT1 B, D, F inhibitor
   2. Medium onset and medium tolerability
   3. **CI:** Cluster headache

B. **eletriptan (Relpax)** except as in the following, identical to sumatriptan
   1. **MOA:** 5-HT1 B, D, F; can be used with MOAI
   2. **C:** CYP3A4 metabolism so do not use within 72 hours of potent CYP 3A4 inhibitors like ketoconazole, itraconazole, clarithromycin, ritonavir, and nelfinavir; not intended to be used with cluster headache

C. **frovatriptan (Frova)** except as below, identical to sumatriptan
   1. **MOA:** 5-HT1 B, D; slow onset and higher tolerability, can be used with MOAI
   2. **C:** Not intended for use with cluster headache

D. **rizatriptan (Maxalt)** except as in the following text, identical to sumatriptan
   1. Fastest onset
   2. **C:** Concomitant propanolol use increases rizatriptan levels by 70%, not intended to be used with cluster headache

E. **sumatriptan (Imitrex)** used for migraine and cluster headache, most variety of preparations (oral, nasal, S.C.)
   1. Fast onset but lower tolerability like all other drugs of this class with two exceptions

2. **MOA:** 5-HT1 D inhibitor, normalize blood vessels in vivo
   3. **C:** Do not use within 24 hours of ergots or other triptans, concomitant use of SSRIs can cause hyperreflexia, weakness, and incoordination
   4. **CI:** May cause vasospasm with uncontrolled hypertension, basilar migraine, hemiplegic migraine, ischemic heart disease, cerebrovascular disease, peripheral vascular disease, concomitant use of MOAI, severe hepatic impairment

X. Multiple Sclerosis

A. **glatiramer (Copaxone)** used in multiple sclerosis; pregnancy category B
   1. **MOA:** Simulates myelin basic protein and acts as a decoy for T cells targeting it
   2. **C:** Thirteen percent of patients will experience a very uncomfortable chest tightness with palpations, anxiety, and difficulty breathing, which lasts about 15 minutes and does not usually recur

B. **interferon beta 1a (Avonex, Rebif)** similar to interferon beta 1b but the data for interferon beta 1b seems more convincing; may benefit those with active clinical disease with reduced disease progression

C. **interferon beta 1b (Betaseron)** for patients with secondarily progressive MS who continue to have relapses and relapsing remitting multiple sclerosis (MS), responders to medication appear to be of the inflammatory type, for secondary progressive MS appears to be beneficial in decreasing relapse related outcomes
   1. **MOA:** Increases suppressor T-cell activity
   2. **C:** Check LFTs at 1, 3, 6 months for autoimmune hepatitis/hepatic failure; flu-like symptoms in a majority of patients; necrosis at injection site; severe psychiatric reactions, even in patients without psychiatric history; increased risk of agranulocytopenia with angiotensin-converting enzyme inhibitor (ACEI), check thyroid stimulating hormone (TSH) every 6 months in patients with history of thyroid problems

D. **mitoxantrone (Novantrone)** for rapidly progressive MS with failed other therapies
   1. **MOA:** Intercalates DNA, inhibits DNA topoisomerase II, may inhibit RNA/DNA synthesis by preventing incorporation of uridine and thymidine
   2. **C:** Check left ventricular ejection fraction (LVEF) at baseline and at each dose (24 months is probably safe), CBC, from cancer data risk of developing secondary acute myelogenous leukemia (AML) is 1% to 2%
   3. **CI:** LVEF of <50% or decrease in LVEF; maximum lifetime dose 140 mg/m^2 due to cardiotoxicity; do not give dose if neutrophil count <1,500/mm^3

E. **natalizumab (Tysabri)** relapsing MS that does not repond to typical MS medication; pregnancy category C
   1. **MOA:** Monoclonal antibody that binds to integrin expressed on all leukocytes except neutrophils
   2. **CI:** Three cases of PML led to temporary withdrawal from market; now can only be prescribed under auspices of a monitoring program called TOUCH

XI. Pain

A. **gabapentin (Neurontin)** used for postherpetic neuralgia, chronic pain, and adjunctively for partial seizures; pregnancy category C
   1. **MOA:** Unknown but structurally related to GABA. In animal models, binds to the $\alpha_2\delta$ voltage gated Ca channel.
   2. **C:** Do not abruptly stop due to increase in seizure frequency

B. **morphine** prototypical opiate
   1. **MOA:** Opiate receptor agonist
   2. **C:** Children younger than 2 years more susceptible to respiratory depression, patients with head injury, asthma, increase smooth muscle tone and spasm, may prolong labor
   3. **CI:** Premature neonate blood–brain barrier not mature (significant respiratory depression)

C. **pregabalin (Lyrica)** structurally similar to gabapentin, same mechanism, same indications, possibly more effective

XII. Psychiatric and Overdose

A. **benzatropine mesylate (Cogentin)** anticholinergic and antihistamine used for all forms of parkinsonianism and extrapyramidal side effects of antipsychotics
   1. **C:** Concomitant use with phenothiazines as can cause fatal paralytic ileus
   2. **CI:** Tardive dyskinesia usually aggravated

B. **diphenhydramine (Benadryl)** anti-emetic, mild sedation, antihistamine; pregnancy category B
   1. **C:** Narrow-angle glaucoma, peptic ulcer, asthma, activates seizures, concurrent use of MAOI, hyperthyroidism
   2. **CI:** Children <9 kg, <1 year old

C. **flumazenil (Romazicon)** benzodiazepine antagonist
   1. **MOA:** Competitive inhibition of benzodiazepine at the receptor
   2. **C:** Concomitant tricyclic overdose, associated with seizures, can cause panic attacks in patients with a history of panic disorder

D. **naloxone (Narcan)** opioid antagonist
   1. **MOA:** Binds competitively to μ opoid receptors to reverse respiratory depression
   2. **C:** May precipitate withdrawal in chronic opiate users

XIII. Other Medications

A. **Intravenous immunoglobulin (IVIG)** used in myasthenia gravis and Guillain-Barré, refractory dermatomyositis/polymyositis
   1. **MOA:** Binds to antibodies in serum
   2. **C:** Anaphylaxis, especially if IgA deficient, aseptic meningitis with doses of 2 g/kg or higher, adequately hydrate due to renal compromise, ? association of thrombotic events and IVIG administration

B. **mannitol (Osmitrol)** osmotic diuretic used to lower intracranial pressure
   1. **MOA:** Osmotic effect expands plasma, increases cerebral blood flow, and draws fluid out of cerebral parenchyma
   2. **C:** Concomitant use of steroids and phenytoin may cause hyperosmolar nonketosis, acute renal failure with high doses

C. **nimodipine (Nimotop)** Ca channel blocker to prevent vasospasm in subarachnoid hemorrhage
   1. 60 mg every 4 hours for 21 days, 1 hour before meals
   2. **MOA:** Unknown mechanism, reduces delayed neurologic deficit if started within 96 hours, with Hunt and Hess grade I-III subarachnoid hemorrhage

D. **oxybate (Xyrem)** is GHB (Gamma hydroxy butyrate) used for sleep apnea
   1. **MOA:** Unknown
   2. **C:** Restricted distribution due to abuse potential and respiratory depression, additional effects of alcohol/CNS depressants may lead to death (one case in clinical trials)

3. **CI:** Concomitant use of sedative hypnotics, enzyme deficiency of succinic semialdehyde dehydrogenase (mental retardation, hypotonia, ataxia)

E. **quinine** cramps/myotonia
   1. **MOA:** Increases the refractory period of muscle, decreases muscle end-plate excitability
   2. **CI:** Myasthenia gravis, pregnancy, glucose-6-phosphate deficiency (G6PD), optic neuritis

F. **riluzole (Rilutek)** amyotrophic lateral sclerosis (ALS), extends time to tracheostomy, survival time by a few months
   1. **MOA:** Inhibits glutamate release and binding
   2. **C:** LFTs every month for 3 months, then every 3 months × 3, more often if see a rise in LFT values
   3. **CI:** Lactation

G. **tizanidine (Zanaflex)** spasticity, spastic paraparesis in ALS
   1. **MOA:** Central α2-adrenergic that inhibits presynaptic motor neurons
   2. **C:** LFTs, Cr monthly for first 6 months

H. **baclofen (Lioresal)**
   1. **MOA:** GABA-B agonist, promotes inhibition in spinal cord; will not help muscle weakness, but can help spacticity
   2. **C:** Diabetes—can cause increase in blood sugar; do not operate machinery until sure of effect

I. **dantrolene (Dantrium)** used in spasticity and malignant hyperthermia
   1. **MOA:** Interferes with the release of Ca from sarcoplasmic reticulum
   2. **C:** With IV use, reports of pulmonary edema; with oral use, reports of aplastic anemia, heart failure, leukemia. Do not combine with verapamil.

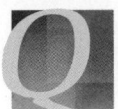 # STUDY QUESTIONS FOR CHAPTER 6

Directions: *Each of the numbered items or incomplete statements in this section is followed by answers or by completions of the statement. Select the ONE lettered answer or completion that is BEST in each case.*

1. A 41-year-old woman is placed on acetazolamide for benign intracranial hypertension. Which of the following is a possible neuro-ophthalmologic side effect of this medication?
(A) retinitis pigmentosa
(B) closed-angle glaucoma
(C) open-angle glaucoma
(D) macular degeneration
(E) serous retinopathy

2. Amantadine is prescribed for a 68-year-old man with Parkinson's disease. Which of the following symptoms may be produced or worsened by this medication?
(A) depression
(B) mania
(C) psychosis
(D) anxiety
(E) obsessive-compulsive disorder

3. Clopidogrel is prescribed as stroke prophylaxis for a 79-year-old man. You check a complete blood count every 2 weeks during the first 3 months of treatment to look for which of the following?
(A) neutropenia and thrombocytopenia
(B) neutropenia and thrombocytosis
(C) anemia and neutropenia
(D) anemia and leukocytosis
(E) neutropenia, anemia, and thrombocytopenia

4. You prescribe memantine for a 73-year-old man with early Alzheimer's disease. The mechanism of action of memantine is:
(A) acetylcholinesterase inhibition
(B) dopamine agonism
(C) γ-aminobutyric acid (GABA) agonism
(D) *N*-methyl-D-aspartate (NMDA) antagonism
(E) selective serotonin reuptake inhibition

5. Lamotrigine is prescribed as seizure prophylaxis for a 23-year-old woman. What is the principal mechanism of action of this medication?
(A) calcium channel agonism
(B) GABA agonism
(C) sodium channel antagonism
(D) carbonic anhydrase inhibition
(E) potassium channel antagonism

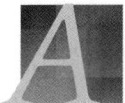# ANSWERS AND EXPLANATIONS

1. B. Acetazolamide can produce closed angle glaucoma, but none of the other listed choices.

2. C. Amantadine can produce psychosis, but does not typically produce the other listed symptoms.

3. A. Clopidogrel may produce neutropenia and thrombocytopenia. It is not associated with thrombocytosis, anemia, or leukocytosis.

4. D. Memantine is an NMDA antagonist. Donepezil is an acetylcholinesterase inhibitor that is effective for early Alzheimer's disease. γ-aminobutyric acid agonism is the mechanism of benzodiazepines. Selective serotonin reuptake inhibitors are effective as antidepressants, but not specifically for Alzheimer's disease.

5. C. The principal mechanism of lamotrigine is sodium channel antagonism.

SECTION II

CLINICAL NEUROLOGY

Cerebrovascular Disease

I. Preliminaries

A. **Epidemiology**
  1. Third most common cause of death, leading cause of adult disability, 750,000 strokes annually
  2. 50% of hospitalized neurology patients will suffer from stroke
  3. 35% risk of stroke recurrence after initial symptomatic stroke

B. **Classification**
  1. Stroke is defined as sudden onset of focal neurologic impairment. Maximum neurologic dysfunction is normally reached rapidly unless there are complicating factors.
  2. The basic differentiation should include whether the stroke is in carotid or vertebrobasilar territories and whether the stroke is hemorrhagic or ischemic.

C. **Pathophysiology**
  1. **Cerebral blood flow** (CBF) normally 50 to 60 mL per 100 g of tissue per minute. When CBF is reduced to 25 mL, there is loss of electrical activity, but tissue remains metabolically active. During infarction, there is core of irreversible tissue damage surrounded by penumbra, where neurologic function ceases but the cells maintain integrity. When oxygen levels decrease to the point that increased oxygen extraction or vasodilation (expansed cerebral blood volume) can no longer compensate, anaerobic metabolism begins, and lactic acid forms, which is neurotoxic.

2. **Physiologic derangements** include glutamate release causing excitotoxic cell injury, binding causing increased intracellular Ca^{++} levels, and through N-methyl-D-aspartate (NMDA) receptors enhanced cellular Na^+ and Ca^{++} plus K^+ efflux entry; anaerobic glucose metabolism causing tissue necrosis; inflammatory cell activation; free radical activation; and cytotoxic and vasogenic edema
3. **Magnetic resonance imaging** (MRI) does not guide utilization of tissue-type plasminogen activator (tPA), but CT to exclude hemorrhage is mandatory.
    a. If the area of perfusion weighted imaging (PWI) is large, denoting low perfusion in a large area, but the area of diffusion weighted imaging (DWI) is small, denoting an area where there is little early ischemic damage, reperfusion is most likely to be beneficial.
    b. If both DWI and PWI are large, the injury has already occurred; reperfusion may be helpful, but the risks of hemorrhage are high.
    c. If PWI is normal, then it is unlikely that reperfusion will be helpful. However, it may be normal in small vessel disease and tPA is effective.

II. Pathogenesis of Stroke

A. **Ischemic stroke**
1. **Atherosclerosis** reduces the vessel lumen and causes artery-to-artery embolism.
    a. **Early plaque** is a fatty streak consisting of low-density lipoprotein (LDL) swollen macrophages.
    b. **Ensuing atherosclerosis** seems to have a predilection for certain sites, notably the initial extracranial portion of the internal carotid artery.
    c. **Concentric atheroma** is nonthrombotic, but eccentric is thrombotic.
    d. **Plaque** is a lipid core surrounded by fibrous rim; if the rim is thin, it can rupture and ulcerate. Platelet-fibrin rich (white) clot forms on irregular ulcerated plaques; this is best treated with antiplatelet agents. Thrombin rich (red) clot forms with slow flow; this is best treated with anticoagulation.
2. **Risk factors** include genetics, excessive LDL, very-low-density lipoprotein (VLDL), low high-density lipoprotein (HDL), excessive saturated fats, inactivity, diabetes with insulin resistance, hyperhomocysteinemia, and, most importantly, hypertension. Moderate alcohol consumption may reduce stroke risk.

B. **Cardiac embolism**
1. **Stagnant blood** induces red clot formation, which fragments and is carried to the cerebral circulation; 20% of cardiac output allocated to brain, so frequently embolizes intracranially; after it dissolves, the infarct can undergo hemorrhagic transformation.
2. **Neurologic deficit** frequently severe as the thrombus lodges in a major artery: branch of middle cerebral artery (MCA), top of basilar, and posterior cerebral artery. Embolism is usually located either in superficial territories or causes large, deep infarcts; infarct is classically wedge shaped.
3. **Imaging** can show infarcts in different vascular territories.
4. **Angiography** is negative unless done early before the clot breaks up.
5. **Cardiac evaluation** is mandatory.
6. **Clinical features:** high risk cardiac disease, systemic embolism, superficial ischemic pattern (isolated Wernicke's, homonymous hemianopia, facial or arm motor deficit), top of the basilar syndrome, no prior transient ischemic attack (TIA), no progression to deficit.
7. **Risk for hemorrhagic transformation** with reperfusion
8. **Risk for embolization** recurrence as high as 1% per day in first 2 weeks.
9. **Stroke risk** 4.5% per year in untreated atrial fibrillation. Secondary prevention with international normalized ratio (INR) of 2.0 to 2.5, unless mechanical heart valve, then INR 3.5 to 4.5. Anticoagulation of patent foramen ovale and interatrial aneurysm controversial. May prescribe tPA.

C. **Lacunar strokes**
 1. **Lacunar strokes** are due to arteriolar disease with microatheromas, lipohyalinosis, and fibrinoid degeneration, causing small and deeply placed infarcts, usually in the internal capsule, basal ganglia, thalamus, corona radiata, and paramedian brainstem.
 2. **Major risk factors** are hypertension and diabetes.
 3. **MRI** > **computed tomography** (CT) in detection; angiography cannot assess arterioles.

D. **Intracranial hemorrhage**
 1. **Hypertension** is major causal factor in Charcot-Bouchard microaneurysm formation. Usually occurs in putamen, thalamus, pons, and cerebellum.
 2. **Nonhypertensive patients** often have lobar hemorrhages; consider vascular malformation, including aneurysm, hypocoagulable state
 3. In the elderly, consider **amyloid** as a cause.

E. **Subarachnoid hemorrhage** (SAH)
 1. **Nontraumatic SAH** usually results from vascular malformation or aneurysm.
 2. **Aneurysms** are congenital (due to absence of arterial wall media) or acquired (from hypertension or smoking). They are located at branch points along the circle of Willis.
 3. **Angiography** is mandatory.

F. **Asymptomatic carotid artery stenosis** (ACAS)
 1. **Arterial bruits** indicate turbulent flow. Bruits should be sought by auscultating in the following places: (i) high in the neck, (ii) bell at upper border of thyroid cartilage to auscultate the common carotid bifurcation, (iii) subclavian fossa
     a. If the noise gets louder as you move to the chest, likely cardiac murmur
     b. If it disappears when recumbent, consider venous hum
     c. Can be heard when arterial crosssection is reduced by more than 50%
 2. **Annual stroke risk** is 1%; 30% will have imaging evidence of silent cerebral infarction
 3. They have increased cardiac risk, as it is a marker of **systemic atherosclerosis**
 4. **ACAS** with >60% stenosis should have carotid endarterectomy, as it reduces 5-year risk of ipsilateral stroke compared to patients with medical treatment at the time the paper was published. Notably, with more recent treatment (statin, ACE, and possibly homocysteine lowering), this may no longer be true.

III. Transient Focal Deficit

A. **Differential**
 1. **Focal seizures**—expect spread, usually over several minutes over involved body region. Also, there should be positive symptoms of clonic jerks, tingling, or paresthesias.
 2. **Migraine** will spread over 10 to 20 minutes: positive visual disturbances of fortification spectrum, scintillating scotoma, followed by contralateral headache.
 3. **TIA**—episodes of focal neurologic dysfunction of sudden onset and duration less than 24 hours occurring in a specific arterial distribution. If it does not resolve within 1 hour, 80% chance that it will not resolve spontaneously.
     a. Stroke will occur in 30% to 35% of untreated TIA patients: about 11% in the first 90 days and 5% in the first 2 days. Stroke should be considered a neurologic emergency.

B. **TIA clinical features**–look for associated features, which can give an idea as to the etiology: palpitations or other cardiac symptoms can point to an embolic source, neck movements with a vertebrobasilar TIA can suggest degenerative cervical spine disease, TIA during arm movement, especially with different blood pressures in the arms could be subclavian steal, ipsilateral blindness and contralateral motor sensory deficit is carotid disease; if precipitated by rapid position changes or exercise likely due to hypotension or cardiac
 1. **Extracranial disease** has two patterns:
     a. **Cortical**—contralateral paresis and sensory deficit, aphasia if dominant hemisphere

        b. Ocular—monocular blurring or amaurosis fugax due to retina ischemia
        c. Search for **internal carotid artery** (ICA) for cardiac etiology
    2. **Subcortical**—isolated motor hemiparesis or hemisensory deficit
        a. Usually small-vessel disease from diabetes or hypertension
    3. **Vetebrobasilar** associated with ataxia, diplopia, dysarthria, drop attacks, and dysphagia; isolated vertigo rarely a TIA.
    4. **Posterior circulation**—both eyes have dimming/graying, scotomas, visual field defects

C. Reversible ischemic neurologic deficit (RIND)
    1. **RIND** is a focal neurologic deficit of vascular origin lasting more than 24 hours but less than 3 days, or, by some definitions, 3 weeks. It is irrational to classify cerebral ischemia by its temporal patterns alone: evaluation and treatment is identical to that of TIA. All versions of a TIA: TIA, RIND, cerebral infarction with transient signs, and "minor stroke" (patients with minimal neurologic dysfunction that remains after several weeks) have a 30% to 35% risk of developing a subsequent major, disabling stroke.

D. Management
    1. For initial labs, see Table 7-1
    2. All patients should be screened with an electrocardiogram (ECG) and CT
    3. It is important to determine if the attack occurs in the carotid or vertebrobasilar system
        a. Carotid—vascular imaging mandatory. Carotid duplex ultrasonography and magnetic resonance angiography (MRA) have a 90% to 95% sensitivity to detect angiographically proven 50% or greater stenosis. Based on the North American Carotid Endarterectomy Study, carotid endarectomy (CEA) is beneficial in all angiographically proven cervical carotids stenosis of >50%. In our practice, we try to have all such patients receive a conventional angiogram to completely assess both intracranial and extracranial circulation. Only conventional angiography allows for detection of both

Table 7-1 *Laboratory Evaluation of a TIA Patient*

All patients should have these tested
1. Complete blood count including platelet count
2. Erythrocyte sedimentation rate
3. Activated partial thromboplastin time and prothrombin time
4. Fasting lipid profile
5. Urine toxicology
6. Syphilis serology
7. Plasma fibrinogen
8. Serum glucose (some use hemoglobin A1c tLo screen for diabetes)
9. Urinalysis (for hematuria or proteinuria)
10. Electrolytes including renal function
11. Hepatic function
12. Homocysteine level

Select patients should have these tested
13. Hemoglobin electrophoresis
14. Protein C, S, antithrombin III levels
15. Lupus anticoagulant and anticardiolipin antibodies
16. Immune complex screening studies including systemic lupus erythematosus and rheumatoid arthritis
17. Serum and whole body viscosity
18. Platelet function studies
19. HIV, Lyme, cysticercosis screening
20. Pregnancy test
21. Serum protein electrophoresis
22. Coagulation factor analysis
23. Chest X-ray for sarcoidosis

symptomatic extracranial ICA stenosis and asymptomatic intracranial ICA aneurysm, where aneurysm treatment would precede CEA.
    b. **Cardiogenic embolic**—anticoagulation indicated in patients with nonvalvular atrial fibrillation, with or without neurologic symptoms; warfarin reduced stroke risk by 70%
    c. **Vertebrobasilar**—transcranial Doppler and angiogram to determine extent of stenosis, occlusion, or blood-vessel wall abnormality
  4. If surgery/anticoagulation not indicated, all patients should be on **antiplatelet agents**.
    a. **Aspirin**—relative risk reduction 30% stroke and 15% cardiovascular/cerebrovascular mortality. Doses from 50 mg to 325 mg all effective for stroke prevention, but low doses avoid gastric irritation by avoiding prostacyclin inhibition.
    b. **Ticlopidine** reduces platelet-fibrin binding within plaque and reduces white clot size; it has no effect on stomach prostaglandins (dosage 250 mg twice daily). Rarely used due to irreversible neutropenia and thrombocytopenia.
    c. **Clopidogrel** similar to ticlopidine but fewer side effects; slightly better than aspirin (ASA) alone.
    d. **Extended release dipyridamole** (200 mg) and ASA (25 mg) is more effective than ASA alone. Side effects: headache, dizziness, chest pain, but no evidence of increased cardiac mortality. In United States, many do not use this combination, because the major trial, ESPS2, has some methodological problems, but in Britain, it is the expectation and is included in the 2005 National Health Service Guideline.
    e. **Warfarin** has been used for stroke prevention in patients who have failed antiplatelet medication; there is no evidence-based medicine (EBM) for this as a rescue strategy, but traditional stroke strategies are hard to change.

IV. Deteriorating Stroke

A. **Most strokes** reach maximum deficit in minutes to hours.

B. **Some progress.** Usually large-vessel disease with artery to artery embolism or distal clot propagation, and lacunar infarct or watershed territory, especially if the patients develop hypotension (or relative hypotension with chronic hypertension). When the stroke is due to intracerebral hemorrhage, this is usually due to continued blood extravasation, vasogenic edema, herniation, or hydrocephalus.

C. **Malignant cerebral edema** with carotid or MCA occlusion, with persistent headache, progressively decreased consciousness, and worsened focal neurologic deficit. Typically occurs 48 to 72 hours after initial presentation.

V. Cerebral Artery Syndromes

A. **Internal carotid artery** (ICA) and MCA syndromes; symptoms depend on the size of territory involved. In either, there is hemiplegia, partial or complete sensory deficit, visual field defects, aphasia/dysphasia if dominant hemisphere, or anosognosia or acute confusion if nondominant hemisphere.
  1. **Motor deficit** with ICA is face, arm (MCA territory), and leg (anterior cerebral artery [ACA] territory). With MCA, leg is either spared or less affected.
  2. **Branch occlusions** can cause isolated syndromes:
    a. Wernicke aphasia with inferior branch MCA occlusion, often initially diagnosed with a psychiatric illness
    b. Broca aphasia without hemiparesis with superior branch MCA
    c. Nondominant temporal lobe can cause isolated acute confusion or lethargy.
  3. **Other hemispheric MCA features:** anosognosia (denial of neglect), unilateral spatial neglect, hemi-inattention with dressing hemiapraxia

4. **Extracranial ICA bifurcation:** ipsilateral blindness, contralateral motor/sensory deficit
5. **Initial portion ICA** is most common site for atherosclerotic disease. MCA occlusion most commonly heart, aortic arch, or ICA embolism, less commonly *in situ* thrombosis.

B. **Anterior cerebral artery** (ACA) syndrome
   1. **Weakness and sensory impairment** of leg with mild or no involvement of upper extremity; mental changes, apraxia, executive function impairment, grasp reflex, suck reflex, and bowel/bladder incontinence are possible
   2. **Isolated acute onset confusion** with bilateral ACA ischemia, usually with both ACAs being supplied with one ICA

C. **Posterior cerebral artery** (PCA) syndrome
   1. **Homonymous hemianopsia** is characteristic. Patients often complain of visual blurring or bumping into objects.
   2. **Hemianesthesia**, impairment of memory, and confusion with hippocampal lesions, alexia, and metamorphopsia (visual distortion) with dominant occipital hemispheric lesion
   3. **Hemiplegia** is unexpected but possible.
   4. **Transient global amnesia** usually isolated, with sudden onset disorientation and inability to form new memories, but no other neurologic signs; it lasts from 15 minutes to 48 hours, and is usually precipitated by exercise, sexual intercourse, or emotional stress. CT/MRI usually negative but can show temporal ischemia; recurrences are rare.

D. **Vertebrobasilar syndromes**
   1. There are more than 30 syndromes with eponyms for infarction of different levels of the brainstem. We list the seven most frequent, with the most common being the lateral medullary syndrome (Wallenberg syndrome; see Table 7-2).
   2. With top of the basilar syndrome, pontine, midbrain, thalamic, and cortical infarction can occur. There can be progression over 24 to 72 hours with clot propagation, which can be prevented with anticoagulation and thrombolysis. Symptoms include impaired consciousness, abnormal eye movements, miotic but reactive pupils, and quadriplegia.
   3. If cerebellum infarcted, compression of the fourth ventricle with ensuing hydrocephalus possible. Removing infarcted cerebellar hemisphere may be necessary to prevent death.

VI. Evaluation and Management

A. Initial evaluation should include the same laboratory tests as for TIA. Patient should have nothing orally (be NPO) except medications, which should include an aspirin.

B. Monitor vital signs and neurologic condition every 2 hours for the first 72 hours to ensure that the patient is hemodynamically stable and that deterioration does not occur.

C. Every patient should get either a formal or bedside swallowing evaluation before initiation of oral intake.

D. **Left ventricular hypertrophy** (LVH) seen on chest x-ray or ECG is most likely a result of cardiovascular disease. Acute cardiac decompensation and T waves can be the result of insular strokes with a transient catecholamine release, which can cause a transient reactive hypertension.

E. **Blood pressure**—the extent to which blood pressure should be lowered is not known at this time. We generally do nothing unless it exceeds 220/120 mm Hg or the patient develops myocardial ischemia, restarting their blood pressure medications on the third day. If tPA is an option, blood pressure must be less than 185/110 mm Hg prior to beginning infusion.

F. Every patient should get an MRI with both PWI and DWI images. If susceptibility and apparent diffusion coefficient (ADC) maps are easily available, they may be helpful.

G. **Reperfusion**
   1. **Thrombolysis** fragments the thrombus and restores flow to the ischemic region, thereby rescuing the penumbra of the stroke.
   2. **Intracerebral hemorrhage** occurs in 6% of thrombolysis; this must be understood and accepted by either the patient, if patient is able, or their surrogate decision maker, if available.
   3. **CT must not show any hemorrhage.** If CT shows hypodensity in greater than one third of the MCA distribution, patient is at high risk for hemorrhagic transformation.
   4. **Always get a focused history** to ensure patient does not have contraindications.
   5. **Give IV** tPA 0.9 mg/kg (maximum dose 90 mg) 10% as bolus, and then the rest over 1 hour, if patient is ready for it within 3 hours. The earlier the tPA administered, the better the outcome. This is a guideline and is expected care.
   6. **If intraarterial thrombolysis is available**, then it may be considered after tPA. The current recommendations are within 6 hours if anterior circulation (ICA/MCA) or 12 to 24 hours if posterior, but this is not the standard of care until further research is completed.
   7. **Give heparin** to those with a cardiac etiology. No evidence for neparin in other stroke, including deteriorating stroke.

H. **Neuroprotection**
   1. Maintain normoglycemia to prevent cytotoxic edema from lactate production.
   2. Treat hyperthermia aggressively.
   3. Monitoring blood gases can be helpful. Hypoxia should be avoided. Hypercarbia should also be avoided to prevent increased intracranial pressure and "reverse CBF steal" (blood is taken from maximally dilated ischemic vessels and shunted to normal vessels, which respond to normal autoregulation)
   4. Cerebral edema—avoid. Always use passive measures: normal saline only and keeping head of bed 30 degrees. Ischemic stroke leads to cytotoxic edema (due to energy failure) >

Table 7-2 *Major Vertebrobasilar Ischemic Stroke Syndromes*

Artery occluded	Ischemic region	Findings
Vertebral or posterior inferior cerebellar	Lateral medullary (Wallenberg syndrome)	Ipsilateral cerebellar ataxia, Horner, facial hemianesthesia, vertigo, horizontal nystagmus, dysarthria, dysphagia, hiccups
Anterior inferior cerebellar	Lateral caudal pons	Ipsilateral cerebellar ataxia, facial anesthesia, facial paresis, horizontal gaze palsy toward lesion, deafness/tinnitus, contralateral pain/thermal hemianesthesia
Paramedian branch of basilar	Inferior medial pons	Horizontal gaze palsy toward lesion (preservation of convergence), ipsilateral abducens and facial paresis, contralateral weakness and tactile and proprioceptive hemianesthesia
Superior cerebellar	Lateral rostral pons and pons–midbrain junction	Ipsilateral cerebellar ataxia, facial hemianesthesia, Horner, contralateral hemianesthesia, skew deviation
Paramedian branch of basilar	Superior medial pons	Internuclear ophthalmoplegia, palatal myoclonus, ipsilateral ataxia, contralateral hemiparesis
Basilar	Pons, midbrain, thalamus, occipital cortex	Abducens paresis, internuclear ophthalmoplegia, impaired horizontal eye movements, ocular bobbing, miotic but reactive pupils, quadriplegia, coma if tegmentum involved, "locked in" if basis pontis involved
Paramedian penetrating midbrain	Medial midbrain (Weber syndrome)	Ipsilateral oculomotor palsy and contralateral hemiplegia

vasogenic edema (due to blood–brain barrier failure). Traditional techniques like mannitol, hyperventilation, or steroids are not effective in reducing cytotoxic edema.
5. Avoid medical complications. Ambulate early if possible. Use deep venous thrombosis (DVT) prophylaxis.

VI. Secondary Prevention

A. **Antihypertensive medication**—there is a clear, direct, and continuous relation between hypertension and cerebrovascular disease. A 6-mm drop in blood pressure may reduce stroke risk by as much as 42%. All types of ant-hypertensives have demonstrated efficacy, but angiotensin-converting enzyme (ACE) inhibitors and ARBs may confer additional protection.

B. **Lipid lowering—depends on the stroke subgroup**
   1. For atherothrombotic strokes, the relation to stroke and dyslipidemia is identical to that of coronary artery disease (CAD). Statin therapy reduces stroke incidence by 25% to 30%, and it has a protective effect even if the lipid profile is normal.
   2. For lacunar stroke and cardiogenic cerebral embolism, the relationship between cholesterol and recurrent stroke has not been shown to be significant.
   3. For intracerebral hemorrhage (ICH), there is a paradoxical effect: stroke risk increases with lowered cholesterol.

C. **Homocysteine lowering**—Elevated homocysteine levels will cause carotid artery intima, media thickening, and an increased risk of stroke. Supplementation with folic acid, vitamin B_{12}, and vitamin B_6 will lower these levels and reduce stroke risk in this case.

D. **Cigarette smoking cessation**—Smoking cessation alone lowers recurrence risk by 50% within one year, and by 5 years the risk is that of the general population.

E. **Diabetes control**—With tight blood pressure reduction and normoglycemia, diabetics have a 44% reduced risk for recurrence.

F. **Antiplatelets and anticoagulation**—see TIA section III.D.4

VII. Nonatherosclerotic Ischemic Stroke

When confronted with the young (<50 year old), nonhypertensive, nondiabetic patient, consider nonatherosclerotic causes. A hypercoagulable work-up is mandatory. Cardiac sources also have to be investigated.

A. Especially if the patient is African American, consider sickle cell disease.

B. In young females, oral contraceptive use and smoking or Takayasu disease

C. If a history of migraine, may be migraine stroke.

D. Giant cell arteritis is possible, but extremely rare before age 60; erythrocyte sedimentation rate (ESR) is always high.

E. Consider venous sinus thrombosis

F. Neurosyphilis

G. Acquired hypercoagulable state, PAPLA syndrome

H. Increased homosysteins

I. There are a myriad of other possibilities not limited to arteritis from collagen vascular disease, carotid artery dissection, fibromuscular dysplasia, atrial myxoma, patent foramen ovale, congenital heart disease, hemoglobinopathies, thrombotic thrombocytopenic purpura, mitochondrial disorders, and illicit drugs.

VIII. Uncontrolled Hypertension and Lacunar Infarcts

A. **Hypertensive encephalopathy**—lethargy, weakness, headache, vomiting with sudden rise in blood pressure followed by seizures and coma; transient focal neurologic findings are rare, but imaging can show reversible posterior leukoencephalopathy.
   1. Lower blood pressure judiciously with labetalol (preferred agent), ACE inhibitors, hydralazine, or minoxidil. Nitroprusside is a last resort because it can cause a temporary increase in intracranial pressure. The longer the blood pressure remains elevated, the higher the risk for ICH. Over aggressive blood pressure correction can lead to stroke, so be careful.

B. **Lacunar infarcts**
   1. **Definition**—They are small (<15 mm), deep infarcts seen in the putamen, pons, thalamus, internal capsule, and caudate.
   2. **For specific classic lacunar** infarcts see Table 7-3.
   3. **Lacunar state**—end stage of longstanding severe hypertension with multiple bilateral lacunes in basal ganglia or pons; neurologic effects due to effect of multiple lacunae; clinical features include bilateral hemiparesis, imbalance, incontinence, shuffling gait, pseudo-bulbar signs, pseudo-bulbar affect, difficulty swallowing and talking, and much higher rates of dementia than the general population; control hypertension aggressively

C. **Binswanger disease**—form of vascular dementia most commonly seen in hypertensive elderly with disorders of cognition, impaired memory and attention, depression, apathy; bilateral corticospinal and corticobulbar signs are usually present; imaging shows subcortical white matter demyelination caused by ischemia, called leukoaraiosis; treatment is aggressive blood pressure control

Table 7-3 *Lacunar Syndromes*

Symptoms	Localization
Pure motor hemiplegia without sensory deficit, aphasia, or cortical sensory deficit	Pons (if spares face), internal capsule, or adjacent corona radiata
Pure sensory stroke	Ventroposterolateral nucleus of the thalamus (most common); also internal capsule/corona radiata, subthalamus, midbrain, medial lemniscus, paramedian dorsal pons. Check spinothalamic modalities—usually preserved in pontine localizations
Usually brainstem syndromes:	
A) Dysarthria–clumsy hand	Basis pontis (most common); also internal capsule and cerebral peduncle. If includes micrographia: genu of internal capsule, putamen
B) Ataxia and hemiparesis involving arm and leg	Pons, midbrain, internal capsule, or parietal white matter
Sensorimotor	Posterior limb of internal capsule (probably most common), thalamus, caudate, putamen
Hemichorea—hemiballismus	Basal ganglia

IX. Hemorrhagic Strokes

A. **Stroke patients** with headaches, nausea, vomiting, altered consciousness, or seizures; hemorrhagic stroke is more likely than ischemic stroke

B. **Hypertensive ICH—most frequent nontraumatic ICH**
   1. Sclerotic and necrotizing changes in lenticulostriate arterioles precede formation of military (arteriolar) aneurysms (Charcot-Bouchard aneurysms), and rupture of military aneurysms believed to be the cause of hypertensive ICH
   2. Usually originate in the putamen, thalamus, pons, cerebellum; can arise from subcortical white matter, but alternative diagnoses must be ruled out
   3. Clinical presentation—initially headaches, nausea, vomiting, altered consciousness, seizures; focal deficit develops suddenly and depends on location (Table 7-4)
   4. Check for other signs of longstanding untreated hypertension like retinal arteriolar changes, left ventricular hypertrophy, and renal impairment.
   5. Treatment—supportive, blood pressure control to prevent ICH enlargement; clearly nonsurgical candidates are those with small hemorrhages (<10 mL blood), minimal neurologic deficits, and patients with Glasgow coma scale (GCS) score of 3 or 4; surgical candidates are young patients with lobar hemorrhage who are clinically deteriorating; prompt surgical evacuation of cerebellar hematoma can prevent brainstem compression and can be effective even with GCS 3 or 4; for all other patients, surgical therapy is unclear; corticosteroid use is not recommended because clinical studies have not shown a benefit; monitoring of intracranial pressure and aggressive treatment are helpful.

C. **Cerebral amyloid (congophilic) angiopathy**—Primary cerebral amyloid angiopathy consists of amyloid infiltration of cerebral blood vessels. Suspect diagnosis in normotensive patients older than 60, or younger if family history. Location is predominantly junction of cortex and white matter in frontal, parietal, and occipital lobes. One third will have a history of previous ICH. Treatment is supportive or surgical evacuation.

D. **SAH caused by saccular arterial aneurysm**
   1. Most frequent cause of primary nontraumatic SAH is **saccular arterial aneurysm**
      a. Asymptomatic aneurysms are found in 5% of the population.
      b. If one is present, there is a 20% chance that there is another.
      c. Mortality 10% from initial hemorrhage, 50% from second hemorrhage
      d. Clinical spectrum:
         i. Asymptomatic—most frequent site of unruptured aneurysms is MCA bifurcation
         ii. Compression of adjacent structures causing, most frequently, third nerve palsy

Table 7-4 *Findings in Hypertensive Intracerebral Hemorrhage*

Cerebellar	Pontine
Nausea, vomiting	Quadriplegia
Ataxia	Pinpoint pupils, eye bobbing
Facial weakness	Absent horizontal eye movement
Coma, decerebrate	Respiratory abnormalities
	Coma

Putaminal	Thalamic
Hemiparesis/plegia	Hemiparesis/plegia
Hemianopia	Hemisensory loss
Eyes look toward lesion	Downward deviation of eyes
	Paralysis of upward gaze
	Small but reactive pupils

Table 7-5: Hunt and Hess Classification of Subarachnoid

Grade	Risk of symptomatic vasospasm	Description
1	22%	Asymptomatic or mild headache (HA) and mild nuchal rigidity
2	33%	Cranial nerve palsy, moderate to severe HA, nuchal rigidity
3	52%	Mild focality, lethargic, confused
4	53%	Stupor, hemiparetic, decerebrate allowed
5	74%	Comatose, decerebrate

Add one grade for systemic disease like hypertension or diabetes, as well as severe vasospasm on angiography

      iii. Rupture—most frequent site is ICA junction with posterior communicating artery, followed by anterior cerebral—anterior communicating artery junction

2. **Symptomatology of ruptured aneurysms**—severe headache maximal at onset, transitory loss of consciousness or weakness of legs; stiff neck not usually found early, but miosis and photophobia are common; focal deficit is not usually found
3. **CT is mandatory.** Due to high rate of mortality, if CT is negative, LP is also mandatory. If CT is positive, no need to do LP. LP may increase transmural pressure and increase bleeding. Get basic labs: blood count, platelets, coagulation panel. Urgent angiogram if aneurysm.
4. **Prognostication for cerebral vasospasm** by Hunt and Hess grading. See Table 7-5.
5. **Treatment depends on Hunt and Hess grade.** Neurosurgeons and neuroradiologists argue, with neurosurgeons presenting evidence that open clipping is superior to endovascular techniques and neuroradiologists showing the opposite. A study in *Lancet* shows the value of coiling. Medical management includes blood pressure management, total bed rest, sedation, laxatives, cardiac monitoring, intake and output measurements, and sodium control. Any headache, nausea, and vomiting are treated. Avoid fluid restriction, since this can induce vasospasm. Calming drugs possibly helpful. Nimodipine (a dihydropyridine L-type calcium channel blocker) 60 mg every 4 hours for 21 days, volume expansion reduces vasospasm; avoidance of intracranial hypertension is necessary; serial CTs for hydrocephalus.

X. Dural and Cortical Venous Thrombosis

A. General information
1. Most commonly involved: superior sagittal, lateral, cavernous, and straight sinus
2. Infectious causes: pyogenic or fungal infections, or as a meningitis complication
3. Noninfectious causes—malnutrition, congenital heart disease, polycythemia, dehydration, head injuries, coagulation disorders
4. Venous sinus thrombosis leads to intracranial hypertension and hydrocephalus
5. In females, associated with pregnancy, postpartum period, and sometimes oral contraceptive use; the latter may be related to concurrent chronic disease states
6. About one fourth will have no risk factor.

B. Clinical features include headache, vomiting, seizures, and focal deficit.

C. Diagnosis: CT may show thrombosed veins; magnetic resonance venography (MRV) for definitive diagnosis

D. Treatment: Heparin is probably the best, although this may cause bleeding with hemorrhagic infarct.

E. Morbidity/mortality: 15% to 25% deaths, survivors: one third have lasting cognitive impairment

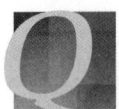 # STUDY QUESTIONS FOR CHAPTER 7

Directions: *Each of the numbered items or incomplete statements in this section is followed by answers or by completions of the statement. Select the ONE lettered answer or completion that is BEST in each case.*

1. A 24-year-old patient with known sickle cell disease comes in with new-onset hemiplegia with sensory deficit in the same location. What is the most likely mechanism for this?
   (A) Intracerebral hemorrhage
   (B) Subarachnoid hemorrhage
   (C) Ischemic stroke
   (D) Malingering
   (E) Hemiplegic migraine

2. A 56-year-old woman is having a conversation with her friend on the phone. Her friend asks her a question and instead of an answer, hears a loud bang. The friend calls 911 and EMTs respond to find an unresponsive patient who is breathing and maintaining a perfusing blood pressure. She is not wearing a medic alert bracelet. You are called for a GCS of 4. What is the initial test to get the diagnosis?
   (A) Complete blood count
   (B) Coagulation profile
   (C) Urine toxicology
   (D) CT of head without contrast
   (E) Lumbar puncture

3. Same patient as in #2. The emergency room physician asks if it would be worthwhile to call neurosurgery. You reply, "While it is never bad to get another opinion, he is likely to say,"
   (A) With GCS 4, surgery is always warranted.
   (B) Surgery is never warranted for Hunt and Hess grade 5.
   (C) With GCS 4, surgery is never warranted.
   (D) Surgery is always warranted for Hunt and Hess grade 5.
   (E) Let's see what the imaging shows us first.

4. A 79-year-old man with diabetes, hypercholesterolemia, and hypertension presents to the emergency room with the sudden onset of right hemiparesis, hemianesthesia, and hemianopia. The most likely location of a stroke would be:
   (A) Left anterior cerebral artery
   (B) Left middle cerebral artery
   (C) Left posterior cerebral artery
   (D) Left anterior choroidal artery
   (E) Left superior hypophyseal artery

5. A 39-year-old woman with Marfan syndrome presents with a right-sided headache, right-sided Horner syndrome, and a left hemiparesis affecting the face and arm. What is the most likely diagnosis?
   (A) Dissection of the right carotid artery
   (B) Dissection of the right vertebral artery
   (C) Infarction of the right middle cerebral artery
   (D) Infarction of the right ophthalmic artery
   (E) Infarction of the right posterior inferior cerebellar artery

6. A neuroradiologist is reviewing a film to "rule out stroke" and notes infarction in the right medial medulla. Which is an expected clinical finding in a patient with a right medial medullary infarction?
   (A) Nystagmus
   (B) Vertigo
   (C) Left hemiparesis
   (D) Paresis of the left side of the tongue
   (E) Loss of taste sensation on the anterior two thirds of the left side of the tongue

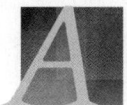 # ANSWERS AND EXPLANATIONS

1. C. Ischemic stroke is the most common intracranial complication of sickle cell disease. Subarachnoid hemorrhage and intracerebral hemorrhage also occur but are less common. Malingering is a common misnomer for sickle cell patients who come into the emergency room complaining of pain. Hemiplegic migraine is not associated with sickle cell disease.

2. D. This is a subarachnoid hemorrhage. CT is used to establish the diagnosis. The other tests should probably be ordered, but they do not establish the diagnosis, unless the CT is negative, then one should do an LP. In this case, with hemorrhage so severe, patient is comatose, it is hard to imagine it would not be positive.

3. C. In a patient with GCS 3 or 4, surgery is never warranted unless there is cerebellar hematoma.

4. D. Infarction of the left anterior choroidal artery classically produces contralateral hemiparesis, hemianesthesia, and hemianopia. Anterior cerebral artery infarctions affect the leg more than the arm. Middle cerebral artery infarctions usually do not affect the leg. Posterior cerebral artery infarctions produce hemianopia but usually not hemiparesis. The left superior hypophyseal artery supplies the anterior pituitary and pituitary stalk and should not produce hemiparesis, hemianesthesia, or hemianopia.

5. A. Dissection of the right carotid artery is most likely to cause a right-sided headache and Horner syndrome. Infarction in the distal right middle cerebral artery is responsible for the face and arm weakness. Dissection of the right vertebral artery would be expected to produce diplopia, dizziness, contralateral hemisensory loss, and neck pain. Infarction of the right posterior inferior cerebellar artery would cause a similar picture, although neck pain would be less likely. Right middle cerebral artery infarction is usually not associated with headache and Horner syndrome. Infarction of the right ophthalmic artery would cause blindness in the right eye.

6. C. Medial medullary infarction would be expected to produce weakness of the ipsilateral tongue and contralateral body. Nystagmus and vertigo are more commonly seen in lateral medullary infarction. Loss of taste on the anterior two thirds of the left side of the tongue would be expected with a left facial nerve lesion.

Chapter 8

Cerebellum

I. Anatomy

A. **Classic Division:** 3 lobes, which contain 10 lobules
   1. **Flocculonodular lobe** = archicerebellum: oldest phylogenetically, inferior, inputs from vestibular nuclei, involved in equilibrium
   2. **Anterior lobe** = paleocerebellum: anterosuperior vermis and paravermian cortex, inputs from proprioceptors of muscles and tendons (spinocerebellum, involved in posture and muscle tone)
   3. **Posterior lobe** = neocerebellum: major portion of cerebellar hemispheres, middle division vermis and lateral extensions, inputs from cerebral cortex via pons (pontocerebellum, involved in coordination, skilled movements)

B. Fissures
   1. **Primary fissure** separates anterior and posterior lobes
   2. **Posterolateral fissure** separates posterior and flocculonodular lobes

C. Longitudinal (sagittal) zones
   1. **Vermian zone**—coordinates movements of the eyes and body
   2. **Lateral zone**—coordinates movements of the ipsilateral limbs
   3. **Intermediate/paravermian zone**—mediates postural tone, movement ipsilateral limb

D. Deep nuclei
   1. **Dentate nucleus**
      a. Function
         i. Involved in initiation of volitional movements
         ii. Neurons shown to fire prior to onset of volitional movements
         iii. Inactivation of dentate neurons produces delayed initiation of movements
      b. Input/output
         i. Afferents premotor and supplementary motor cortices, via lateral zone cerebellum
         ii. Efferents—to the ventrolateral thalamus then motor cortex
   2. **Interpositus nucleus** (globose and emboliform)
      a. Function: fire in relation to a movement once it has started, responsible for making volitional oscillators or alternating movements, dampens physiologic tremor, cells fire in tandem with these actions, inactivation of interpositus neurons impair the regularity and amplitude of alternating movements; may also play a role in intention tremor
      b. Input/output
         i. Afferents cerebrocortical projections via pontocerebellar system, spinocerebellar projections from Golgi tendon organs, muscle spindles, cutaneous afferents, and spinal interneurons via intermediate zone of cerebellar cortex, via intermediate zone of cerebellum

ii. Efferents to contralateral red nucleus
3. **Fastigial nuclei**
   a. Function: controls antigravity and other muscle synergies in standing and walking, ablation significantly impairs gait and balance
   b. Input/Output
      i. Afferents from flocculonodular lobe and vermis
      ii. Efferents to vestibular nuclei

E. **Neuronal organization**
   1. **General information:** cerebellum comprises 10% of total weight and volume of the brain but contains half of the brain's neurons; 40% more afferent than efferent axons; stereotyped three-layered structure with five types of neurons
   2. **Layers**
      a. Molecular layer—outermost
         i. Stellate cells—inhibitory
         ii. Basket cells—inhibitory
         iii. Dendrites of Purkinje cells
      b. Purkinje cell layer—somites of Purkinje cells—inhibitory
      c. Granular layer—innermost
         i. Granule cells—densely packed, inhibitory
         ii. Golgi interneurons—fewer, inhibitory
         iii. Glomeruli—synaptic connections mossy fibers with granule/Golgi cells; Tables 8-1, 8-2
   3. **Peduncles:** Superior cerebellar peduncle, middle cerebellar peduncle, inferior cerebellar peduncle
   4. **Vascular supply**
      a. **Posterior inferior cerebellar artery (PICA)**, branch of vertebral artery: supplies posterior inferior surface cerebellar hemispheres, cerebellar tonsils, inferior vermis, posterior lateral medulla (Wallenberg syndrome), choroid plexus fourth ventricle

Table 8-1 *Cells of the Cerebellum*

Cell type	Stellate	Basket	Purkinje	Granule	Golgi interneuron
NT	GABA	GABA	GABA	glutamate	GABA
E/I	I	I	I	E	I
Input	granule		stellate/granule		granule
Efferent	Purkinje	Purkinje	cerebellar, vestibular nuclei	parallel fiber	granule

Excitatory, E; GABA, γ-aminobutyric acid; Inhibitory, I; NT, neurotransmitter.

Table 8-2 *Afferent Fibers*

Fiber Type	Mossy	Climbing	Aminergic	Parallel
Parent cell	spinal cord, Vestibular pontine nuclei	inferior olivary nuclei	(1) raphe nuclei (2) locus ceruleus	granule cell
Efferent Target	granular layer-granule dendrites	molecular layer-Purkinje	(1) granular & molecular (2) all 3 layers	molecular layer basket, Purkinje dendrite Golgi cell stellate
E/I	E	E	E	excitatory
NT	aspartate	aspartate	(1) serotonin (2) norepinephrine	glutamate

b. **Anterior inferior cerebellar artery (AICA)**, branch of basilar artery supplies anterolateral surface cerebellar hemispheres, middle cerebellar peduncle, flocculus, cranial nerves VI, VII, VIII
c. **Superior cerebellar artery (SCA)**, branch of basilar prior to bifurcation of PCAs, supplies entire superior surface cerebellar hemispheres and vermis, deep cerebellar white matter, dentate nucleus

II. Clinical Features

A. **Clinical signs and symptoms**
   1. Incoordination of volitional movement: dysmetria/dyssynergia, dysdiadochokinesia, dysarthria (slurring, scanning), ataxia ipsilateral to side of lesion
   2. Ocular: gaze paretic nystagmus, saccadic dysmetria, catch-up saccades
   3. Characteristic tremor: "rubral tremor," titubation of head/trunk
   4. Disorders of equilibrium and gait: hemispheric lesion produces extremity problems affecting arm, leg, and trunk; if vermal produces truncal and leg instability sparing arms
   5. Decreased muscle tone, especially with acute lesions
   6. Cognitive dysfunction
   7. "Pendular" deep tendon reflexes

B. **Clinical syndromes according to anatomic lobe**
   1. **Flocculonodular lobe lesion:** disturbances equilibrium with positional nystagmus, limbs relatively unaffected
   2. **Anterior lobe lesion:** increased shortening and lengthening reactions, exaggerated postural reflexes
   3. **Posterior lobe lesion:** ipsilateral clumsiness, hypotonia, if dentate, marked symptoms

C. **Vascular syndromes**
   1. **PICA infarct**: Wallenberg syndrome: "crossed sensory" with ipsilateral face/contralateral body decreased pain/temp, vertigo/nausea, nystagmus, hoarseness, dysphagia, dysarthria, ipsilateral Horner, ipsilateral ataxia limbs, partial Wallenberg common
   2. **AICA infarct:** vertigo/nausea/vomiting, *tinnitus with occasional ipsilateral deafness, ipsilateral facial weakness, cerebellar ataxia, Horner; contralateral decreased pain/temp body, if proximal—can hit corticospinals and produce hemiplegia, if distal can get cochlear/labyrinthine infarction
   3. **SCA infarct:** nausea/vomiting, dysarthria, ipsilateral cerebellar ataxia, contralateral decreased pain/temp body

D. **Neoplasm**
   1. **Primary neoplasms:** medulloblastoma, hemangioblastoma, astrocytoma, ganglioneuroma of Lhermitte-Duclos
   2. **Metastatic disease**: more common in adults: lung and gastrointestinal neoplasms, especially colon
   3. **Paraneoplastic disease:** Subacute cerebellar degeneration—anti-Yo, anti-Purkinje antibody, usually secondary to lung or breast cancer, subacute onset of cerebellar disease that can predate diagnosis of cancer. Causes pancerebellar syndrome with vermal and hemispheric involvement.

E. **Infectious disease**
   1. **Acute cerebellitis**
      a. Acute ataxia of childhood—most often associated with chickenpox, but also seen with enteroviruses, Epstein-Barr virus (EBV), mycoplasma, cytomegalovirus (CMV), Q fever, and a number of vaccines; pathology is infectious or postinfectious
      b. In adults—EBV and mycoplasma most common

c. Work-up is usually normal: cerebrospinal fluid (CSF) shows mild pleocytosis and protein may be elevated.
 2. **Whipple disease**, pathogen is *Tropheryma whippleii*
    a. Ataxia develops in 20%; may see neurologic symptoms without systemic features
    b. Typical case is middle-aged man with fever, steatorrhea, abdominal pain, arthralgias, hyperpigmentation, and weight loss
    c. "Oculomasticatory myorhythmia" rhythmic myoclonus/spasm in eyes/jaw/face with supranuclear gaze paresis—pathognomic for CNS Whipple
    d. Diagnosis is made by periodic acid—Schiff (PAS positive organisms in jejunal mucosa biopsy)

F. **Metabolic**
 1. **Alcohol** men > women, vermal syndrome
    a. Wide-based stance and gait, truncal instability > than ataxia of limbs, tremor
    b. Nystagmus/dysarthria infrequent
    d. Anterior superior vermian atrophy
    e. Likely secondary to nutritional deficiency rather than direct toxicity
 2. **Hypothyroid**
    a. Ataxic gait, dysarthria associated with myxedema
    b. With primary or secondary hypothyroidism
    c. Same pathologic changes as seen with alcohol abuse and malnutrition
 3. **Hyperthermia**
    a. Disproportionately affects cerebellum
    b. After acute phase of coma, seizures, shock, renal failure often, residual symptoms of pure cerebellar dysfunction
 4. **Sprue**
    a. Usually after several years of enteropathy see progressive cerebellar ataxia of gait and limbs, occasionally associated with polymyoclonus
    b. Often with peripheral neuropathy, occasionally with myelopathy and encephalopathy
 5. **Jejunal bypass** episodic cerebellar ataxia associated with lactic acidosis
 6. **GM2** gangliosidosis

G. **Hereditary**
 1. **Metabolic**
    a. Abetalipoproteinemia—Bassen-Kornzweig acanthocytosis: Autosomal recessive (AR), onset 6 to 12 years of age, weakness of limbs with areflexia and sensory ataxia later with cerebellar ataxia, impaired fat absorption in small intestine that leads to abnormal cell membranes, diagnosis by acanthocytes on blood smear—thorny red blood cells (RBCs), decreased low-density lipoproteins (LDLs)
    b. **Familial hypobetalipoproteinemia:** Autosomal dominant (AD), similar to abetalipoproteinemia
    c. **HARP**: hypocholesterolemia, acanthocytosis, retinitis pigmentosa, pallidal atrophy
 2. **Channelopathies** covered in 13.VIII.D.19,20
 3. **Degenerative** covered in 13.VIII.D,E.

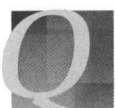 STUDY QUESTIONS FOR CHAPTER 8

Directions: *Each of the numbered items or incomplete statements in this section is followed by answers or by completions of the statement. Select the ONE lettered answer or completion that is BEST in each case.*

1. A 67-year-old man is referred to your clinic for evaluation of an abnormal MRI of his brain. Prior to his visit, you are able to review the MRI, which demonstrates a contrast-enhancing lesion in the flocculonodular lobe of the cerebellum. What are the primary inputs to this part of the cerebellum?

(A) Basal ganglia
(B) Cerebral cortex
(C) Muscle spindle afferents
(D) Pons
(E) Vestibular nuclei

2. You are called to the emergency department to see a 78-year-old man with sudden onset of hearing loss in his left ear. When you examine him, there are no other neurologic abnormalities. Infarction of what arterial territory would most likely produce a stroke with these symptoms?

(A) Left anterior inferior cerebellar artery
(B) Left posterior inferior cerebellar artery
(C) Left superior cerebellar artery
(D) Left vertebral artery
(E) Basilar artery

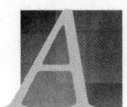 ANSWERS AND EXPLANATIONS

1. E. The primary inputs to the flocculonodular lobe are the vestibular nuclei. Cerebral cortex and the pons project mainly to the cerebellar hemispheres, whereas the muscle spindle afferents project mainly to the vermis.

2. A. The anterior inferior cerebellar artery supplies the eighth cranial nerve, and infarction in this territory can produce ipsilateral sudden-onset hearing loss. Infarction of the left posterior inferior cerebellar artery is more commonly associated with Wallenberg syndrome. Superior cerebellar artery strokes usually produce nausea, vomiting, dysarthria, ataxia, and sensory changes, but do not produce hearing loss. Vertebral and basilar artery infarctions may produce hearing loss as one symptom, but other symptoms including dysarthria, ataxia, sensory changes, diplopia, and nystagmus would also be expected.

CHAPTER 9

Spinal Cord

We will organize by the mnemonic VITAMINS (see Table 9-1).

I. V for Vascular

1% of strokes are spinal in origin.

A. Myelomalacia (sequelae of infarction of spinal cord)—less common than brain (spinal arteries are not susceptible to atherosclerosis)
  1. **Anterior spinal artery** most common vessel: presentation based on level of infarct, pain with bilateral motor paralysis, loss of pain/temperature sensation below level of lesion, develop within 1 to 2 hours; causes: disease of aorta or collateral artery, polyarteritis nodosa, aortic surgery; the most important artery supplying the anterior circulation is the artery of Adamkiewicz, which enters the spinal cord usually on left between T9 and L2; diagnosis: magnetic resonance imaging (MRI); treatment: supportive
  2. **Watershed infarct** especially T6 to T8

B. Dissecting aortic aneurysm—triad of sensory loss below T6; brachial artery obstruction causing sensorimotor neuropathy of arm; leg/sphincter paralysis

C. Hemorrhage into spinal cord/canal—rare; causes: trauma, vascular malformation, complication of spinal tap; bleeding disease; diagnosis: blood/xanthochromic in cerebrospinal fluid (CSF); treatment: emergent surgical evacuation

D. Vascular malformations of spinal cord—venous angioma with arteriovenous (AV) fistula—acute cramping pain in sciatic distribution; weakness/numbness/paresthesia legs; episodic over days/weeks; worse supine; treatment: surgical occlusion of feeding artery

E. Fibrocartilaginous embolism—spinal apoplexy; healthy individual, acute pain back/neck then signs of transverse cord lesion; evolves over minutes to hour; may be preceded by strenuous activity/trauma; CSF: normal

F. Spinal subdural or epidural hemorrhage—severe thoracic pain, stiff neck/headache; no myelopathy; causes: obscure, trauma/anticoagulation; CSF: dark yellow–brown fluid, red blood cell (RBC); computed tomography (CT)—subdural collection, MRI can also clearly show blood; treatment: sedation/analgesia, surgical evacuation

Table 9-1	*Vitamins*

V—vascular
I—inflammatory
T—toxic, traumatic
A—autoimmune
M—metabolic
I—infection
N—neoplastic
S—systemic*

*Some use vitamin D with D for degenerative, but systemic covers that and more.

II. I for Inflammation

Myelitis of neurons/meninges/gray and/or white matter or infection

A. Viral—includes coxsackie, polio, herpes simplex virus (HSV), human immunodeficiency virus (HIV)

B. Vacuolar myelopathy with AIDS—asymmetrical limb weakness; onset 4 to 6 months prior to death; diagnosis: lipid-laden macrophages/vacuoles in white matter of spinal cord
  1. Often obscured by neuropathies associated with HIV, associated cognitive impairment
  2. Tropical spastic paraparesis due to human T-cell lymphoma/leukemia virus (HTLV)-I—chronic infective/inflammatory disease of spinal cord; slowly progressive paraparesis, loss of sphincter control; paresthesias, ⇓ vibratory/position sense, ataxia, ⇑ deep tendon reflexes and Babinski; diagnosis: CSF- ⇑ T lymphocytes, ⇑ immunoglobulin G (IgG); serum antibodies to HTLV-I; MRI-gradient echo hyperintensity, multiple punctate/nodular T2 hyperintensity without mass effect, periventricular white matter, subcortical white matter
  3. Myelitis due to bacterial/fungal/parasitic/granulomatous disease—multiple presentations depending on which portion of column is affected; MRI initial test to define presence of lesion; CSF to establish etiology.
  4. Acute transverse myelitis—disordered immune response to infection/immunization/vasculitis causes demyelination/necrosis of spinal cord; symptoms evolve over 6 to 24 hours; impaired motor/sensory/autonomic; CSF ⇑ protein, lymphocytes, oligoclonal bands; MRI T1 hypointensity, T2 hyperintensity, with possible enhancement; prognosis variable
  5. Postinfectious/postvaccinal myelitis—status post infection/vaccination; asymmetrical extremity weakness/numbness; patient usually afebrile; causes: rubella, rubeola, varicella, Epstein-Barr virus (EBV), cytomegalovirus (CMV), hepatitis B virus (HBV), mycoplasma; smallpox vaccine; CSF ⇑ protein/lymphocytes/polymorphonuclear cells; treatment: supportive
  6. Demyelinative myelitis similar to postinfectious but symptoms evolve over 1 to 3 weeks; painless numbness/weakness of feet/anterior thighs/trunk; possible leg paralysis; CSF normal; usually resolves; treatment: corticosteroids
  7. Acute necrotizing myelitis (Foix-Alajourine syndrome)—acute onset persistent/profound flaccidity of limbs; areflexia; bladder atony; sensory loss
  8. Paraneoplastic myelitis (subacute necrotic myelitis)—painless, rapidly progressive motor/sensory loss; CSF/imaging normal; diagnosis: search for primary; treatment: none; with unknown primary, test for anti-Hu (small cell lung and neuroblastoma)

C. Spinal arachnoiditis (chronic adhesive arachnoiditis)—onset between 40 and 60 years, bilateral burning/stinging pain lumbofemoral region; causes: repeated disk surgery, syphilis, introduction of medications/contrast into subarachnoid space; "candle gutting" on myelogram; treatment: corticosteroids (early), limited success with surgery

D. **Infection**
   1. **Spinal epidural abscess**—presentation/diagnosis: small/innocuous injury to back seeds into epidural space or vertebrae; fever with local tenderness; rapidly progresses to paraparesis and sensory loss; most common cause *Staphylococcus aureus*; CSF: ⇑ protein, neutrophilic leukocytosis; CT/MRI to determine level; treatment: laminectomy and drainage (if no neurologic signs can use antibiotics only; antibiotics for *S. aureus* PCN resistant)
   2. **Subacute pyogenic infection/granulomatous infection in subdural space**—less dramatic/painful than abscess; diagnosis: CT myelogram and MRI; treatment: antibiotics
   3. **Spinal cord abscess**—rare; similar presentation to that of epidural abscess; causes: septicemia/endocarditis, contiguous skin abscess; diagnosis: MRI

E. **Neurosyphilis** caused by *Treponema pallidum*, central nervous system (CNS) invasion, meningitis in one fourth of all cases of syphilis, later stage vascular syphilis: paresis, tabes dorsalis, optic atrophy, psychosis possible
   1. **CSF** is helpful with lymphonuclear pleocytosis, elevated protein up to 200 mg/dL, oligoclonal banding, positive CSF serology; serology is unreliable in later syphilis, so antigen tests fluorescent treponemal antibody absorption (FTA-ABS) or Treponema pallidum immobilization (TPI) must be performed
   2. **Pathology**—frontal and temporal lobes with perivascular lymphocytic, monocytic invasion, and rod-shaped microgliacytes; iron can be found in the mononuclear cells; granular epididymitis and meningeal fibrosis are common

F. **HIV**—protean manifestations of HIV in the spinal cord; the most common appear to be sensory axonal polyneuropathy, likely second most is a painful mononeuritis multiplex, chronic demyelinating polyneuropathy (CIDP), polyradiculitis; others have been described, rarely diffuse infiltrative lymphocytosis syndrome producing similar protean manifestations, but specific to HIV

III. T for Trauma

A. **Mechanism**
   1. **Flexion**—bony damage causing cord trapping/dislocation
   2. **Whiplash/recoil injury**—usually just injury of tissues (ligament, tendon, muscle, joint), but if recoil is bad enough can cause spinal cord concussion
   3. **Spinal cord concussion**—high velocity impact to vertebral column can cause shock waves down cord; reversible paralysis happens for 1 to 2 days; falls flat on back from ladder/contact sports
   4. **Vulnerability to injury** can increase with spondylosis or stenosis of vertebrae
   5. **Cord** can be damaged without radiographic evidence of fracture

B. **Clinical effects** of spinal cord injury (SCI)
   1. **Spinal shock/areflexia** stage occurs initially and lasts 1 to 6 weeks: loss of motor/sensation/reflexes below injury, bowel/bladder atony, gastric atony, autonomic nervous system (ANS) loss (systemic hypotension, dry/pale skin, sphincter contraction secondary to loss of inhibition from CNS centers, overflow incontinence)
   2. **Heightened reflex activity** stage emerges as the initial stage recedes: reflex responses to stimulation return (flexion reflexes with Babinski first); eventually becoming exaggerated; may have sensory return below lesion (often pain/burning)
   3. **Mass reflex** emerges after several months—mild stimulation leads to flexor spasms and ANS (sweating, piloerection, incontinence)
   4. **Autonomic dysreflexia** also after several months—mild stimulation leads to norepinephrine, epinephrine release; increased sweating above lesion, cutaneous flushing, hypertension, headache, reflex bradycardia
   5. **Central cord syndrome:** motor loss, upper limbs > lower; most severe in hands; bladder dysfunction; minimal sensory loss, retroflexion head/neck

C. **Acute spinal cord injury**—in localizing level: lesions of lower cervical cord may have preserved sensation to nipple line from C3/C4 cutaneous branches of cervical plexus
   1. **Treatment:** Immediate cervical immobilization, methylprednisolone 30 mg/kg bolus followed by 5.4 mg/kg every hour for 23 hours; use if presents <8 hours.
      a. Vertebral dislocation with SCI treat with halo brace for 4 to 6 weeks then rigid collar
   2. **Recovery prognosis** more favorable if movement or sensation elicited in first 48 to 72 hours
   3. ⇑ mortality first 7 to 10 days to gastric dilation, ileus, shock, infection; ⇓ after first 3 months
   4. **Aftercare:** supportive management for bladder (intermittent cath; watch for infection), fecal incontinence (suppositories, periodical enemas), chronic pain (nonsteroidal anti-inflammatory drugs [NSAIDs], local anesthetic injections), spasms (baclofen, diazepam, tizanidine), physical rehabilitation

IV. A for Autoimmune

A. **Acute myelitis** seen in association with systemic lupus erythematosus (SLE); there are both rapidly evolving and subacute presentation forms; etiology seems to be spinal cord microvasculitis

B. **Multiple sclerosis** please see chapter 11.II

V. M for Metabolic

A. **Vitamin E deficiency** a disorder of children
   1. **Inherited form** 8q, α-tocopherol transfer protein abnormal, so vitamin E can not be incorporated into very-low-density lipoprotein (VLDL)
   2. **Ataxia**, decreased or absent deep tendon reflexes, decreased sensation and proximal strength, elevated creatine phosphokinase (CPK) level, ophthalmoparesis from posterior column, spinocerebellar tract, and sensory root degeneration
B. **Vitamin B_{12}**
   1. **Symptoms: initial**—constant, progressive paresthesias hands > feet; progression—stiffness, weakness legs > arms, ataxia
   2. **Signs**—position, vibratory loss legs > arms, proximal leg weakness and spasticity, gait eventually becomes spastic
   3. **N_2O** (nitrous oxide) effects on vitamin B_{12} impairs metabolism of vitamin by inactivating methionine synthetase, affects those patients that are subclinically B_{12} deficient, classic history: patient wakes up from surgery at dentist with ataxia, or anesthesiologist has worsening ataxia due to chronic nitrous exposure.
   4. **Related problems:** methylmalonic aciduria—2 types
      a. **D-Methylmalonyl coenzyme A (CoA)** mutase apoenzyme deficiency—D-methylmalonyl CoA cannot be made into propionyl CoA, so it accumulates; treatment: low protein diet, and L-carnitine supplementation
      b. **Adenosylcobalamin and methylcobalamin**—necessary cofactor for preceding reaction, homocystinuria appears as well; treatment: as previously described but add hydroxocobalamin 1mg once per week
      c. **Symptoms**—normal birth. 1 week for methylmalonyl mutase deficiency (MMD), and 1 month for adenosylcobalamin; lethargy, recurrent vomiting, anemia, intracranial hemorrhage. Most patients with MMD die by 2 months of diagnosis; those that survive with mental retardation
   5. **Pathology**—initial swelling of myelin sheaths with intramyelin vacuoles, especially in posterior columns of lower cervical and upper thoracic spinal cord; later vacuolar degeneration similar to HIV and gliosis

VI. I for Iatrogenic

Radiation injury to spinal cord (status post radiation treatment [RTX] to areas around cord)

A. Transient myelopathy "early": 3 to 6 months after radiation treatment; paresthesias in extremities

B. Delayed progressive radiation myelopathy "late": 6 months to years after radiation treatment; insidious onset of paresthesias/dysesthesias then rapidly progressive weakness in extremities; CSF: normal; MRI: abnormal intensity; treatment: prevention (maintain XRT at recommended doses); steroids provide temporary improvement

VII. N for Neoplastic causing Compression Injury

Note that most lesions can cause compression injury.

A. Cauda equina syndrome, below L3 causes early radicular pain worsened by Valsalva; later symptoms include asymmetric sensory loss in the saddle region, peripheral paraplegia, absent Achilles reflex, uncommon sphincter dysfunction, absent Babinski

B. Conus medullaris syndrome
1. **Lesions:** sphincter dysfunction, pelvic floor paralysis, autonomous neurogenic bladder (usually with saddle anesthesia), constipation, erectile/ejaculatory dysfunction, pain may occur later, positive Babinski
2. **Tethered cord syndrome** or low conus medullaris syndrome most commonly present with foot numbness, asymmetric atrophy of calf or thigh muscles, bowel and bladder dysfunction, and cutaneous manifestations of spinal dysraphism; this is a defect of secondary neurulation with defect in closure of posterior neuropore

C. Tumors: much less frequent than brain tumors; usually benign, effect by compression; gradual onset asymmetrical motor or sensory deficit and back pain
1. **Lesions** are described as extradural (think metastasis) versus intradural; intradural lesions are divided into extramedullary (meningioma) versus intramedullary (syrinx)
2. **Extramedullary** most common (neurofibromas, meningiomas); diagnosis: CSF, CT/MRI to help localize; treatment: specific to tumor type; can usually be removed surgically
3. **Radicular-spinal cord syndrome**—cord compression causes knifelike pain, radiates away from spine, increased pain with cough/sneeze
4. **Syringomyelia**—chronic progressive degenerative disorder of cord; associated with type I Chiari malformation; cavitation of central part of spinal cord (syrinx); can also be acquired from surgery/radiation
   a. **Types I/II** (with and without foramen magnum obstruction); sporadic; onset age 25 to 45, M=F, insidious onset/irregularly progressive; presentation depends on size/location syrinx; segmental weakness/atrophy of hands/arms with decreased tendon reflex; cape distribution, loss of pain/temperature sensation
   b. **Syringobulbia:** bulbar equivalent; occur with syringomyelia but can be independent; unilateral nystagmus, analgesia, dysarthria, dysphagia, hoarseness
   c. **Type III** (with other spinal cord disease); suspect if sensorimotor abnormalities extend over whole body; also post SCI or with Von Hippel Lindau
   d. **Type IV** (pure hydromelia); usually known hydrocephalic with weakness in cape distribution; diagnosis: MRI brain/cord; contrast myelography with delayed CT exposes syrinx; treatment: I/II: surgical decompression relieves pain but most sensorimotor symptoms persist; III: excise tumor/mass; IV: ventriculoperitoneal (VP) shunt for hydrocephalus usually treats

VIII. S for Systemic: Arthritic

A. Cervical spondylosis with myelopathy—degenerative disease of cervical spine narrows canal; compression/injury of cord/roots; triad: painful/stiff neck, brachialgia and numb hands, spastic leg weakness and unsteady gait; diagnosis: distinguish from multiple sclerosis; CSF: normal, MRI/CT: cord flattening and CSF space obliteration; treatment: laminectomy

B. Lumbar stenosis—older men; hypertrophy of facets/disk degeneration; compress roots; numb/weak legs; minimal pain; aggravated by standing/walking (neurologic claudication); diagnosis: lumbar spine radiographs, electromyogram (EMG), rule out metabolic cause; treatment: NSAIDS, surgery

C. Ankylosing spondylitis—rheumatologic condition; fused/rigid spine; increased susceptibility to fracture; can lead to cauda equina syndrome

D. Paget disease (osteitis deformans)—enlargement of vertebrae causes narrowing of spinal canal; diagnosis: increased alkaline phosphatase level; treatment: surgical, NSAIDs, calcitonin, cytotoxic drugs

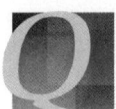 STUDY QUESTIONS FOR CHAPTER 9

Directions: *Each of the numbered items or incomplete statements in this section is followed by answers or by completions of the statement.* Select the ONE lettered answer or completion that is BEST in each case.

1. A 21-year-old man is brought to the emergency room after being thrown from his motorcycle one hour earlier. He is immobilized in a hard collar and intubated. Neurologic examination shows that he is awake and has normal eye movements and pupillary reactions. His limbs are flaccid and his reflexes are absent. He shows no response to noxious stimuli in his extremities. What is the most appropriate next treatment?

(A) Cervical spine MRI
(B) Emergent laminectomy
(C) Methylprednisolone
(D) Cervical spine x-ray
(E) Traction

2. An 88-year-old woman presents to the emergency room with the acute onset of flaccid weakness in her lower extremities. On examination, her upper extremities are of normal strength and her lower extremities are flaccid with absent reflexes. Sensory examination shows decreased pinprick and cold sensation with preserved joint position and vibration perception below the umbilicus. What is the most likely mechanism of her neurologic dysfunction?

(A) Infarction of the spinal cord
(B) Herniated thoracic disk
(C) Metastasis to the thoracic spinal cord
(D) Spinal subdural hemorrhage
(E) Dissecting aortic aneurysm

3. While playing basketball, a 19-year-old man developed acute mid-back pain and weakness in his lower extremities. The symptoms progressed over 2 hours. He has no other medical problems and has been in good health. Of the following choices, which is the most likely mechanism of injury?

(A) Direct trauma to the thoracic spine
(B) Transverse myelitis
(C) Fibrocartilaginous embolus
(D) Lumbar disk herniation
(E) Epidural abscess

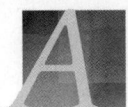# ANSWERS AND EXPLANATIONS

1. C. This man has an acute traumatic spinal cord injury and should receive methylprednisolone as a 30 mg/kg bolus followed by 5.4 mg/kg every hour for the following 23 hours. Although cervical spine MRI and x-ray may be helpful to establish a diagnosis, he should receive the methylprednisolone first. Emergent laminectomy and placement in traction are not appropriate treatments.

2. A. Acute onset flaccid lower extremity weakness with loss of pinprick and cold sensation and preservation of joint position and vibration sensation is most consistent with spinal cord infarction. The dissociation of the sensory findings is not typical of the other listed conditions.

3. C. The most likely mechanism of injury is fibrocartilaginous embolus. This usually occurs in otherwise healthy people and is characterized by the sudden onset of pain and leg weakness. Direct trauma to the thoracic spine is not likely to produce his symptoms. Transverse myelitis typically progresses over a longer time frame. Lumbar disk herniation would be expected to produce lower back pain rather than mid-back pain. An epidural abscess is unlikely if he has been in good health.

Peripheral Nerves

I. Symptomatology and Definition of Peripheral Nerve Disease

A. **Definition**—peripheral nerves have myelin derived from Schwann cells
  1. All cranial nerves (CNs) (except for CN I and II, which have oligodendrocytes), spinal, sensory, and autonomic nerves
  2. About 95%: congenital, diabetes, renal, or alcohol-nutritional; worldwide, leprosy is most common

B. **Motor signs**
  1. All peripheral nervous system (PNS) disease is associated with atrophy except for three circumstances: pseudohypertrophy, hypertrophy associated with myotonia, and compensatory hypertrophy
     a. Muscle volume normally decreased by no more than 25% to 30%
  2. Weakness is usually hypotonic.
     a. Weakness can develop acutely with compression (Saturday night or crossed leg palsy), penetrating trauma, crush injury, vascular infarction (diabetic femoral neuropathy or ophthalmoplegia), or vasculitis (polyarteritis nodosa)
     b. Subacute (less than one month) Guillain-Barré
     c. Chronic—distal wasting, hereditary or toxic-metabolic

C. **Sensory signs** are either positive or negative
  1. **Positive signs**—aberrant sensation in absence of stimulation; usually seen in acquired neuropathy
     a. Paresthesias are usually acquired
     b. Dysesthesia (normal sensation unpleasant), allodynia (pain from stimuli that are not normally painful), partial nerve injury or during recovery
     c. Burning/hyperesthesia diabetic, alcoholic neuropathy, multiple myeloma
     d. Causalgia—persistent burning pain that radiates distally along nerve trunk; if accompanied by autonomic dysfunction it is reflex sympathetic dystrophy
  2. **Negative signs**—no sensory response from adequate stimulation most common as sole sign in congenital neuropathy
     a. Numbness usually congenital neuropathy, but can be early or only sign of a peripheral neuropathy
     b. Loss of all modalities in distal distribution then gradual return is demyelination
     c. Loss of touch, vibration, proprioception is large fiber loss seen in tabes dorsalis, diabetic neuropathy, Friedreich ataxia
     d. Loss of pain and temperature is small myelinated sensory fiber loss, seen in leprosy and some hereditary sensory neuropathies

D. **Autonomic signs**—usually diabetic or amyloid
   1. Most consistent early abnormality is orthostatic hypotension without pulse change
   2. Diarrhea, heat intolerance, hyperhidrosis in unaffected areas with anhidrosis in affected areas, difficulty voiding, sexual impotence, decreased tearing, papillary abnormalities, retrograde ejaculation can all be seen.

E. **Symptoms**
   1. Decreased or loss of tendon reflexes: except axonal neuropathies; Babinski is not expected and would need to be explained (think of combined system disease. B_{12})
   2. Fasciculations/cramps/spasms/myokymia
   3. Deformity and trophic changes: secondary to uneven atrophy and denervation
   4. About 95% are caused by one of: congenital diabetes, renal, alcohol/nutritional (We will continue to use the VITAMINS mnemonic as is in Chapter 9 because it is useful here.)

II. Vascular Arteritis of Small/Medium-Sized Vessels Causing Neuropathy

A. **Polyarteritis nodosa:** either diffuse, symmetrical due to small nerve infarction or mononeuropathy multiplex: abrupt, pain/numbness followed by sensory loss in any peripheral n. distribution; treatment: steroids/cyclophosphamide for several months if local, methotrexate if systemic; may have no recovery

B. **Nonsystemic vasculitic neuropathy:** isolated necrotizing vasculitis of PN; usually indolent multiple mononeuropathy; treatment: high dose steroids

C. **Sarcoidosis:** subacute/chronic polyneuropathy; asymmetric; can cause facial nerve palsy, muscle lesions, central nervous system (CNS) involvement; myelitic syndrome; cerebrospinal fluid (CSF) increased cells, protein, immunoglobulin (IgG), oligoclonal bands; magnetic resonance imaging (MRI): nodular lesions, enhancement surrounding meninges

D. **Lyme disease**
   1. **Acute phase:** painful radiculitis in dermatome around bite; then cauda equina sign, headache, fever; neuropathy in affected patients 1 to 3 weeks after tick bite
   2. **Disseminated stage:** paresthesias/weakness of limb/buttock, facial palsy
   3. **Late stage:** chronic adrenal polyneuropathy, diagnosis: serologic; treatment: doxycycline or amoxicillin + probenecid (early); ceftriaxone if CNS involved

E. **Sjögren-sicca syndrome:** sensory polyneuropathy; prior to keratoconjunctivitis and sicca; diffuse sensory loss including trunk; decreased kinesthetic sense (movement on skin); limb/gait ataxia; autonomic nervous system (ANS) dysfunction; diagnosis: anti-nuclear antibody; monoclonal immunoglobulin; treatment: symptomatic; steroids/cyclophosphamide if vascular/renal/pulmonary involvement

F. **Migrant sensory neuritis of Wartenberg:** searing/pulling sensation of small area of limb upon extension, residual numb patch; resolves over weeks/months; episodic over many years

III. Inflammatory/Infectious

A. **Guillain-Barré syndrome (acute inflammatory polyneuropathy):** no age/sex predominates; nonseasonal; nonepidemic; associated with *Campylobacter jejuni*; mild respiratory or gastrointestinal infection 1 to 3 weeks prior; symmetrical ascending paresthesias, weakness over days to 2 weeks, afebrile; decreased ankle reflexes; CSF: acellular, protein increase at 4 to 6 weeks; nerve conduction studies (NCS): decreased CMAP amplitude, conduction velocity (but may be normal);

treatment: ADMIT to observe for respiratory decline or autonomic (cardiac) disturbance; follow pulmonary function tests (PFTs) every 3 to 4 hours to evaluate inspiratory force and expiratory vital capacity (VC) (better assessment than dyspnea/arterial blood gases [ABG]); intensive care unit (ICU) if VC decreased to 20 mL/kg endotracheal tube (ET) intubation if VC decreased to 15 mL/kg; intravenous (IV) immune globulin for 5 days or plasma exchange (within 2 weeks for maximum effect; institute once walk or breathing is effected); prognosis: 3% to 5% mortality from cardiac/respiratory arrest; most recover completely; do not use steroids
   1. **Acute axonal form of Guillain-Barré syndrome:** clinically similar but with muscle atrophy in early stage; prolonged recovery/poor resolution

B. **Churg-Strauss and hypereosinophilia:** granulomatous disease with diffuse subcutaneous nodules, eosinophilia, asthma; neuropathy with fever/weight loss, acute painful mononeuritis multiplex; diagnosis: cytoplasmic antineutrophil cytoplasmic antibody (c-ANCA)

C. **Idiopathic eosinophilic syndrome:** eosinophilia with infiltration of organ systems; painful sensorimotor neuropathy or mononeuritis multiplex; treatment: high dose corticosteroids or immunosuppressive medications for refractory

D. **Wegener:** similar polyneuropathy to Churg-Strauss but cranial nerve involvement usually prominent

E. **Diphtheric polyneuropathy:** local, acute effects of diphtheria first; 5 to 8 weeks later: progressive limb weakness/paresthesias, distal loss vibratory/position sense; CSF: increased protein; treatment: diphtheria antitoxin (must be given within 48 hours of infection); respiratory support if progresses; prognosis: full recovery if respiratory supported

F. **Chronic inflammatory demyelinating polyradiculopathy:** widespread polyradiculopathy with an insidious relapsing course and enlarged nerves somewhat similar to Guillain Barré syndrome; a key difference is the responsiveness to steroids
   1. **Multifocal motor neuropathy:** multiple focal sites of motor block without sensory involvement, high likelihood of anti-GM1
   2. **Multifocal conduction block:** block of sensory and motor nerves at a single site.
   3. **Treatment:** intravenous immunoglobulin (IVIG) or plasmapheresis, steroids second line—most needing regular treatment every 4–24 weeks

G. **Leprous polyneuritis:** *Mycobacterium leprae* infection; painless skin lesion from cutaneous nerve invasion; may evolve to epithelial granulomas or widespread organ involvement (lepromatous leprosy) with symmetrical pain/temperature loss over body; eventual motor loss; treatment: dapsone, rifampin, and clofazimine

IV. Trauma

The main thing to know here is Sneddon and Sunderland classification of nerve injuries (Tables 10-1, 10-2). Plexopathies when they occur are commonly traumatic occurrences.

A. **Brachial plexus neuropathies:** unilateral; two to trauma/compression injury/idiopathic; presentation based on location; diagnosis: electromyogram (EMG); MRI to localize lesion
   1. **Infraclavicular lesions of vessels:** presentation based on location; cause: hematoma from small puncture wound; humeral trauma
   2. **Disease:** (neuralgic amyotrophy, brachial neuritis, Parsonage-Turner syndrome): abrupt onset, healthy individual, or postinfection/vaccine/surgery/heroin/childbirth; minor ache in neck/shoulder; rapid increasing pain 3 to 10 days; weakness/sensory impairment arm/shoulder muscles; possible paralysis; no fever/leukocytosis; recover usually 6 to 12 weeks with return to baseline
   3. **Brachial neuropathy after radiation therapy:** usually for breast cancer; weakness/sensory loss in hand/fingers up to 3 years after radiation

Table 10-1 Sneddon Classification

	Type of injury	Affect on nerve	Recovery
Neurapraxia	Mild	No wallerian degeneration	Within months
Axonotmesis	Crush	Axon/myelin sheaths broken Wallerian degeneration	Depends on axonal regrowth
Neurotmesis	Transection	Nerve severed	Surgery needed

Table 10-2 Sunderland Classification

Classification	Pathology	Prognosis
1st	Demyelination or ischemia Normal EMG/NCV	Excellent
2nd	Axonal loss, EMG/NCV show denervation	Good depends on distance
3rd	Endoneurial tube disruption fibrillations	Moderate
4th	Perineurium disrupted	Poor without surgery
5th	Epineurium severed	None without surgery

EMG, electromyogram; NCV, nerve conduction velocity.

B. **Brachial mononeuropathies**
   1. **Causalgia**—post trauma; severe, persistent burning pain; increases with heat/cold/noise, trophic changes to skin, treatment: short-term pain relief with prolonged cooling or guanethidine injection

C. **Lumbosacral plexus:** unilateral weakness/sensory loss; decreased reflexes; pain with straight leg raising (Lasègue sign) or hip movement; common causes: abdominal/pelvic surgery, childbirth, aortic aneurysm, tumors
   1. **Lumbosacral plexitis**: similar to brachial; treatment: immunosuppressive drugs

V. Autoimmune

A. **Rheumatoid arthritis (RA):** patients with severe RA >10 years have pressure neuropathies secondary to thickened tendons/joint changes; some get ischemic necrosis/demyelination; seropositive for rheumatoid factor

B. **Lupus:** usually advanced stages, symmetrical/progressive, sensorimotor paralysis in feet/legs spread to arms over several days/weeks; also progressive or relapsing forms; peripheral nervous involvement less common than CNS involvement

C. **Cryoglobulinemia:** IgM or IgG agglutinin disease may have associated peripheral neuropathy; distal, symmetrical pain/paresthesias leading to weakness/wasting; insidious development; may have Raynaud; treatment: corticosteroids, chlorambucil, cyclophosphamide, plasma exchange (improve symptoms but recovery incomplete)

VI. Metabolic

A. **Inherited sensory polyneuropathies**
   1. **Mutilating sensory neuropathies:** present as insensitivity to pain, eventual foot/hand abrasions to chronic ulcers; autosomal dominant (AD) variant: onset in teens, pain/

sensory loss in feet: calluses/ulcers, osteomyelitis, decreased reflexes; autosomal recessive (AR) variant: onset in infancy, delayed walking, toe/finger ulcerations, sensation loss limbs/trunk; no reflexes; treatment: prevention of stress fractures/infection
2. **Also:** Friedreich ataxia, Riley-Day

B. **Inherited mixed polyneuropathies**
   1. **Peroneal muscular atrophy (Charcot-Marie-Tooth [CMT]):** chronic degeneration peripheral nerves feet/legs; eventual weakness/atrophy; sensory ataxia; painful; "stork like" appearance; CSF: normal; treatment: none; stabilization of ankles/legs
      a. CMT1A autosomal dominant 17p11.2 affects PMP22, onset first or second decade with absent reflexes, legs involved before hands, nerve conduction studies: prolonged
      b. CMT1B autosomal dominant 1q21 affects Po protein, same symptoms as CMT1A
      c. CMT2 autosomal dominant 1p35p36; onset second decade with leg > hand weakness if autosomal recessive onset in infancy with severe global peripheral weakness, wheelchair bound by the second decade
   2. **Hypertrophic neuropathy of infancy (Dejerine-Sottas disease):** onset infancy; delayed/impaired walking; pain/paresthesias feet; symmetrical weakness/atrophy limbs; enlarged ulnar, median, radial, personal nerves visible through skin; treatment: none; wheelchair bound at young age
   3. **Hereditary areflexic dystasia (Roussy-Lévy syndrome):** onset infancy; benign course; sensory ataxia/areflexia in lower legs/hands; atrophy; EMG: denervation
   4. **Chronic polyneuropathy with hereditary spastic paraplegia:** children with slowly progressive spastic paraplegia; atrophic legs

C. **Inherited polyneuropathies** with metabolic disorders
   1. **Refsum disease:** onset late childhood/teens; triad of retinitis pigmentosa, cerebellar ataxia, chronic polyneuropathy (symmetrical, distal, sensorimotor, legs > arms, no reflexes); diagnosis: ⇑ phytanic acid in serum and urine; CSF: ⇑ protein; infantile variant presents with failure to thrive/mental retardation/diarrhea
   2. **Metachromatic leukodystrophy:** cerebral deterioration, hyporeflexia, atrophy
   3. **Anderson-Fabry:** onset childhood; pain/paresthesias fingers/toes; treatment: nonspecific; phenytoin, carbamazepine
   4. **Others (rare):** abetalipoproteinemia, Tangier disease

D. **Amyloid neuropathies:** peripheral neuropathy common manifestation amyloidosis
   1. **Familial type**—AD; "Portuguese Type" onset 25 to 35 years, slowly progressive; numbness/paresthesias/pain feet/legs; ANS dysfunction; fatal; treatment: liver transplant; note: other familial variants affect specific peripheral nerves
   2. **Primary amyloid neuropathy**—amyloid deposits in organs, some have sensory peripheral neuropathy; numbness/paresthesias/pain then weakness feet/then hands/arms; ANS dysfunction; rapid progression (mean survival 1 to 2 years); diagnosis: paraprotein in serum/urine, amyloid on nerve biopsy; treatment: none, poor prognosis

E. **Acute uremic polyneuropathy**—end-stage renal disease (ESRD) patients; generalized weakness and distal paresthesias over few weeks until bedridden; treatment: transplant
   1. **Chronic uremic polyneuropathy:** painless, progressive, symmetrical sensorimotor paralysis of limbs; evolves over months; in patients with chronic renal failure (CRF); peritoneal dialysis better than hemodialysis (HD) for improvement; recovery after renal transplant

F. **Porphyric polyneuropathy**—Severe, rapidly advancing, symmetrical polyneuropathy; associated with abdominal pain, psychosis, convulsions; occurs during porphyria attacks; diagnosis: urine increased production/excretion porphobilinogen and δ-aminolevulinic acid (δ-AVA); treatment: may regress on own, or respiratory support, IV glucose (suppress heme biosynthesis), pyridoxine; prevention (avoid porphyrinogenic drugs: sulfa, estrogens, barbiturates, phenytoin, anticonvulsants)

VII. Iatrogenic Mainly Drugs

A. **Isoniazid (INH):** 3 to 35 weeks posttreatment; symmetrical numbness toes/feet; may spread upward; decreased tendon reflexes; treatment: pyridoxine with INH (disulfiram: similar to INH in presentation)

B. **Antineoplastic drugs—vincristine:** paresthesias to fingers/wrists then spreads proximally; dose related; cisplatin/Taxol: sensory neuropathy weeks after treatment completion; impaired proprioception/vibratory sense, color change fingertips/toes

C. **Antimicrobials:** include metronidazole, chloramphenicol, dapsone, stilbamidine, nitrofurantoin, trichloroethylene

D. **Amiodarone:** motor sensory neuropathy in 5%

E. **Also:** phenytoin, colchicines, clioquinol, thalidomide, tryptophan

F. **Also HIV drugs** (if drugs begins with "d," may cause neuropathy)

VIII. Neoplastic

A. **Paraneoplastic:** distal, symmetrical sensory polyneuropathy, weakness/atrophy, ataxia, sensory loss; over several weeks/months; may occur before tumor appearance; with cancer, lymphoma, multiple myeloma; also multiple polyneuropathies with non-Hodgkin; CSF: increased protein, acellular, anti-Hu antibody; treatment: corticosteroids may help; poor prognosis; recovery parallels tumor recovery

B. **Paraproteinemia neuropathy:** occurs in multiple myeloma, POEMS syndrome (polyneuropathy, organomegaly, endocrinopathy, ⇑ M-protein, skin pigmentation),

C. **Monoclonal gammopathy of undetermined significance:** paraproteinemia with no multiple myeloma (MM) or malignancy; 50 to 60s, insidious onset numbness/paresthesias feet/hands, then symmetrical wasting; slowly progressive; some have Raynaud or action tremor; CSF: increased protein; treatment: plasma exchange as in GBS; if myelin associated glycoprotein antibody present include immunosuppression or cyclophosphamide

D. **Macroglobulinemia:** elderly; subacute or chronic fatigue/weakness, bleeding diathesis; hyperviscosity/slowed cerebral circulation causing confusion/strokes; ⇑ IgM; CSF ⇑ protein, globulin fraction

IX. Systemic—Normally Subacute Sensorimotor Paralysis (Symmetrical)

A. **Nutritional deficiency:** lack of thiamine/pyridoxine/pantothenic acid/folic acid; usually associated with alcoholism in Western countries

B. **Arsenical polyneuropathy:** painful; acute: 1 to 3 weeks after ingestion; resemble GBS; chronic present as nutritional polymyopathy but may be focal

C. **Lead neuropathy:** adults with impaired motor upper extremities (usually radial nerve, wrist drop); diagnosis:, anemia, basophilic stippling, lead line in gingiva, constipation, lead levels >70 µg/dL, history of exposure; treatment: penicillamine, end exposure (kids get encephalopathy, not neuropathy)

D. **Diabetic** subacute asymmetrical and multifocal polyneuropathy:
   1. Acute diabetic mononeuropathy: most common is ophthalmoplegia (CN III), also femoral and sciatic; secondary to infarction of nerve; recovery possible but many months
   2. Multiple mononeuropathy and radiculopathy: older patients, acute painful, asymmetrical, usually low back spreading down leg/knee; deep ache; worse at night; eventual atrophy/sphincter involvement; recovery months to year; may recur on opposite side
   3. Distal polyneuropathy: symmetrical sensory loss; numbness/tingling stocking distribution; ⇓ ankle/patellar; may cause ulcers/neuropathic joints; diabetic pseudotabes: sensory loss/ataxia/bladder atony
   4. Autonomic neuropathy: includes papillary/lacrimal dysfunction; sweating; nocturnal diarrhea; gastrointestinal/bladder atonicity; impotence; orthostatics; treatment: prevention with glucose control; antidepressants/neurontin may be used to treat

E. Elderly: "burning feet of elderly" chronic benign polyneuropathy; slowly progressive burning/numbness feet to calves; treatment: poor success; antidepressants, capsaicin cream

X. What is the Role of Neurophysiologic Testing in PNS disease?

A. Localize diffuse/unclear disease, help identify plexopathy

B. Give likelihood of differing possibilities of differential diagnosis

C. Confirm a tentative diagnosis

D. Classify nerve injury

E. Muscle biopsy is typically reserved for myositis

F. For further details, see Chapter 4

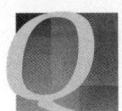# STUDY QUESTIONS FOR CHAPTER 10

Directions: *Each of the numbered items or incomplete statements in this section is followed by answers or by completions of the statement. Select the ONE lettered answer or completion that is BEST in each case.*

1. A 32-year-old man is admitted in January to the neurology service with 2 weeks of lower back pain, paresthesias, and weakness that has progressed from his lower extremities to now involving his hands. On examination he has a temperature to 101°C, flaccid weakness in the lower extremities, mild weakness in his small hand muscles, and absent reflexes. His CSF shows 0 white blood cells (WBCs)/mm^3, 28 protein mg/dL, and 67 mg/dL glucose. Which of the features of his presentation is atypical for Guillain-Barré syndrome?

(A) Onset of symptoms in the winter months
(B) Low-back pain
(C) Fever
(D) Absent reflexes
(E) Normal CSF protein

2. An otherwise healthy 39-year-old woman is admitted to the hospital with rapidly progressive polyneuropathy. She has a history of several unexplained attacks of severe abdominal pain in the last several years. While in the hospital, she has a generalized-tonic-clonic seizure. What is the most likely diagnosis?

(A) Acute uremic polyneuropathy
(B) Diphtheric polyneuropathy
(C) Porphyric polyneuropathy
(D) Arsenic polyneuropathy
(E) Lead neuropathy

3. A 56-year-old man is referred by his rheumatologist for a chronic polyneuropathy with bilateral facial palsy. Which of the following is the most likely diagnosis?

(A) Polyarteritis nodosa
(B) Churg-Strauss syndrome
(C) Wegener granulomatosis
(D) Systemic lupus erythematosus
(E) Sarcoidosis

4. A 7-year-old boy is brought to your office for falls, clumsiness, and difficulty walking. On examination, you find retinitis pigmentosa and signs of a distal, sensorimotor polyneuropathy with absent reflexes. Which is the most likely diagnosis?

(A) Refsum disease
(B) Metachromatic leukodystrophy
(C) Fabry disease
(D) Abetalipoproteinemia
(E) Tangier disease

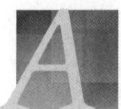

ANSWERS AND EXPLANATIONS

1. C. Fever is not a typical feature of Guillain-Barré syndrome (GBS). There is no seasonal predilection for development of this condition. Patients with GBS often have low back pain. Absent reflexes are the rule for a patient with GBS. CSF protein may be normal at 2 weeks into the disease course; the protein is typically elevated at 4 to 6 weeks.

2. C. A rapidly progressive polyneuropathy associated with unexplained attacks of abdominal pain and seizures is most consisted with polyneuropathy. Patients with acute uremic polyneuropathy should have other signs of uremia. Diphtheric polyneuropathy is typically a descending process preceded by an upper respiratory infection and is not associated with seizures. Arsenic and lead neuropathies are not associated with seizures.

3. E. Of the choices listed, sarcoidosis is the one that most often produces a polyneuropathy and bilateral facial palsy.

4. A. Although all the choices can produce a polyneuropathy, only Refsum disease is associated with retinitis pigmentosa.

CHAPTER 11

Demyelination

I. Basics of Myelin

Proteolipids form the insulation of axons; produced by oligodendrocytes in central nervous system (CNS) and Schwann cells in peripheral nervous system (PNS); loss of myelin results in slowed conduction velocity and conduction block; sometimes imaging is helpful in differentiating different etiologies of demyelination (Table 11-1)

II. Multiple Sclerosis

A. **Pathogenesis**
   1. Chronic recurrent autoimmune inflammatory disorder of the CNS with genetic and environmental factors; not peripheral nervous system
   2. T lymphocytes react against myelin (molecular mimicry)
   3. Decreased suppressor T lymphocyte activity
   4. Injury to the CNS myelin sheaths > oligodendrocytes >> axons and nerve cells
   5. Plaques of demyelination and inflammation lead to sclerotic glial scars

B. **Epidemiology**: prevalence is 0.1%; female to male ratio is 2:1; incidence rises until age 35 and then declines; first degree relative greater than 3% to 5% lifetime risk; prevalence of multiple sclerosis increases with distance from the equator; if migration before age 15 years, the risk is that of the new area

C. **Most common presenting symptoms of MS include:** sensory disturbances, cranial nerve dysfunction, bilateral INO due to MLF involvement, pyramidal tract dysfunction, autonomic dysfunction, cerebellar dysfunction, and cognitive/psychiatric disturbance; other symptoms/signs include Lhermitte sign (electric sensation running down the back with passive neck flexion), Uhthoff phenomenon (worsening of symptoms in warm environment), and fatigue

D. **Diagnosis:** to rule in for definite multiple sclerosis, use McDonald criteria
   1. **Clinical evidence**
      a. Two or more deficits separated by neuroanatomic space and time
      b. Includes symptoms referable to the optic nerves and spinal cord
   2. **MRI evidence:** white matter lesions on T2 and FLAIR with prominent periventricular distribution; acute plaques often enhance with paramagnetic contrast (gadolinium)
   3. **Electrophysiologic evidence:** slowed conduction velocities on somatosensory evoked potential (SSEP) and visual evoked potential (VEP); SSEP, usually testing the posterior tibial nerves due to length; VEP, sensitive for silent optic nerve demyelination; brainstem auditory evoked potential (BAER or BAEP) for brain stem lesion

Table 11-1	MRI of Demyelination
MS	T2 white matter hyperintensities highly variable in character. Most frequently located in periventricular white, internal capsule, corpus callosum, and pons. Linear or ovoid lesions perpendicular to the lateral ventricle are classic. Called Dawson fingers. Lesions often enhance if active disease.
Optic neuritis	Suggest asking for T2 fast spin echo with fat suppression and FLAIR with short inversion times. T1 hyperintensity, some signs may be helpful, like tram track enhancement (can be normal variant, sarcoid, other things as well). Nerve can show eccentric enlargement, which would help distinguish MS from meningioma, glioma.
Transverse myelitis	Relatively easy to differentiate from the others with T1 hypointensity and T2 hyperintensity. Cord can show enlargement. With contrast, there can be nodular or patchy areas of enhancement.
ADEM	Looks almost identical to MS, can have large lesions without mass effect. Lesions can enhance but do not have to.
Central pontine myelinolysis	Central pontine T2 hyperintensity with rim of normal appearing parenchyma. Except in extreme cases, will spare the corticospinal tracts. Can have enhancement along periphery. Also does not have to be in the pons.
PML	Ill-defined hyperintensities in the subcortical white matter, most often parietal. Can cause mass effect. Usually does not enhance; about 10% will have faint peripheral enhancement. About one half of patients will have some gray matter involvement.

ADEM, acute disseminated encephalomyelitis; MS, multiple sclerosis; PML, progressive multifocal leukoencephalopathy.

   4. **Cerebral spinal fluid (CSF) evidence:** presence of oligoclonal bands (sensitivity of 85% but poor specificity) and myelin basic protein; elevated immunoglobulin G (IgG) index, synthesis rate (most specific test)—needs serum for IgG and albumin; mononuclear pleocytosis (<50 cells)
   5. **Rule-out diagnoses include:** lupus, vasculitis, vitamin B_{12} deficiency, neurosyphilis, human T-cell lymphoma/leukemia virus (HTLV)–associated myelopathy, neurosarcoidosis, Lyme disease, metachromatic leukodystrophy, adult-onset white matter degenerative disorders, conversion reaction

E. Clinical types of multiple sclerosis
   1. **Relapsing-remitting multiple sclerosis** (RRMS): self-limited attacks over days to weeks, followed by variable recovery over several weeks to months; patient stable between attacks
   2. **Secondary progressive multiple sclerosis** (SPMS): begins as RRMS, but at some point there is progressive loss of neurologic function and fewer individual attacks
   3. **Primary progressive multiple sclerosis** (PPMS): progressive function from onset without acute attacks
   4. **Progressive-relapsing multiple sclerosis** (PRMS): progressive loss of neurologic function from onset with occasional acute attacks
   5. **Clinically isolated syndromes:** optic neuritis, transverse myelitis, bilateral INO. If MRI positive, then high risk of MS, if negative, low risk.

F. Treatment of acute exacerbations
   1. **Glucocorticoids:** speed functional recovery from acute attacks, no evidence that they affect the long-term functional recovery methylprednisolone/Solu-Medrol 1,000 mg per day (can be divided b.i.d.) for 3 to 5 days with or without a prednisone taper over next 7 to 10 days
   2. **Plasmapheresis:** can be tried if unresponsive to high-dose steroids

G. Prevention of multiple sclerosis attacks
   1. Interferon β-1a (Avonex) intramuscularly once per week or Rebif 44 μg subcutaneously thrice per week (tapered up from 8.8); Rebif significantly worse side effect profile, but relative risk (RR) of relapse 37% lower at 6 months; interferon β-1b (Betaseron) given subcutaneously once every other day

a. Side effects include injection site reactions, flulike symptoms, mild liver enzyme elevation, lymphopenia, and depression
   b. Interferon β-1b > interferon β-1a, possible development of neutralizing antibodies to interferon β; possibly better than Avonex (level of evidence 2b)
  3. Glatiramer acetate (Copaxone) given subcutaneously once per day
  4. Each reduces attack rate, disease severity by magnetic resonance imaging (MRI), slow sustained disability
  5. Natalizumab (Tysabri)—new medication, high risk of PML when used in combination with avonex, monoclonal antibody given 300 mg IV every 4 weeks; registry for use

H. **Prevention of multiple sclerosis progression**
  1. Very limited evidence in support of interferon β, glatiramer acetate, in progression prevention
  2. Methotrexate, azathioprine, cyclosporine, mitoxantrone for progressive multiple sclerosis, but there are no large studies confirming effectiveness of treatment; mitoxantrone for tumefactive multiple sclerosis but is limited by cardiomyopathy: an echo should be checked every 6 months

III. Multiple Sclerosis Variants

A. **Neuromyelitis optica (NMO)/Devic disease:** optic neuritis + transverse myelitis
  1. Possibly a distinct disease that is rare in United States
  2. Monophasic or polyphasic, often fulminant
  3. Seen in association with multiple sclerosis, acute disseminated encephalomyelitis (ADEM), lupus, Sjögren, and postinfectious (usually in children) after Epstein-Barr virus (EBV), varicella, HIV, and tuberculosis
  4. CSF shows increased protein, pleocytosis, and less commonly oligoclonal bands (OCBs)

B. **Marburg/tumefactive:** rapidly progressive disease that can present like a mass lesion/tumor; can be distinguished from a tumor by MR spectroscopy or biopsy

C. **Schilder:** fulminant disease seen in children

D. **Concentric sclerosis of Balo:** seen in children, characterized pathologically by concentric rings of demyelination

E. **Isolated syndromes:** optic neuritis, transverse myelitis, brainstem bilateral internuclear ophthalmoplegia (INO)

IV. Optic Neuritis

A. Inflammatory demyelinating disorder of the optic nerve

B. Mean age of onset is in the 30s, onset after age 45 is rare; 2:1 female-to-male ratio

C. Eye pain with movement; onset is acute or slowly progressive over days to weeks

D. Monocular visual problems include: monocular central scotoma, decreased visual acuity, impaired color vision (detected by testing for red desaturation). Loss of color vision is most sensitive and long-lasting effect of ON.

E. Exam of pupils reveals ipsilateral relative afferent pupillary defect (RAPD)—dilation of affected pupil on swinging flashlight test

F. Funduscopic examination reveals swollen optic disc (papillitis) if bulbar; normal optic disc if retrobulbar; optic disc pallor suggests prior episodes. Retrobulbar neuritis: patient sees little;

clinician sees little on examination. Optic papillitis: patient sees little but clinician sees much on examination.

G. VEPs: measure the responses of the visual cortex to pattern-reversal visual stimuli (normal positive [P] wave latency is 100 msec = P100)
   1. Very sensitive (nearly 100%), but not specific, test for optic neuritis
   2. Prolonged latency with preserved amplitude consistent with *prior* demyelination
   3. Reduced/lost P100 amplitude is consistent with *acute* optic neuritis
   4. Abnormal in 70% to 80% with multiple sclerosis with no history of optic neuritis or visual symptoms

H. Differential diagnosis of monocular visual loss includes optic neuritis, optic disease (major refractive error, lens and media opacities, glaucoma, and retinopathies), ischemic lesion of the optic nerve (anterior ischemic optic neuropathy), neoplasm (meningioma, optic glioma, lymphoma, and metastasis), and inflammatory process (sarcoidosis and Lyme disease); therefore, requires additional work-up
   1. MRI of the brain with or without gadolinium to rule out an infiltrative or compressive lesion of the optic nerve and as part of the evaluation for multiple sclerosis
   2. Lumbar puncture is indicated as part of the evaluation for multiple sclerosis
   3. Atypical features include age older than 45 years, no eye pain, bilateral symptoms, and lack of recovery, and warrant further work-up with erythrocyte sedimentation rate (ESR), Lyme titer, syphilis serologies, EBV, HIV, B_{12}, folate, and antinuclear antibody (ANA).

I. Treated with high-dose steroids as in multiple sclerosis flare

J. Prognosis: near complete recovery common by 6 to 8 weeks; some permanent visual loss possible; 33% relapse rate; 50% with isolated optic neuritis develop multiple sclerosis

V. Transverse Myelitis

A. Epidemiology and presentation
   1. Focal inflammatory disorder of the spinal cord
   2. Incidence is 1 to 4 million people per year; no sex or familial predisposition
   3. Individuals of all ages are affected, bimodal peaks: ages 10 to 19 years and 30 to 39 years
   4. Characterized by acutely or subacutely (4 hours to 21 days) evolving symptoms and signs of neurologic dysfunction in motor, sensory, and autonomic nerves and nerve tracts referable to the spinal cord; symptoms are almost always bilateral, but asymmetric
   5. Often a clear rostral border of sensory dysfunction

B. **Differential diagnosis of acute noncompressive myelopathy:** multiple sclerosis related, systemic disease (e.g., systemic lupus erythematosus [SLE], anti-phospholipid syndrome, Sjögren disease), parainfectious (enteroviruses, herpes simplex virus [HSV], varicella-zoster virus [VZV], EBV, cytomegalovirus [CMV], HIV, and HTLV-I), delayed radiation myelopathy, spinal cord infarct, and idiopathic myelopathy

C. **Spinal MRI** often shows evidence of acute inflammation
   1. Increased cord signal on T2 and FLAIR; gadolinium enhancement of acute lesions
   2. *Must* exclude an extraaxial compressive lesion

D. **CSF analysis** often shows evidence of acute inflammation with pleocytosis and elevated IgG index

E. **Treatment** is generally high-dose steroids

F. **Prognosis:** one third recover with little or no sequelae, one third are left with moderate permanent disability, one third have severe disabilities; rapid progression of symptoms, back pain, and spinal shock predict poor recovery
   1. Can be the presenting feature of multiple sclerosis; when associated with multiple sclerosis, symptoms are more likely asymmetric with predominantly sensory symptoms, lesions extend over fewer than two spinal segments, brain MRI is abnormal, and OCBs are present in the CSF
   2. If brain MRI is consistent with demyelinating lesions, 83% chance of multiple sclerosis over the next 10 years; if brain MRI is normal, 11% chance of MS over the next 10 years

VI. Acute Disseminated Encephalomyelitis (ADEM)

A. **Monophasic inflammatory demyelinating disorder** usually children by 6 weeks of infection or immunization caused by autoreactive T lymphocytes reacting against MBP, characterized by rapid development of multifocal or focal neurologic deficits

B. **CSF findings** can look just like those for multiple sclerosis; distinguished from multiple sclerosis by multifocal involvement at onset; focal neurologic symptoms are often associated with encephalopathy, stupor, coma, meningismus, seizures, and persistence of OCBs in CSF

C. **Treated** with high-dose steroids, plasmapheresis, or intravenous immunoglobulin (IVIG)

VII. Central Pontine Myelinolysis (CPM)

A. **Symmetrical noninflammatory demyelination** in the base of the pons +/−extrapontine sites caused by rapid correction of hyponatremia (>12 mEq/L/day)

B. **Classic presentation of CPM** is pseudobulbar palsy and spastic quadriparesis

C. **Correction of chronic hyponatremia** is more likely to produce neurologic injury than is correction of acute hyponatremia

VIII. Progressive Multifocal Leukoencephalopathy (PML)

A. **Subacute progressive demyelinating disease** of the CNS that most commonly occurs in people with AIDS with CD4 count usually <100, but can occur posttransplantation

B. **Usually presents** with headache, visual field deficit, subacute onset of focal neurologic deficits, and seizures

C. **Solitary or multiple nonenhancing white matter lesions** on imaging; lesions most often in parietooccipital region

D. **CSF polymerase chain reaction** (PCR) for JC virus is sensitive (74% to 92%) and specific (92% to 96%)

E. **No effective treatments**; average life expectancy is usually months; however, can spontaneously remit, so regard treatment results with a jaundiced eye.

IX. Hereditary Disorders

A. Alexander disease: cytoskeletal disorder caused by mutation in *GFAP* gene with megalencephaly, seizures, developmental deficits, and spasticity
  1. **Histology:** Rosenthal fibers and demyelination predominantly in the frontal lobes

B. Canavan disease: autosomal recessive with macrocephaly, seizures, severe developmental deficits, spasticity, optic atrophy; histology diffuse spongiform white matter lesions

C. Krabbe's globoid cell leukodystrophy: lysosomal disorder due to galactocerebrosidase deficiency, which presents at 3 to 6 months with seizures, irritability, spasticity, and fever and progresses to blind decerebrate vegetative state

D. Metachromatic leukodystrophy: autosomal recessive lysosomal disorder due to sulfatase A deficiency, onset usually during infancy or early childhood with cognitive and neurologic cumulative deficits due to demyelination of CNS and PNS

E. Adrenoleukodystrophy: X-linked recessive peroxisomal disorder causing demyelination and adrenal cortex dysfunction; very long chain fatty acids accumulate; also an autosomal recessive form
  1. Usually presents in children with cognitive dysfunction, then cumulative neurologic deficits, death; in adults, presents in third decade with spasticity and spinal cord dysfunction
  2. Bone marrow replacement may prevent progression of disease

F. Pelizaeus-Merzbacher disease: X-linked recessive disorder, presents in infancy with nystagmus, involuntary head movements, progresses to ataxia, spasticity, and choreoathetoid movements

DEMYELINATING DISEASES OF THE PERIPHERAL NERVOUS SYSTEM

X. Guillain-Barré Syndrome—Acute Inflammatory Demyelinating Polyneuropathy

Subtypes include: acute inflammatory dysmyelinating polyradiculoneuropathy (AIDP), acute inflammatory axonal polyradiculopathy (AIAP), acute motor axonal neuropathy (AMAN), and acute motor-sensory axonal neuropathy (AMSAN)

A. Pathogenesis and pathophysiology
  1. Autoimmune disease (activated T lymphocytes) involving peripheral nerve myelin; the myelin sheath is the specific target structure (motor and autonomic nerves more likely involved than sensory)
  2. Multifocal lesions consisting of discrete areas containing inflammatory cells (lymphocytes and macrophages) and demyelination throughout the PNS
  3. Predilection for nerve roots and distal peripheral nerve fibers

B. Epidemiology: 1 to 2 cases per 100,000 population; most common cause of acute flaccid paralysis; West Nile virus may present with this
  1. Occurs worldwide, affects all races and all ages; males more than females
  2. Most cases are sporadic; the acute axonal form occurs principally in epidemics, during the summer months, and typically affects children and young adults

C. Risk factors: two thirds have preceding illness (influenza, HSV, CMV, EBV, hepatitis, HIV, *Campylobacter jejuni*, *Mycoplasma pneumoniae*, spirochetal, *Borrelia burgdorferi*), vaccination (rabies and vaccinia), or surgery 1 week to 1 month before onset.

D. **Clinical features**
   1. *Cardinal features*: weakness, paresthesias, diminished or absent muscle stretch reflexes, begins in feet and legs
   2. Flaccid (decreased tone) weakness varies in severity and distribution.
   3. Often involves all four extremities, the respiratory muscles, and cranial nerves.
   4. 30% require mechanical ventilation
   5. Deep pain is commonly present in the shoulder girdle, back, and posterior thighs.
   6. Associated with syndrome of inappropriate antidiuretic hormone (SIADH) and hyponatremia
   7. Autonomics with cardiac arrhythmias

E. **Physical examination** reveals symmetric weakness, decreased tone, minimal loss of sensation, diminished or absent reflexes
   1. **Autonomic dysfunction (50%):** cardiac dysrhythmias, orthostatic hypotension, hypertension, paralytic ileus, bladder dysfunction, abnormal sweating

F. **Diagnosis**
   1. **CSF albuminocytologic dissociation:** elevated protein (may be normal early in the course) and few cells (generally $<20/\mu L$) with normal pressure
   2. **Electrophysiologic testing:** slowing of nerve conduction velocity, conduction block, and temporal dispersion (suggestive of demyelination), and prolonged or absent F-waves (suggestive of proximal segment dysfunction); may be normal in early phase

G. **Differential diagnosis** of acute flaccid paralysis (Table 11-2)

H. **Treatment**
   1. Indications for admission to the intensive care unit (ICU) include rapid progression less than 7 days, inability to raise head against gravity, bulbar dysfunction, bilateral facial weakness, significant autonomic dysfunction, aspiration
   2. Indications for mechanical ventilation (20, 30, 40 rule): Vital capacity <20 mL/kg, maximum inspiratory pressure <30 cm H_2O, or maximum expiratory pressure <40 cm H_2O
   3. IVIG 2 g/kg, given 0.4 g/kg per day for 5 days; simpler to administer, costs less than plasmapheresis, less complications than plasmapheresis; risk of acquiring viral infections because it is made from plasma pooled from thousands of donors; contraindicated for IgA deficiency due to anaphylaxis; produces hyperviscous state and associated with stroke; can cause aseptic meningitis, headaches, neutropenia, anemia, pseudohyponatremia, and renal failure
   4. Plasmapheresis—two plasma volume exchanges on days 1, 3, 5, 7 ± 9 (150 to 250 mL/kg over 4 to 5 treatments); plasma is replaced with albumin; fresh frozen plasma (FFP) is given

Table 11-2 *Differential Diagnosis of Acute Flaccid Paralysis*

- Brainstem infarction (locked-in)
- Acute myelopathies
- Poliomyelitis
- Rabies
- Diphtheria
- Enteroviruses
- Transverse myelitis
- Cord compression
- Peripheral neuropathies
- Heavy metals: arsenic, thallium, Ag, Pb
- Alcohol
- Organophosphates
- Conversion reaction or malingering
- Acute intermittent porphyria
- Hexacarbons
- Drugs including steroids
- Lyme disease
- Critical illness
- Vasculitis
- Neuromuscular disorders
- Botulism
- Tick bite paralysis
- Myasthenia gravis
- Snake or sea urchin venom
- Hyper- or hypokalemia
- Hypermagnesemia
- Muscle disorders
- Hypophosphatemia

if there are bleeding complications; results: less mechanical ventilation required; decreased ICU and hospitalization time; risks: infection from central line and coagulopathy
- **a.** The effects of plasmapheresis and IVIG are thought to be equivalent; sequential treatment with plasmapheresis followed by IVIG is not recommended.
- **b.** Corticosteroids not recommended for GBS; they may worsen the condition.
5. Do not forget to prevent complications including: fatal arrhythmia, cardiovascular collapse, aspiration, atelectasis, gastric and skin ulcers, deep venous thrombosis (DVT), urinary tract infection (UTI); treat aggressively with physical therapy (PT), occupational therapy (OT), and speech therapy (SP), antidepressants, and analgesics when indicated.

I. **Prognosis:** The majority (70% to 75%) of patients will recover completely; 15% to 25% of patients are left with mild weakness that does not interfere with routine activity; 5% to 10% of patients are left with permanent disabling weakness. 3% to 8% will die despite ICU care for acute respiratory distress syndrome (ARDS), sepsis, thromboembolic disease, and cardiac arrest; factors associated with a poor outcome include age, severe or rapidly progressive disease, prolonged (>1 month) mechanical ventilation, and preexisting lung disease. Worse prognosis with axonal involvement.

J. **Guillain Barré variants**
1. **AMAN:** motor axonal loss without demyelination; associated with *C. jejuni* and autoantibodies to GM-1
2. **AMSAN:** motor and sensory axonal loss without demyelination
3. Miller-Fisher syndrome—ophthalmoparesis, gait ataxia, and areflexia, associated with *C. jejuni* infection and autoantibodies to GQ1b

XI. Chronic Inflammatory Demyelinating Polyradiculoneuropathy (CIDP)

A. **Pathogenesis and pathophysiology:** autoimmune disease that targets the myelin sheaths of peripheral nerves; has a predilection for proximal nerve segments

B. **Epidemiology:** prevalence of 1 to 7.7 per 100,000; peak incidence fifth and sixth decades

C. **Clinical features and diagnostic studies**
1. Weakness must be present for at least 2 months; steadily progressive, stepwise progressive, chronic monophasic, or recurrent patterns
2. Sensory loss in stocking-glove distribution and occasionally there are palpable hypertrophic peripheral nerves
3. May be associated with HIV infection, lupus, monoclonal gammopathy of unknown significance (MGUS), and plasma cell dyscrasias
4. Testing: CSF shows cytoalbuminologic dissociation, nerve conduction studies show decreased nerve conduction velocity, conduction block, temporal dispersion, prolonged or absent F waves

D. **To distinguish CIDP from GBS:** CIDP rarely caused by an antecedent infection, immunization, or surgery; extended period of progressive symptoms; more pronounced sensory disturbance; symptoms respond to steroids

E. **Associated with prolonged neurological disability**; 60% remain ambulatory after 7.5 years, 28% are confined to a wheelchair or bed, and 4% recover

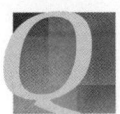# STUDY QUESTIONS FOR CHAPTER 11

Directions: *Each of the numbered items or incomplete statements in this section is followed by answers or by completions of the statement. Select the ONE lettered answer or completion that is BEST in each case.*

1. A 28-year-old man develops acute burning sensation across his shoulders and tingling in his left leg. Over the next several hours, he has numbness and pins-and-needles sensations of both of his arm and his left leg. He has difficulty rising from the sofa where he was watching football and is unable to walk due to weakness in his leg and poor balance. He is brought to the emergency room where is found to have normal vital signs, general medical examination, and mentation. On neurologic examination, his cranial nerves are intact; he has weakness in left shoulder abduction, bilateral grip, and left hip flexion and dorsiflexion. He has diffusely brisk reflexes and a Babinski sign on the left. He has multimodal patchy sensory loss and hyperesthesias up to his neckline. He has a markedly abnormal Romberg sign and is unable to ambulate without hand held assistance. With assistance, he has a staggering gait. What diagnostic test should be done immediately?

   (A) CSF examination
   (B) Cervical spine x-ray
   (C) MRI of cervical and thoracic spine
   (D) MRI of brain

2. Patient has an evaluation for possible multiple sclerosis including a detailed medical history, CSF examination, MRI of the brain, and evoked potentials. Which of the following would not support clinically or laboratory-supported definite multiple sclerosis?

   (A) History of few weeks of double vision with brainstem hyperintensity on T2 MRI
   (B) No prior history of neurologic symptoms with elevated IgG index and synthesis rate. Normal MRI of the brain.
   (C) No prior history of neurological symptoms with elevated IgG index and synthesis rate and T2 MRI of the brain revealing multiple hyperintense lesions in the periventricular region
   (D) Prior history of painful monocular visual blurring, a relative afferent papillary defect, and prolonged NCV on VEP

3. A 4-month-old infant has persistent fever, generalized rigidity, and myoclonus in response to auditory stimuli. What is the most likely diagnosis?

   (A) Globoid cell leukodystrophy
   (B) Metachromatic leukodystrophy
   (C) Lipogranulomatosis
   (D) Spongy degeneration of infancy

4. A 24-year-old man develops subacute loss of vision in his left eye over a period of 3 days. His examination discloses 20/200 acuity in the left eye and 20/20 acuity in the right eye. The remainder of his examination is normal. A lumbar puncture is performed. Which of the following CSF findings is most suggestive for multiple sclerosis?

   (A) Oligoclonal bands
   (B) Myelin basic protein
   (C) Elevated IgG index
   (D) Elevated protein
   (E) Neutrophilic pleocytosis

5. You admit a 41-year-old man to the intensive care unit with Guillain-Barré syndrome. Which of the following would prompt you to treat this man with plasmapheresis rather than with intravenous immunoglobulin (IVIG)?

   (A) History of previous ischemic cerebral infarction
   (B) History of von Willebrand disease
   (C) Increased likelihood of improvement with plasmapheresis
   (D) Lower complication rate with plasmapheresis
   (E) Illness of greater severity

6. A 21-year-old woman presents with double vision and clumsiness for a week. She is noted to have complete ophthalmoparesis, areflexia, and limb ataxia. Which autoantibodies would you expect to find?

   (A) GM1
   (B) GQ1b
   (C) Hu
   (D) dsDNA
   (E) Ro

139

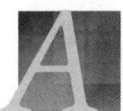ANSWERS AND EXPLANATIONS

1. C. MRI of cervical and thoracic spine. This patient's symptoms are all referable to the cervical spinal cord. May involve ± caudal levels. A spinal cord compression must be excluded! The most likely diagnosis is transverse myelitis involving the cervical spinal segment. (D) MRI brain does not provide for evaluation of the cervical spinal cord. Both (A) CSF and (B) cervical x-ray do not provide nearly as much detail as MRI.

2. B. All but (B) would qualify for clinically or laboratory supported definite multiple sclerosis. (A) fulfills the criteria for two attacks, clinical evidence of one lesion, and paraclinical evidence (MRI finding) of a second lesion. (C) fulfills the criteria for abnormal CSF with one attack, clinical evidence of one lesion, and paraclinical evidence (MRI finding) of a second lesion. (D) fulfills the criteria of two attacks and clinical evidence of two separate lesions, but this may represent neuromyelitis optica/Devic disease, especially if the MRI of the brain is not suggestive of multiple sclerosis.

3. A. Globoid leukodystrophy is first characterized by generalized rigidity, loss of head control, spasms induced by stimulation often with myoclonic spasms with auditory stimulation. (B) Metachromatic leukodystrophy has an onset in the second year of life. (C) Lipogranulomatosis occurs in the first weeks of life with a characteristic hoarse cry and respiratory distress. (D) Spongy degeneration of infancy or Canavan disease has onset at about 3 months with characteristic rapid degeneration of function, optic atrophy, and macrocephaly.

4. C. Elevated IgG index is the most specific CSF finding for multiple sclerosis. Oligoclonal bands, increased myelin basic protein, and elevated protein are less specific for multiple sclerosis. The pleocytosis of multiple sclerosis is mononuclear rather than neutrophilic.

5. A. IVIG may produce a hyperviscous state and is associated with stroke. Plasmapheresis may be a better treatment in this setting. Von Willebrand disease predisposes the patient to bleeding complications, and the central line placement that would be required with plasmapheresis may complicate the procedure. IVIG and plasmapheresis have similar likelihoods of improving the clinical conditions of patients with GBS. Plasmapheresis has a higher complication rate than IVIG. Severe GBS should be treated with IVIG or plasmapheresis, but does not clearly favor one treatment over the other.

6. B. The patient has the Miller-Fisher variant of Guillain-Barré syndrome. Autoantibodies to GQ1b are most likely. GM1 autoantibodies are seen in multifocal motor neuropathy with conduction block. Anti-Hu antibodies are seen in paraneoplastic neurological syndromes. dsDNA is characteristic of systemic lupus erythematosus and anti-Ro antibodies are seen in Sjögren syndrome and other rheumatologic conditions.

CHAPTER 12

Muscle

Myopathies are diseases that primarily affect the muscles and are usually characterized by weakness, fatigue, stiffness, and/or pain. The complaints of fatigue are usually referable to the changes in life state caused by weakness. We include disorders of the neuromuscular junction in which physical fatigue is the most prominent feature.

I. Muscular Dystrophies

These are hereditary disorders of muscles characterized by progressive muscle degeneration that manifest by progressive skeletal muscle weakness, associated with late joint contractures and variable cardiac muscle and brain involvement. The diagnosis is based on the clinical features (phenotype); family pedigree that may define the inheritance pattern; peripheral blood for genomic DNA analysis; serum muscle enzymes (creatine kinase [CK]); electromyographic findings, and muscle biopsy with immunostains and Western blot analysis (immunoblotting). The genomic DNA analysis, when available, is an accurate test, is specific, and confirms the diagnosis before doing more invasive tests.

A. Dystrophinopathies: These include Duchenne, Becker, and manifesting carriers of Duchenne muscular dystrophy. These X-linked inherited disorders are caused by deletions (60%), duplications (5% to 10%), or point mutations on the Xp21 *DMD/BMD* gene. The dystrophin gene is the largest gene identified in humans and consists of 79 exons expanding 2.4 million base pairs in Xp21, which explains the high rate (30%) of new mutations. The *DMD/BMD* gene encodes the dystrophin protein. The protein mediates the connection among the extracellular membrane, the muscle membrane, and the cytoskeleton. Its integrity is important to preserve the integrity of the muscle membrane during muscle contraction. There is phenotype–genotype correlation, but immunostaining, and, more specifically, the Western blot analysis can differentiate among Duchenne, Becker, and manifesting carrier state.
  1. **Duchenne muscular dystrophy** is the most common dystrophy in children.
     a. **Clinical features:** boys are delayed in reaching developmental milestones followed by toe walking and frequent falls with difficulty getting up from the floor that require the use of the hands to push themselves up (Gower sign). The waddling gait is due to weakness of the gluteal muscles that support the pelvis.
     b. **Phenotype:** exaggerated lordosis, protuberant abdomen, enlarged and firm (pseudohypertrophic) calf muscles, weak proximal limb muscles, and variable mental impairment.
     c. **Clinical course:** progressive weakness that requires the use of wheelchairs between the ages of 4 and 8 years, followed by kyphoscoliosis and joint contractures, and respiratory muscle involvement and cardiomyopathy leading to cardiac failure are late and fatal.

d. **Laboratory tests:** The serum CK is invariably elevated and the genomic DNA test is diagnostic in approximately 70% of the patients. The muscle biopsy in the negative DNA cases shows dystrophic changes and with the use of immunostaining and immunoblotting can differentiate between the different types of dystrophinopathies.
e. **Treatment:** No effective treatment is available at the present time. However, 0.75 mg/kg of prednisone daily during the first 10 days of each month preserves motor function in ambulatory patients. Physical and occupational therapy are important to prevent contractures. Braces are useful to prolong ambulation and prevent contractures. Scoliosis surgery may be needed for select patients.
2. **Becker muscular dystrophy** is less common and less severe than the Duchenne type.
   a. **Clinical features:** mean age of onset is about 11 years with long survival. Calf hypertrophy is a prominent feature. Cardiac and mental involvement is rare.
   b. **Laboratory tests:** CK is elevated and genomic DNA analysis shows mutations/deletions maintaining the reading frame or proximal rod deletions. The muscle biopsy shows dystrophic changes with reduced dystrophin by immunohistochemistry (IHC). If results are inconclusive reduced dystrophin by immunoblotting analysis confirms the diagnosis.
3. **Manifesting carriers.** Most female carriers of Duchenne/Becker muscular are asymptomatic. Only 5% to 10% of female carriers manifest the disease and show clinical features similar to the Becker type.
   a. **Laboratory tests:** CK is elevated and the genomic DNA test may be confirmatory. In negative DNA cases the muscle biopsy shows mosaicism in dystrophic expression; immunoblots show normal but decreased dystrophin.

B. **Congenital muscular dystrophies** (CMDs) are heterogeneous autosomal recessive disorders (affecting both genders) that manifest at birth by floppiness, variable degree of joint contractures, and brain abnormalities. There are four types of CMD: pure or classic (occidental) form, the Fukuyama type, muscle-eye-brain (MEB) disease, and the Walker-Warburg syndrome. The last three are associated with severe structural brain abnormalities.
   1. **Merosin (laminin α2) deficiency:** Has been identified in 40% to 50% of the pure occidental cases of congenital muscular dystrophies. Mutations in the *LAMA2* gene (6q22–23) encoding laminin α2 result in merosin deficiency. Laminin α2 is an extracellular matrix protein that links the extracellular space to the membrane cytoskeleton through its specific membrane receptors dystroglycan and integrin α7β1.
   2. **Total merosin deficiency** produces severe muscle weakness at birth that partially improves with time but not to the extent that the patients are able to walk. They usually have normal mentation with variable abnormal white matter signals on the MRI. Some patients require tracheotomies and feeding tubes.
      a. **Partial deficiency:** produces a milder phenotype such that most patients are able to walk unsupported. The mentation is normal but the MRI shows abnormal white matter signals in all cases.
      b. **Laboratory tests:** The CK is elevated; the muscle histochemistry shows severe dystrophic changes. Immunostaining and genomic DNA analysis confirm the diagnosis.
   3. **CMC with abnormal brain development and mental retardation:** The Fukuyama type is an autosomal recessive form of congenital muscular dystrophy associated with severe brain abnormalities as the cause of mental retardation. The genomic DNA analysis shows point mutations in 9q31–33 that encode a highly glycosylated α-dystroglycan protein deficient in these patients. Dystroglycans are muscle membrane complexes that form a link between the dystrophin glycoproteins and the basal lamina. Mutations in genes encoding other glycotransferases are the cause of MEB disease and the Walker-Warburg syndrome.

C. **Limb-girdle muscular dystrophies** (LGMDs) are a heterogeneous group of myopathies that affect the proximal girdle muscles. The age of onset is variable but most start in adolescence or early adulthood and the progression is very slow. The weakness begins in the hip, quadriceps, and hamstring muscles. Striking features of the disease consist of waddling gait, back kneeing, and modified Gower sign. Shoulder weakness usually follows the hip weakness but is usually less

striking. Hypertrophy of the gastrocnemius muscles, and heart and respiratory involvement can be seen in some cases.
- a. **Laboratory tests:** the CK is invariably elevated and the muscle biopsy show dystrophic changes. Immunostaining, immunoblotting, and genomic DNA can differentiate among more than 15 different genotypes. However, mutations in the same protein can produce different phenotypes. The encoded proteins span the muscle membrane; 90% of the cases are autosomal recessive (LGMD2) and the rest are autosomal dominant (LGMD1).
- b. **Autosomal recessive types LGMD2**
    - i. LGMD2A calpain 3q15.1–q21.1
    - ii. LGMD2C λ-sarcoglycan 12q13
    - iii. LGMD2E β-sarcoglycan 4q12
    - iv. LGMD2G-telethonin 17q-11q12
    - v. LGMD2J titin 2q31
    - vi. LGMD2B dysferlin 2p13.1–p13.3 Miyoshi myopathy
    - vii. LGMD2D α-sarcoglycan 17q21 adhalin
    - viii. LGMD2F δ-sarcoglycan 5q33–34
    - ix. LGMD2I Fukutin 19q3.3
- c. **Autosomal dominant types LGMD1**
    - i. LGMD1 dysferlin distal myopathy
    - ii. LGMD1B 1q11–21 laminin A/C Emery-Dreifuss
    - iii. Bethlem myopathy 21q22.3 and 2q37
    - iv. LGMD1A 5q22.3–31.3 myotilin
    - v. LGMD1C 3q25 Caveolin-3

D. **Emery-Dreifuss muscular dystrophy** is an X-linked (Xq28) or autosomal dominant inherited disorder. Early onset of elbow, ankle contractures, even before a significant weakness, are the most prominent clinical features. DNA analysis confirms diagnosis.

E. **Facioscapulohumeral muscular dystrophy** (FSH) is as an autosomal dominant inherited disorder due to short strings of repeated sequences of DNA in an area designated as D4Z4 on 4q35, but the specific gene has not been identified. Deletions and rarely point mutations are diagnostic of the disease.
1. **The infantile form** is noticed in the first 2 years of life with facial diplegia associated with deafness and severe limb weakness. Many children are using wheelchairs by the end of the first decade of life.
2. **The adult form** is first noticed in the teens or twenties; features include difficulty raising the arms above the head and winging of the scapula. Weakness of the facial muscles is variable but not as severe as in the infantile form. The neck and proximal shoulder muscles, including the biceps and triceps, are atrophic, with preservation of the arm muscles giving the "Popeye" appearance. The deltoid muscles are usually spared. The hip muscles are affected later and are associated with a dorsal lordosis and waddling gait. The weak abdominal muscles produce a prominent abdomen. Weaknesses of the peroneal muscles produces a slapping gait.
3. **Laboratory tests:** Serum CK is invariably elevated, the genomic DNA test is diagnostic, and muscle biopsy shows dystrophic changes with prominent inflammation or denervation features in some cases.

F. **Oculopharyngeal muscular dystrophy**: Progressive bilateral ptosis (in late 30s) and dysphagia (in late 40s) characterize a late-onset autosomal dominant inherited disorder. Facial and palate weakness is mild. Ophthalmoplegia and hip muscle weakness appear late but may progress to incapacitate the patients.
1. **Laboratory tests:** The CK is mildly elevated, and the muscle biopsy may show rimmed vacuoles and inclusion bodies. The definite diagnostic genetic test detects short GCG triplet repeat expansion in the 14q11.3q13 that encodes the polyadenylate-binding (PABPN2) protein.
2. **Treatment:** Surgical eye treatment consists of a frontal suspension or frontal sling to improve the ptosis and myotomy of the cricopharyngeal muscle to improve the swallowing. Esophageal dilations and Botox injections of the cricopharyngeal muscle are other available options.

G. **Distal myopathies** are rare disorders that are inherited as autosomal dominant or recessive, are usually of late onset, and have different clinical presentations.

H. **Myotonic muscular dystrophy:** dystrophia myotonica (DM) or Steinert disease is the most frequent type of muscular dystrophy in adults and includes the myotonic dystrophy type 1 (DM1), the congenital myotonic dystrophy (CmyD) and the proximal myotonic myopathy or PROMM (DM2). Myotonic dystrophy is an autosomal dominant inherited disorder with onset in the late teens or early adulthood.
1. **Clinical features:** myotonia or painless inability to relax the muscles after contraction is associated with distal muscle weakness and atrophy. There is facial weakness with mild ptosis, boldness and weak neck flexor muscles. The hip muscles are affected later as well as the distal leg muscles. The voice becomes nasal and the speech is dysarthric and rapid. Mental changes are frequent and consist of low intelligence with demanding and frequent hostile personality. Dysphagia, abdominal pain, and constipation are frequent and are associated with hypomotility and dilation of the esophagus and colon. Cholelithiasis and diabetes mellitus are frequent. Cardiac abnormalities caused by lesions in the conduction system are frequent and are the cause of sudden death in some patients. Testicular or ovarian atrophy and diabetes mellitus are frequent. Eye abnormalities consist of early cataracts, retinal degeneration, and low intraocular pressure.
2. **Laboratory tests:** In MD1 the CK is normal or mildly elevated. The EMG shows myotonic discharges and the muscle biopsy shows dystrophic changes with an increased number of internal nuclei, presence of ring fibers, and type I fiber atrophy. The DNA test confirms the diagnosis by showing expansions of CTG repeats in the 3'-untranslated region of myotonin protein kinase (*MDPK*) gene (19q13.3). In genetic *anticipation* the disease becomes symptomatic at a younger age with each generation and the symptoms are accentuated. In anticipation the genetic defect grows larger during recombination at the time of fertilization.

I. **CmyD** is present at birth in children born of an affected mother. The child is severely hypotonic at birth and has facial diplegia associated with an open triangular, tent-shaped mouth ("fish mouth") with high arch palate. The children have difficulty sucking and swallowing associated with talipes and other joint contractures. No evidence of myotonia is seen at birth, but the floppiness improves with age only to be transformed into myotonia. Developmental motor milestones are delayed and mental retardation is frequent.

J. **The proximal myotonic myopathy** (DM2), or PROMM, is rare, has a similar phenotype to that of DM1, and the gene is located in 3q21.

II. Inflammatory Myopathies

Inflammatory myopathies are a heterogeneous group of disorders characterized by distinct pathogenic mechanisms. Some bacteria can invade large skeletal muscles in drug addicts and produce *pyomyositis*. Fungal infections (candidiasis, aspergillosis, mucormycosis) parasitic infections (trichinosis, cysticercosis, toxoplasmosis), and viral infections can produce myositis. However, the most frequent inflammatory myopathies are caused by immunodysfunctions. Although inclusion body myositis is not an inflammatory disorder it will be discussed. Clinical and histopathologic features of dermatomyositis, polymyositis, and inclusion body myositis are delineated in Tables 12-1 and 12-2.

A. **Dermatomyositis:** is an autoimmune disorder produced by deposition of membrane attack complexes (MACs) in the endomysial microvasculature. Vasculitis is a prominent finding, along with perifascicular fiber necrosis and atrophy. Inflammation is not a prominent feature. The disease has an acute or subacute severe onset of weakness associated with a skin rash that affects the eyelids (heliotrope) and dorsal surfaces of the joints. The adult form of the disease may be associated with cancer and screening for neoplasm is warranted. Calcinosis is more frequent in

TABLE 12-1	Inflammatory Myopathies: Clinical Features			
	Age	Site of weakness	Calcinosis	Malignancy
DM	5–14 40–60	Proximal and neck Proximal and neck	Present Absent	No In 20% of patients
PM	40–60	Proximal and neck	Absent	Rare
IBM	After 50	Quadriceps and hands	Absent	No

children than in adults. Dysphagia is a frequent complaint. The disease usually responds well to immunosuppressant therapy (Tables 12-1, 12-2).

B. Polymyositis: is due to activated CD8 (cytotoxic suppressor) T cells that invade nonnecrotic fibers. The disease has an insidious onset and a slow progression which does respond to steriods. May recur and initial finding may be elevated CK before muscle weakness. Inflammation is a prominent component of the muscle biopsy. *Inclusion body myositis* affects predominantly males after 50 years and has an insidious onset and a slow progression. The presence of amyloid in the rimmed vacuoles seen in the muscle fibers suggests a senescence of myofiber repair process. Inflammation is mild and angulated atrophic fibers are frequent. This responds poorly if at all to steroids.

III. Congenital Myopathies

Congenital myopathies are heterogeneous hereditary disorders of muscle transmitted in different hereditary patterns. Although they are called congenital and frequently appear early in life as floppiness or delayed motor development, muscle weakness may appear later (in childhood) or even in adulthood. The earlier the age of onset the worse the motor deficit will be. The muscle mass is constantly small and there can be associated dysmorphic features. CK and electromyogram (EMG) are usually normal.

A. Central core disease (CCD) and malignant hyperthermia are autosomal dominant or recessive allelic disorders caused by mutations in the *ryanodine* receptor gene in chromosome 19q13.1. Patients with CCD have a high risk of malignant hyperthermia (MH) during general anesthesia. However, not all patients with MH have CCD. There is no specific phenotype; the CK and EMG are usually normal.

B. Nemaline myopathy (NEM) is a heterogeneous disorder transmitted as an autosomal dominant or recessive pattern and encodes to different genes including
    1. NEM1: 1q21–23 alpha tropomyosin (TPM3); NEM2: 2q21.1–22 nebulin

TABLE 12-2	Inflammatory Myopathies: Histopathology		
	Arteries and arterioles	Capillaries	Muscle fascicles
DM	Vasculitis and immune complex deposition	Decreased	Perifascicular fiber atrophy or necrosis and microinfarcts
PM	Perivascular inflammation	Normal	Single fiber necrosis and regeneration; T-cells around normal or necrotic fibers
IBM	Normal	Increased	Rimmed vacuoles, amyloid inclusions, angulated fibers, and inflammation

2. **NEM3:** 1q42.1 sarcomeric actin (ACTA1); **NEM4:** 9q13.2 beta tropomyosin (TPM2)
3. The symptoms can appear in the neonatal period with severe hypotonia, facial diplegia, deafness, and joint contractures. When the symptoms appear in childhood the weakness is slow or nonprogressive and is associated with skeletal deformities and dysmorphic facial features. The adult onset type has variable weakness and the patients have a *Marfan-like* phenotype. The muscle biopsy shows subsarcolemmal rods. The CK and EMG are usually normal.

C. **Centronuclear (myotubular) myopathy** includes a neonatal and a late onset form. Floppiness, dysmorphic facial features, and skeletal abnormalities characterize the neonatal X-linked form. The myotubularin protein encodes the X28q gene. The adult form is characterized by elongated face with ptosis and variable muscle weakness. No gene has yet been found. The muscle biopsy shows round fibers with large centrally located nucleus giving the appearance of a fried egg. The EMG and CK are usually normal.

IV. Metabolic Myopathies

Metabolic myopathies are rare hereditary muscle diseases caused by enzymatic defect, endocrine dysfunction, or a metabolic abnormality; are associated with transitory or permanent muscle weakness as part of a multisystem disease or a primary muscle disorder.

A. **Glycogen storage myopathies:** are inborn errors of metabolism due to enzymatic defects and characterized by glycogen accumulation in the muscle fibers.
1. **Myophosphorylase deficiency:** glycogenosis type V or McArdle disease is an autosomal recessive genetic defect of the muscle isoform of glycogen phosphorylase. The (*PGYM*) gene is located on chromosome 11 and more than 30 different mutations have been identified. The most frequent mutation R49X can be screened in blood. Clinical features include exercise induced cramps, fatigue, and, in some patients, muscle necrosis and myoglobinuria that can lead to renal failure. The CK is elevated and the muscle biopsy shows subsarcolemmal vacuoles with absent or decreased myophosphorylase activity. High protein diet seems to help.
2. **Phosphofructokinase (PKF) deficiency:** glycogenosis type VII or Tauri disease is an autosomal recessive genetic defect caused by mutations in chromosome 1. Clinical features include exertional fatigue, muscle cramps, and exercise-induced myoglobinuria. The muscle biopsy shows subsarcolemmal vacuoles. High protein diet may help.
3. **Debranching enzyme deficiency:** glycogenosis type III or Cori-Forbes disease due to mutation 1p21. Clinical features are mild and involve the liver; the disease is rarely incapacitating.
4. **Acid maltase deficiency: glycogenosis type II or Pompe disease** is an autosomal recessive genetic defect cause by mutations of the lysosomal hydrolase acid alphaglucosidase (*GAA*); gene traced to 17q21–23. The *infantile* type appears as a floppy baby with cardiomegaly and liver and spleen enlargement. *Childhood* type presents as proximal muscle weakness and *adult* type presents as respiratory failure. Muscle biopsy shows vacuolar myopathy; final diagnosis is by biochemical analysis of tissue.
5. **Disorders of lipid metabolism** include several rare disorders that are diagnosed by biochemical determination on the muscle biopsy. L-Carnitine deficiency responds to L-carnitine supplementation. In carnitine palmitoyltransferase (CPT) deficiency, myoglobinuria not preceded by muscle cramps is the usual presentation.

V. Mitochondrial Myopathies

Mitochondrial myopathies are a heterogeneous group of disorders due to defects in the oxidative phosphorylation (OXPHOS) system. Although the mtDNA encodes only 13 polypeptide subunits, more than 100 proteins are necessary for the system's function. When a diagnosis of mitochondrial myopathy is suspected all the medical information including the phenotype and family pedigree needs to be forwarded to a specialized laboratory for detection of mitochondrial deletions. In most mitochondrial myopathies the muscle histologic abnormalities include the presence of *ragged fibers* on modified Gomori trichrome stains and cytochrome oxidase (COX) deficiency. Electron microscopy of the muscle can show crystalline or paracrystalline inclusions ("parking lot" appearance).

A. Chronic progressive external ophthalmoplegia (CPEO) is *the* most frequent manifestation of the mitochondrial myopathies. The onset of the symptoms is in the second or third decade of life and usually has a benign clinical course without any other organ involvement. It is characterized by slowly progressive bilateral ptosis followed months to years later by paralysis of the extraocular muscles. Diplopia is rare but retinitis pigmentosa and skeletal muscle weakness may occur late. mtDNA rearrangements are frequent.

B. Kearns-Sayre syndrome is characterized by onset before age 20, progressive external ophthalmoplegia, pigmentary degeneration of the retina, cardiac conduction defects, cerebellar ataxia, deafness, variable limb weakness, and diabetes mellitus. Brain MRI shows lucent cerebellar lesions. Elevated cerebrospinal protein and peripheral neuropathies have also been described. Spongy degeneration of the brain has been found in autopsied cases. mtDNA rearrangements are found in most patients.

C. Mitochondrial myopathy, encephalopathy, lactic acidosis, and strokelike episodes (mitochondrial myopathy, encephalopathy, lactacidosis, stroke [MELAS]) begins in childhood or adolescence with episodes of vomiting and headache leading to somnolence and coma. Some episodes lead to seizures, hemiparesis, cortical blindness or hemianopsia. Dementia, ataxia, diabetes mellitus, and deafness are frequent. Strokes in young patients may be the first manifestation of the disease. Cardiomyopathy may occur late. A to G mutation in the tRNA gene is frequent. Check serum lactic acid level; muscle biopsy shows "ragged red fibers," magnetic resonance spectroscopy shows lactic acid peak in involved brain region.

D. Myoclonic Epilepsy with Ragged Red Fibers (MERRF) can occur at any age but occurs most frequently in childhood and adolescence. The first symptom may be cerebellar ataxia or myoclonus followed by generalized seizures. Sensorineural deafness, muscle weakness, and ptosis are common. Cardiomyopathy can develop late.

VI. Diseases of the Neuromuscular Junction (NMJ): Myasthenic Disorders

A. Congenital myasthenic syndromes (CMSs) are rare and occur early in life with ocular and generalized weakness. Autosomal recessive disorder frequently seen in gypsy families. The antibodies against AChR are negative; weakness responds poorly to anticholinesterase medication. The neuromuscular junction defects can occur in presynaptic, synaptic, and postsynaptic areas. Exact diagnosis is difficult and requires specialized laboratories.

B. Toxic myasthenic syndrome: Botulism is a paralytic illness caused by a nerve toxin produced by the bacteria *Clostridium botulinum*. The disease can be acquired by eating contaminated food, by a wound infection, and in infants by eating the spores of the bacteria. The toxin produces descending paralysis, blurred vision, diplopia, and other autonomic symptoms. Penicillamine can produce a *drug induced* myasthenia gravis.

C. Immune disorders: The Lambert-Eaton syndrome is an acquired autoimmune myasthenic syndrome of presynaptic neuromuscular transmission. The antibodies bind to and induce a downregulation of voltage-gated calcium channels (VGCCs) that reduce the calcium-dependent release of ACh from motor terminals. Fatigable muscle weakness affecting predominantly the proximal limbs without or with minimal ocular involvement characterizes the disease. There is loss of muscle stretch reflex that returns after exercise and is frequently associated with autonomic dysfunction. It is frequently but not always associated with a small dark-cell cancer of the lung. More than 90% of the patients have serum antibodies (P/Q type) to VGCCs. The repetitive nerve stimulation shows an initial decrement of the muscle contraction followed by a striking incremental response. Common drymouth and impotence in men. Removal of the tumor and immunosuppression are the treatments of choice but usually with poor response. Treatment includes pyridostigmine and 3,4-diaminopyridine (with IRB and FDA approved protocol)

D. Acquired autoimmune myasthenia gravis (MG) is the most common disorder of neuromuscular transmission due to antibodies that target the postsynaptic muscle membrane. In MG, postsynaptic muscle membrane is distorted, simplified by losing its folded normal shape. Characterized by fatigability, MG involves the most active muscles including muscles of eyes, speech, chewing, and swallowing. Symptoms worsen during the day and improve with rest and cold temperatures. In 40% of cases, onset is purely ocular and the disease remains confined to eyes in 16%; 87% of generalizations within 13 months. The pure ocular form is more frequent in children and elderly patients with partial response to treatment. Generalized form without thymoma and onset in patients younger than age 40 affects females predominantly, shows intermediate elevation of AChR-AB, and responds well to treatment. Onset in patients 40 years of age and older without thymoma, affects predominantly males, shows low AChR-AB, and shows high striated muscle antibodies. Onset in patients 40 and older with thymoma shows no sex predilection, high AChR-AB, high striated muscle antibodies, high Titin antibodies, and absent muscle specific receptor tyrosine kinase MuSK antibodies.

E. Transient neonatal MG in 12% of infants born of myasthenic mothers, symptoms appear in first day of life, last for 18 days, expect complete recovery without recurrences

F. The diagnosis of MG is confirmed by reproducing objective fatigability that improves dramatically after intravenous (IV) injection of edrophonium chloride and finding decremental response to the repetitive nerve stimulation. Elevated AChR binding antibodies can also confirm the diagnosis. Other antibodies include: Titin antibodies found in patients with thymoma and in half of older non-thymoma patients. These patients have a more severe disease and are less responsive to treatment. MuSK plays a central role in agrin-mediated signaling at the neuromuscular junction and is essential for the development, maintenance, and clustering of the neuromuscular junction. Patients with elevated MuSK antibodies tend to have a more bulbar than limb weakness and usually do not respond to thymectomy and immunosuppressive therapy. A group of medications can exacerbate or worsen the myasthenic symptoms.

G. Treatment
  1. Treatment of MG has to be tailored to the patients' needs. Symptomatic treatment consists of the use of anticholinesterase medication (pyridostigmine [Mestinon]) that can be used as needed. Thymectomy is recommended in most patients, except for elderly patients without thymoma and MuSK-AB and with other medical contraindications. Best result to thymectomy is seen in young females without thymoma. In patients with thymoma the response to treatment is not good. Immunosuppressant treatment consists of the use of prednisone, azathioprine, and CellCept. Plasmapheresis and IVIG is use in MG crisis and is an adjuvant to immunosuppression.
  2. In patients who present with crisis, usually after taking medication that worsens n-m transmission or respiratory infection, do the following:
      a. Stop Mestinon; not do Tensilon
      b. Diagnose offending medication
      c. Admit patient to ICU for swallowing and respiratory assessment
      d. Determine need for intubation or trach
      e. Plasma exchange and/or steroids, or IVIG

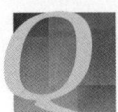# STUDY QUESTIONS FOR CHAPTER 12

Directions: *Each of the numbered items or incomplete statements in this section is followed by answers or by completions of the statement. Select the ONE lettered answer or completion that is BEST in each case.*

1. A 19-year-old man is brought to your clinic with the recent onset of weakness in the hips, quadriceps, hamstrings, and shoulder muscles. A muscle biopsy shows dystrophic changes. What is the most likely pattern of inheritance of this disorder?

(A) Autosomal dominant
(B) Autosomal recessive
(C) Mitochondrial
(D) Sporadic
(E) X-linked

2. You follow a 26-year-old woman with facioscapulohumeral muscular dystrophy. Which of the following muscles is most likely to be spared by this disease process?

(A) Biceps
(B) Deltoids
(C) Triceps
(D) Tibialis anterior
(E) Abdominal muscles

3. A 27-year-old man with myotonic dystrophy is under your care. Which of the following endocrine conditions is he most likely to develop as a consequence of this disorder?

(A) Acromegaly
(B) Adrenal insufficiency
(C) Diabetes
(D) Hypothyroidism
(E) Hyperthyroidism

4. A 57-year-old man with a 6-month history of painless muscle weakness and a heliotrope skin rash is referred to your care. In order to confirm the diagnosis of dermatomyositis, you request a muscle biopsy. What are the most likely findings of this study?

(A) Normal
(B) Endomysial inflammation
(C) Fiber splitting
(D) Perifascicular fiber necrosis
(E) Target fibers

5. You are asked to see a 38-year-old man with the sudden onset of stiffness and high fevers during general anesthesia for an appendectomy. What mutation is most likely to be present in this patient?

(A) Alpha tropomyosin
(B) Calpain
(C) Merosin
(D) Myotilin
(E) Ryanodine receptor gene

149

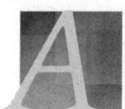# ANSWERS AND EXPLANATIONS

1. B. The clinical vignette is most suggestive of limb girdle dystrophy. In 90% of cases this disorder is inherited in an autosomal dominant fashion.

2. B. The deltoids are characteristically spared in facioscapulohumeral dystrophy. The muscles that are affected by this autosomal dominant disorder include the facial muscles, neck muscles, biceps, triceps, abdominal muscles, hip muscles, and tibialis anterior.

3. C. Diabetes is the endocrine disorder most commonly associated with myotonic dystrophy.

4. D. The most likely biopsy findings of dermatomyositis are vasculitis with perifascicular fiber necrosis. Endomysial inflammation is characteristic of polymyositis. Fiber splitting is prominent in limb-girdle dystrophy. Target fibers are seen in denervation.

5. E. The ryanodine receptor gene mutation, which can cause central core disease, is frequently associated with malignant hyperthermia. Alpha tropomyosin is mutated in nemaline myopathy. Calpain mutations are the cause of limb-girdle muscular dystrophy 2A. Myotilin mutations are found in limb-girdle muscular dystrophy 1A. Merosin deficiency is seen in congenital muscular dystrophies.

CHAPTER 13

Movement Disorders

I. Characterization of Movement Disorders

A. **Hyperkinetic disorders,** that is, increased movement (spontaneous involuntary movements or abnormal movements superimposed over voluntary ones); hypokinetic disorders, that is, decreased movement (characterized by rigidity, slow volitional movements, and impairments of gait and postural reflexes)
   1. **Hyperkinetic:** tremor, tic, dystonia or athetosis, myoclonus, chorea or ballismus
   2. **Hypokinetic:** dopaminergic disorders consist predominantly of the parkinsonisms

B. **Protein accumulation, neurodegeneration, and movement disorders**
   1. Neurodegeneration or neuronal damage caused by toxic effects from accumulation of certain aggregation-prone proteins; damaged or unusable proteins typically cleared by ubiquitin-dependent proteasome protein degradation system
   2. Many movement disorders have abnormalities in synthesis, folding, or degradation of alpha-synuclein and tau proteins (synucleinopathies and tauopathies, respectively) and in pathways involving proteins with expanded polyglutamine tracts (polyQ disorders).
   3. The synucleinopathies include Parkinson disease (PD), diffuse Lewy body disease (LBD), and multiple system atrophy (MSA).
   4. The tauopathies include progressive supranuclear palsy (PSP), corticobasal degeneration (CBD), frontotemporal dementia with parkinsonism-chromosome 17 (FTDP), postencephalitic parkinsonism (PEP), posttraumatic parkinsonism, and Lytico-Bodig or amyotrophic lateral sclerosis-parkinsonism dementia complex of Guam (ALS-PDC).
   5. The polyQ disorders include Huntington disease (HD), dentatorubral-pallidoluysian atrophy (DRPLA), and spinocerebellar ataxias (SCA).

II. Primary Parkinsonian Disorders

A. **Parkinson disease (PD)**
   1. Chronic, progressive neurodegenerative disorder; >80% of all parkinsonisms; likely results from variety or combination of genetic and environmental factors
      a. Medication effect also common, especially with antipsychotics/antiemetics
   2. Prevalence 300/100,000 all ages; 40 years or younger <5/100,000; >500/100,000 for those 70 or older; incidence 50,000 to 60,000 new cases per year
   3. Pathology: degeneration of dopaminergic neurons, pigmented cells in SNc; eosinophilic cytoplasmic inclusions, Lewy bodies in surviving SNc (substantia nigra pars compacta) neurons
   4. Diagnosis: two thirds cardinal features (asymmetrical rest tremor, bradykinesia, and rigidity); exclusion other neurodegenerative disorders secondary causes of parkinsonism; PD with tremor is an easy diagnosis, without about one fourth diagnostic error rate; need more than just the tremor, as could be mistaken for essential tremor

5. Presence of asymmetrical rest tremor/rigidity/bradykinesia; significant improvement following L-dopa supplementation and absence of other known causes of parkinsonism has been reported to carry PPV of 92% and sensitivity of 90% for PD.
6. Hemiparesis, spasticity, autonomic dysfunction, and early dementia suggest may not be PD; 20% of cases no tremor, need to consider other diagnoses, especially supranuclear palsy
7. Initial presentation—70% tremor, 20% stiffness/ slowness, 13% loss of dexterity or handwriting disturbance (micrographia), 12% gait disturbance, 8% muscle pain/cramps
8. Differential includes idiopathic PD, PSP, DLB, CBD, MSA; and, Lytico-Bodig (ALS-PDC), HD, SCAs, Wilson, Hallervorden-Spatz, Lubag (X-linked dystonia-parkinsonism affecting Philippine adult men), and mitochondrial cytopathies. If patient has resting tremor, risk of misdiagnosis is low; if no tremor, carefully consider the alternative diagnoses. Autopsy studies suggest about 20% diagnosed with ideopathic PD actually have a related disorder.
9. Secondary causes include drug induced (neuroleptics, metoclopramide, reserpine, tetrabenazine, lithium, calcium channel blockers), metabolic (hypoxia, hepatocerebral degeneration, hypocalcemia), structural (tumor, hydrocephalus, subdural, trauma), toxic (carbon monoxide, manganese, MPTP), vascular, infectious (AIDS, subacute sclerosing panencephalitis, postencephalitis, prion disease).
10. As PD progresses, it is increasingly difficult to control symptoms because of both progression and medication effect. Most common med effects are motor complications (motor fluctuations, dyskinesias). Motor fluctuations refer to unanticipated loss of effect of a given dose of levodopa ("wearing off"); may suddenly switch from "on" (symptoms controlled) to "off" (symptoms return). Dyskinesias are involuntary movements that occur when dopamine levels are too high. The goal of treatment is to maintain constant level during fluctuations.
11. Workup: complete blood count (CBC), blood chemistries, liver function tests (LFTs), and thyroid function tests; if patient is younger than 50 years, serum ceruloplasmin, 24 hour urine copper, and slit-lamp exam for Kayser-Fleisher rings to rule out Wilson's disease; magnetic resonance imaging (MRI) of brain if atypical features (especially if no tremor), at least CT for everyone.
12. Treatment includes: Amantadine (improves all early PD symptoms; duration varies; may improve dyskinesias caused by other medications); selegiline (central monoamine oxidase B [MAOB] inhibitor; may prolong benefit of L-dopa; can improve all cardinal features; do not use with selective serotonin reuptake inhibitors [SSRIs]); anticholinergics (trihexyphenidyl, benztropine may improve rest tremor, drooling; avoid in older patients); dopaminergic agents (L-dopa is precursor to dopamine and better absorbed; carbidopa included to increase the effectiveness of L-dopa and minimize nausea and vomiting; side effects include nausea, dizziness, confusion, hallucinations, and dyskinesias); dopamine agonists (pergolide, pramipexole, bromocriptine, and ropinirole act directly on dopamine receptors; no conversion step/storage needed as with levodopa; less effective/more side effects than L-dopa; delays onset of dyskinesias; side effects of nausea (should take with/after meals), dizziness, postural hypotension, leg edema, sedation; catechol-O-methyltransferase (COMT) inhibitor (entacapone and tolcapone increase availability/transfer of levodopa into brain by decreasing elimination; decreased "off" time, increased "on" time)
    a. Some patients begin treatment with Sinemet, and others with a dopamine agonist. Sinemet gives a better response but has more side effects.
13. Surgical treatments are effective for medically intractable and disabling tremor. Thalamotomy is rarely used now. Globus pallidus interna (GPi) surgery improves or may abolish permanently contralateral dyskinesias. Subthalamic nucleus (STN) surgery improves all motor symptoms. Typically use deep brain stimulation, as this can modify strength of effect.

B. **Primary parkinsonian disorders—atypical**
   1. **Dementia with Lewy bodies** (DLBs)
       a. Second most prevalent degenerative dementia after Alzheimer disease (AD).
       b. Progressive dementia, symmetrical parkinsonism, profound disturbances of attention/alertness, fluctuating cognitive impairment; and delusions, visual hallucinations, apathy, and agitation are often significant features.

c. Shares clinical and pathologic features with both AD and PD; onset approximately 40 years of age, younger than both AD and PD
d. Diffuse alpha-synuclein aggregates, neuronal Lewy inclusions, appear more prominent in cortex in DLB than in PD. Neurofibrillary tangles similar to that seen in AD.
e. Keys to diagnosis: Age, prominent early cognitive, psychiatric and behavioral symptoms (including visual hallucinations), early and frequent axial features, dementia and parkinsonism often present together within 1 year of onset, suboptimal response to levodopa and heightened sensitivity to neuroleptics. Hallucinations and clinical fluctuations are common.
f. Computed tomography or MRI may show frontotemporal atrophy.
g. Treatments not very effective; cholinesterase inhibitors may improve cognition but worsen parkinsonism; dopaminergics may increase hallucinations

2. **Multiple system atrophy** (MSA)
   a. Group of steadily progressive, atypical parkinsonisms with variable onset, distribution, and severity of cerebellar, extrapyramidal, and autonomic features.
   b. Subtypes named for predominant manifestations. Parkinsonism MSA (MSA-P) replaced striatonigral degeneration. Cerebellar MSA (MSA-C) replaced olivopontocerebellar atrophy. Autonomic MSA (MSA-A) replaced Shy-Drager syndrome.
   c. The combination of autonomic insufficiency, speech or bulbar dysfunction, absence of dementia, postural instability with falls, poor response to dopaminergic medication, and absence of levodopa-induced confusion gave a diagnostic sensitivity and specificity greater than 90%.
   d. Mild restriction of downgaze in 10%; anal sphincter EMG (90% have an abnormality) is sensitive and specific; classic rest tremor is uncommon (29%); cerebellar signs in 54% and upper motor neuron signs in 49%; severe dementia uncommon
   e. CT or MRI may show cerebellar/pontine atrophy, putaminal atrophy; T2 pontine hyperintensity "hot cross bun" sign
   f. Levodopa effective for bradykinesia and rigidity in one third of patients; moderate duration; may worsen orthostatic hypotension, treated with fludrocortisone or midodrine

3. **Progressive supranuclear palsy** (PSP)
   a. Rare, progressive, atypical parkinsonism, prevalence estimates range 1.39 to 6.4/100,000.
   b. Men > women, onset in fifth to sixth decades, almost never before 40 years.
   c. Tauopathy: 4-repeat tau protein aggregates in cytoplasm, forming neurofibrillary tangles, and in glia; causes neuronal loss, gliosis; accumulates in cell body of oligodendrocytes as "coiled bodies" and forms "threads" around axons, astrocytic tuft
   d. Symmetrical parkinsonism with prominent akinesia and axial rigidity; distinct appearance, retrocollic neck dystonia, wide-eyed stare, paucity or absence of blinking, furrowing of forehead, deepening of facial creases, fixed facial expression; tremor not present
   e. Presents profound postural instability, frequent falls, especially first year of symptoms
   f. Slowing of vertical saccades precedes vertical supranuclear gaze palsy; impaired volitional upward and pursuit gaze can be overcome by doll's head maneuver
   g. Pseudobulbar palsy with dysarthria and dysphagia combined with spasticity, hypokinesia, and ataxia; may have severe impairment of speech and swallowing
   h. Prominent frontal lobe symptoms (apathy, significant executive dysfunction, decreased verbal fluency, impulsivity and poor judgement, "imitation" behavior) and frontal release signs typically seen earlier or more severely than in other parkinsonians
   i. CT or MRI midbrain, frontal atrophy involving subcortical region, dilation of third ventricle
   j. Drugs: L-dopa, amantadine, amitriptyline, desipramine, and yohimbine; no dramatic or long-lasting benefit; botulinum toxin used for blepharospasm (eyelid spasms) and other dystonias; artificial tears prevent drying of eyes due to decreased blinking

4. **Corticobasal degeneration** (CBD)
   a. Prevalence 3/100,000; <3% cases of parkinsonism in movement disorders clinics
   b. Male = female; onset 50s to 70s and never before the age of 45
   c. Tauopathy; 4-repeat tau accumulates in cytoplasm as neurofibrillary tangles; accumulates in glia and cell body of oligodendrocytes; astrocytic plaque

d. Unilateral or asymmetrical, levodopa-resistant parkinsonism; akinetic-rigid syndrome with cortical signs such as apraxia, cortical sensory loss or neglect, and alien limb syndrome most commonly recognized presentation; magnetic apraxia, approach behavior with groping and manipulation, is sign of CBD. Others may present with bilateral parkinsonism and incontinence; frontal lobe behavior, aphasia, attention disorders presenting features in some
   e. Dystonic arm and hand posturing common. Action tremor rather than rest tremor.
   f. Saccadic pursuit, difficulty initiating saccades more prominent than supranuclear palsy
   g. CT or MRI may show unilateral or asymmetrical frontoparietal atrophy
   h. Tremor and myoclonus may be improved with clonazepam; baclofen may reduce rigidity; levodopa, other dopaminergic drugs used in PD may help some

III. Dystonia

A. **Sustained muscle contractions** usually produce twisting and repetitive movements, abnormal postures; dynamic disorder changes in severity depending on activity and posture

B. Prevalence varies depending on study methods, populations; generalized 3 to 4/100,000 in a U.S. study; 6.8/100,000 among Ashkenazi Jews; focal 30/100,000 (6 to 225/100,000) incidence of focal approximately 24/million/year and generalized 2/million/year; misdiagnosis, inadequate screening may account for wide variations

C. Categorized based upon age of onset; body distribution; and, etiology
   1. Age of onset: young onset <27 years, typically begins lower extremities, progresses to generalized; adult onset >26 years, usually begins upper body, rarely progresses to generalized
   2. Distribution: focal if single body region; segmental if contiguous regions; generalized if both legs and at least one other body region; multifocal if noncontiguous body regions; hemidystonia if one half of the body is involved; cervical dystonia (torticollis, retrocollis, antecollis) may result from neuroleptics; may be confused with psychiatric conversion disorders
   3. Etiology: primary if dystonia is only sign; may be sporadic or inherited; secondary if associated with a defined etiology or associated with other neurologic abnormalities

D. **Genetics:** 13 genetic forms of dystonia described; loci designated *DYT1* to *DYT13*; all but *DYT2* (AR); *DYT3* (X-linked recessive), one of the two *DYT5* loci (AR, AD) are inherited as AD

E. Benzodiazepines for focal, segmental, and generalized; baclofen for spasticity, some dystonia; anticholinergics (trihexyphenidyl, diphenhydramine) to treat focal, segmental, generalized (may be better tolerated by children than other medications); dopa-blocking/-depleting agents (benefit a paradox since may cause dystonia); surgery considered for severe dystonia not responsive to medications: thalamotomy, pallidotomy. Botulinum toxin type A or B for cervical dystonia; type A approved for patients ages 12 and older affected by strabismus, blepharospasm. Torticollis resulting from neuroleptics rapidly responds to parenteral Benadryl.

IV. Myoclonus

A. Involuntary, sudden, brief, shocklike movements; may be "positive" or "negative"; positive myoclonus from contraction of a muscle or multiple muscles; negative myoclonus due to brief loss or inhibition of muscle tone

B. **Classification** based upon observable symptomatology or clinical presentation; nervous system focus or loci; and, cause or etiology

C. **Presentation** according to distribution, relation to provocation, and pattern of movements

1. Distribution: focal (limited to specific muscle, group of muscles of body part), segmental (areas adjacent to or near each other, contiguous); multifocal (two or more areas not adjacent to each other, anatomically separate); generalized (one or more major muscle groups)
2. Spontaneous myoclonus—without provocation; reflex myoclonus—response to stimulus; action myoclonus—during voluntary movements or intention to move
3. Can be rhythmic, regular pattern; irregular without set pattern; repetitive, or oscillatory with fast tremor quality; same pattern as tonic-clonic seizures

D. **Nervous system origin** designated as being cortical, subcortical, spinal, or peripheral; most commonly caused by metabolic impairment including hypotoxic-ischemic disorder

E. **Genetics**
1. Myoclonus dystonia: 7q21–*DYT11, SCGE;* 18p11–*DYT15*
2. Myoclonic epilepsy: 8q24—familial adult myoclonic epilepsy; *G8363A* mutation—MERRF; 21q22.3—*CSTB* gene, Unverricht-Lundborg disease; 6p24, *EPM2A, EPM2B*—Lafora progressive myoclonic epilepsy
3. Other: PRNP H187R—hereditary Creutzfeldt-Jakob disease; 3242A > G-MELAS 22q11—DiGeorge syndrome

F. **Myoclonus** 1.3/100,000 and prevalence 8.6/100,000; secondary myoclonus 72% of cases, most associated with Lance Adams syndrome, AD, and Creutzfeldt-Jakob disease; myoclonic epilepsy 17% of cases; essential myoclonus 11%

G. **Blood electrolytes**, glucose, kidney and liver functions, screening studies for drugs, toxins, antibodies; imaging to help identify underlying disease etiologies (cortical myoclonus, reticular myoclonus); MRI of brainstem for symptoms associated with palatal myoclonus; electroencephalogram (EEG) used to identify myoclonus of cortical origin and symptomatic syndromes such as Creutzfeldt-Jakob disease; motor and somatosensory evoked potentials (SEPs) to assess characteristics of myoclonus

H. **Primary drugs** used include levetiracetam, clonazepam, valproic acid, primidone, piracetam, and acetazolamide; opsoclonus–myoclonus in children treated with immunosuppression (adrenocorticotropic hormone [ACTH], azathioprine, corticosteroids, IVIG)

V. Tremor

A. **Most common type of movement disorder**; rhythmic, oscillatory back-and-forth movement; may be only manifestation/monosymptomatic entity; can belong to symptom complex indicating particular disease or syndrome; can result from exogenous cause

B. **Primarily designated as rest tremor or action tremor**
1. Rest tremor occurs when affected body part not voluntarily moved or activated; supported against gravity (resting hand in the lap)
2. Action tremor produced while actively contracting a muscle; postural tremor when affected part is maintained against gravity; kinetic tremor during voluntary movement; if tremor occurs during nontargeted/directed movement, considered a simple kinetic tremor; if movement is target directed and tremor increases in amplitude at end of movement, considered intention tremor; task-specific tremor occurs or worsens during specific activities or can be position-specific (writing tremor); isometric tremor from contraction of muscle, force against stationary object (push hand against wall); tremor may involve voice, neck movement for "yes" (side-to-side) or "no" (forward-backward); intention tremor may interfere with activities of daily living; resting tremor does not diagnose, but is the "calling card" of PD
3. Syndromic classifications: physiologic, essential, dystonic, parkinsonian, cerebellar, palatal, drug-induced/toxic, neuropathic, psychogenic

4. Mild tremor may not need treatment. If specific illness such as PD or Wilson disease, tremor will improve with therapy of underlying disease. Tremor may be treated with propranolol, primidone, or benzodiazepines, neurontin, topiramate.

VI. Tics

Tics are repetitive, stereotypic movements or behaviors; motor or vocal, simple or complex; primary disorder or secondary to identifiable etiology; transient or chronic

A. May be suppressed for variable periods but causes mounting anxiety, a need to allow tic to occur; patients feel relief or lessened anxiety from performing tics

B. Simple motor tics involve single body part (eye blinks, shoulder shrugs); simple vocal tics are brief noises (sniffing, throat clearing)

C. Complex motor tics resemble semipurposeful movements; complex movement often involve more than one muscle group; complex vocal tics are words/phrases that may intrude into normal speech, out of context (echolalia, palilalia, coprolalia)

D. Transient motor/vocal tics last <1 year; chronic motor or vocal tics persist >1 year but do not meet diagnostic criteria for Tourette syndrome (GTS)

E. Onset often before 21 years of age, usually childhood or adolescence, males > females

F. Reported prevalence varies; transient motor tics 3% to 19% school-aged children; chronic motor tics 2% to 5% children; 0.1% to 3% school-aged children meet criteria of GTS

G. Diagnostic criteria for GTS: both multiple motor and one or more vocal tics present, not necessarily at same time; occur many times/day most days for at least 1 year; tic-free periods are <3 months; location, number, frequency, type, complexity, severity change over time; onset before 21 years of age; witnessed by reliable examiner or a video recording at some time during the illness; no other etiologies identified as cause of tics

H. Obsessive compulsive disorder (OCD) in 45% to 65%, attention deficit hyperactivity disorder (ADHD) in 50% to 75% of GTS; may reveal relatives with OCD (especially female kin) and add with/without motor symptoms

I. Likely polygenic; suggested autodominant with variable expression

J. Secondary causes: infections, drugs, toxins, developmental/chromosomal abnormalities, head trauma, stroke, psychotic disorders, and neurodegenerative diseases

K. Treatment: low dose neuroleptics reduce frequency/intensity of tics. *Botulinum* toxin (BTX) into involved muscles may alleviate abnormal movements/premonitory sensations/urges; clonazepam or antidepressants for behavioral symptoms; clonidine or guanfacine for ADHD/impulsivity; SSRIs for OCD

VII. Chorea

Chorea is rapid, arrhythmic, purposeless/semipurposeful, flowing motor jerks; seem to move from one body part to another; can affect limbs, trunk, face

A. Reduced inhibitory output from striatum/indirect pathway leads to excessive inhibition of STN by external segment of globus pallidus (GPe); excitatory outflow from STN to internal segment of globus pallidus (GPi)/substantia nigra (SN) reduced, less inhibition of thalamus by

GPi/SN, leads to increased thalamocortical activity; thus, increase in extraneous movements; later, degeneration of direct pathway leads to reduction of chorea/increased parkinsonism, causes greater akinesia/less prominent chorea

B. **May be brief, random** as in HD; tardive-repetitive, stereotyped; ballismus-large amplitude, proximal movements; hemichorea/hemiballismus suggest focal lesion, contralateral subcortical structures

C. **Involuntary, rapid, irregular, jerky movements** of face, arms, legs, or trunk. Mild chorea may make patient appear restless or fidgety. Patient may be unaware of symptoms.

D. **HD neurodegenerative**; characterized by emotional, behavioral, psych abnormalities; loss of acquired intellectual/cognitive functioning; movement/motor disturbances
   1. Prevalence 4 to 10/100,000; autodominant; onset third to fifth decades; begins insidiously but progressively devastating until death on average 17 years after onset
   2. PolyQ disorder; unstable CAG repeat; *IT15* gene 4p16.3; regulates or "encodes" production of Huntingtin protein; mutant Huntingtin longer than normal polyQ tract, resists degradation by ubiquitin-dependent proteasomal proteolytic system; normal 9–29 repeats; HD 36–121 CAG repeats; 30–39 incomplete penetrance; >40 complete penetrant
   3. Number of repeats often correlates inversely to age of onset; >60% juvenile onset; >80 onset first decade; anticipation, paternal transmission associated with earlier onset
   4. Classic signs include chorea, impairment of memory, abstract thinking, and judgment; disorientation; agitation; personality changes (personality disintegration)
   5. Gait wide-based, lurching, dipping/bobbing, frequent falls; saccadic eye movements
   6. Treatment symptomatic relief, features that affect function/quality of life; neuroleptics will suppress chorea and psychoses but not alter outcome of illness

E. Other causes of chorea include Syndeham, tardive dyskinesia, medication effect, basal lacunar infarction, and many others.

VIII. Ataxia

A. **Inability to maintain normal posture/smoothness of movement**; defective muscular coordination, usually more pronounced with voluntary movements

B. **Many variations** from pure cerebellar dysfunction to mixed patterns reflecting extrapyramidal, brainstem, and cerebral cortical involvement

C. **Interruption of afferent, efferent paths** spinocerebellar system results in broad-based/ataxic gait, scanning dysarthria, explosive speech, intention tremor, dysdiadochokinesia, dysmetria, abnormal eye movements (ocular dysmetria, nystagmus)
   1. **Dysmetria:** abnormal force/magnitude of movement; patient points beyond/short of examiner's target finger during finger to nose test
   2. **Dysdiadochokinesia:** rapid alternating movements clumsy, not fluid
   3. **Pure cerebellar cortical atrophy:** familial and sporadic; clinical features: insidious onset ataxia gait, truncal instability, tremor of hands, head, dysarthria; pathology: symmetric atrophy of vermis > hemispheres, loss Purkinje cells, granule cells, inferior olivary nuclei

D. **Autosomal-dominant cerebellar ataxias:** large group; most present with ataxia, cerebellar dysfunction; chronic/progressive with/without other neurologic abnormalities; many with identifiable biochemical defects; DNA testing available for many
   1. **Spinocerebellar ataxia (SCA-1)** onset third to fourth decades; CAG repeat; 6p22–p23; protein ataxin-1; gait/limb ataxia, dysarthria, dysmetria, nystagmus, muscle wasting; dystonia, ophthalmoplegia, bulbar signs later stages

2. **Spinocerebellar ataxia (SCA-2)** onset third to fourth decades; ataxia, facial fasciculation, lid retraction, early reduced ocular saccadic velocity, myoclonus, polyneuropathy; CAG repeat; 12q23–q24; protein ataxin 2
3. **Spinocerebellar ataxia (SCA-3)** allelic to Machado-Joseph disease; onset after fourth decade; ataxia, pyramidal/extrapyramidal signs, amyotrophy, facial/lingual fasciculations, ophthalmoplegia, exophthalmos; CAG repeat; 14q24–q32; ataxin 3
4. **Spinocerebellar ataxia (SCA-4)** 16q22.1; mutation unknown; onset second to fourth decade; late onset ataxia, sensory axonopathy; degeneration of cerebellar Purkinje cells, dorsal root sensory ganglion neurons, and ascending posterior columns
5. **Spinocerebellar ataxia (SCA-5)** locus is 5 cM candidate region on chromosome 11 in open reading frame of unknown gene; cerebellar ataxia, facial myokymia, impaired vibration sense; very slow progression; onset variable, ages 10 to 68 years; first family described descending from Abraham Lincoln's grandparents
6. **Spinocerebellar ataxia (SCA-6)** CAG repeat; 19p13; mutation affects calcium channel *CACNL1A*; onset fourth to sixth decades; ataxia, nystagmus, dysarthria, loss of vibration/proprioception; loss of Purkinje cells, granule cells, neurons of inferior olive nucleus, dentate nucleus; progressive pancerebellar dysfunction without involvement of cognitive, pyramidal, or extrapyramidal function; slow progression over 20 to 30 years
7. **Spinocerebellar ataxia (SCA-7)** 3p21.1–p12; CAG repeat; ataxin-7; ophthalmoplegia, dysarthria, pyramidal/extrapyramidal signs, impaired vibration sense; visual loss/macular retinal degeneration (unique finding in this disorder)
8. Spinocerebellar ataxia (SCA-8) not translated CTG repeat; 13q21; onset age 18 to 65 years; dysarthria, gait instability often initial symptoms; spastic dysarthria, nystagmus, spasticity, limb/gait ataxia, and diminished vibration perception; slow progression
9. **Spinocerebellar ataxia (SCA-10)** 8.8 cM candidate region 22q13; ATTCT repeat; onset third to fifth decades; pure cerebellar ataxia, nystagmus, dysarthria, dysphagia, hypotonia, generalized and/or complex partial epilepsy
10. **Spinocerebellar ataxia (SCA-11)** 15q14–q21.3; mutation unknown; mild disorder, pure ataxia a major feature; normal life span; onset 15 to 70 years; retained ambulation
11. **Spinocerebellar ataxia (SCA-12)** CAG repeat; 5q31–q33 brain-specific regulatory subunit of phosphatase PP2A; early tremor; later pure spinocerebellar ataxia, dementia
12. **Spinocerebellar ataxia (SCA-13)** unknown mutation; chromosome 19; onset early childhood; limb ataxia, mental retardation, dysarthria, nystagmus
13. **Spinocerebellar ataxia (SCA-14)** reported in single Japanese family; unknown mutation; chromosome 19; onset 12 to 42 years; tremor, axial myoclonus and ataxia
14. **Spinocerebellar ataxia (SCA-15)** linkage, mutation not identified; pure cerebellar ataxia; onset mid-childhood to middle age; cerebellar vermis atrophy
15. **Spinocerebellar ataxia (SCA-16)** unknown mutation; 8q22; onset 20 to 66 years; pure cerebellar gait/limb ataxia, dysarthria, nystagmus; head tremor found rarely
16. **Spinocerebellar ataxia (SCA-17)** CAG/CAA repeat of TATA-binding protein gene; chromosome 6; third decade; gait ataxia; later dementia, bradykinesia, dysmetria, dysdiadochokinesia, and hyperreflexia
17. **Spinocerebellar ataxia (SCA-19)** unknown mutation; 1p21–q21; 20 to 45 years of age with mild ataxia, myoclonus, cognitive impairment and slow postural tremor
18. **Spinocerebellar ataxia (SCA-21)** unknown mutation; 7p21.3–p15.1; 6 to 30 years of age; slowly progressive gait/limb ataxia; variable extrapyramidal signs, hyporeflexia, cognitive impairment, and akinesia
19. **Episodic ataxia I (EA1)** rare auto-dominant channelopathy; point mutations affect voltage-gated potassium channel gene; 12p13; continuous myokymia between attacks; partial epilepsy; sudden episodes of ataxia precipitated by movement, startle, or emotion; electromyogram (EMG) shows continuous motor unit activity in all patients; partial responses to acetazolamide, carbamazepine, phenytoin, and phenobarbital
20. **Episodic ataxia 2 (EA2)** autodominant; mutations affect calcium channel (*CACNA1A*) gene; 19p13; allelic to familial hemiplegic migraine and SCA6; headache, intermittent midline cerebellar dysfunction, ataxia, nystagmus, dysarthria lasting minutes to hours, vertigo; no myokymia; provoked by stress, exercise, fatigue; may respond to acetazolamide

21. **Dentatorubropallidoluysian atrophy (DRPLA)** 12p triplet-repeat; autodominant with anticipation; mutation may affect protein product atrophin −1; includes serine repeat and variable polyglutamine repeat; nerve cell loss, gliosis affect dentate nucleus, red nucleus, pallidum, subthalamic nucleus of Luys; age of onset varies with ataxia, dementia, polymyoclonus, and chorea; no treatment is available

E. **Autosomal recessive ataxias**
  1. **Hartnup disease** defective intestinal transport, renal tubular reabsorption of neutral amino acids (primarily tryptophan) leads to niacin deficiency; locus is 11q13; incidence 1/30,000; intermittent ataxia, cerebellar signs; neuropsych dysfunction; pellagralike rash induced by sunlight; normal intelligence, most have no neurologic signs; excessive urine monoamino-monocarboxylic amino acids; urinary indoxyl derivatives; treatment high-protein diet; niacin reverses skin/neuropsychiatric manifestations; tendency for spontaneous improvement
  2. **Fatty acid oxidation** defects affect mitochondrial beta-ox; episodic vomiting, intermittent weakness, lethargy; ataxia; coma; neuro symptoms induced by fasting
  3. **Urea cycle defects:** defects of five urea cycle enzymes and one of its activators described; hyperammonemic coma in neonate; five urea cycle enzymes are carbamyl phosphate synthetase, ornithine transcarbamylase (X-linked inheritance), argininosuccinate synthetase, argininosuccinate lyase, arginase; four of five deficiencies (excepting ornithine transcarbamylase) autorecessive; behavioral problems (self-abuse); episodic hyperammonemia, ataxia, spasticity; protein intolerance with intermittent vomiting; adults: migraine-like episodes, confusion, visual impairment, hallucinations, neuropsychiatric symptoms reported; hyperreflexia, papilledema, decerebrate/decorticate posturing; argininemia may mimic spastic diplegic cerebral palsy
  4. **Ataxia with selective vitamin E deficiency:** mutation affects gene for alpha-tocopherol transfer protein; phenotypically similar to Friedreich ataxia (FRDA); head titubation, spinocerebellar ataxia, areflexia, proprioception loss; xanthelasmata and tendon xanthomas; onset age 2 to 52 years, usually younger than 20 years; slowly progresses over decades; vitamin E 400–1200 IU per day improves neurologic function; should be taken for life
  5. **FRDA** first recessive condition with triplet repeat; 96% FRDA1 9q13 *X25* gene. 7–38 repeats in normal alleles; 66 ⇒ 1700 triplets in disease-causing alleles (most > 600); remaining cases are compound heterozygotes for GAA expansion and frataxin point mutation; appears to have more than 1 locus; the mutation leads to formation of the abnormal protein termed frataxin; the cells carrying this mutation appear to be sensitive to oxidative stress; great phenotype variance exists, even within the same family
      a. Late-onset FRDA (LOFA, onset 25 to 39 years) and very-late-onset FRDA (VLOFA, onset >40 years). Deep tendon reflexes retained; progresses slowly, particularly Acadians
      b. Variable age of onset when younger than 20 years
      c. Initial ataxic gait and clumsy hands followed by cerebellar ataxia, dysarthria, nystagmus, uncoordinated limb movements, hypoactive knee, ankle reflexes, Babinski sign, impaired position/vibratory sense; symmetric, concentric, hypertrophic cardiomyopathy (>50%); congestive heart failure; and subaortic stenosis; pes cavus, scoliosis, hammer toe; abnormal glucose tolerance test, diabetes mellitus, and diabetic ketosis
      d. Abnormal electrocardiogram, echocardiogram, sensory nerve conduction absent or reduced; MRI—cerebellar atrophy, thin spinal cord
      e. Iron accumulation within mitochondria of FRDA fibroblasts subjected to oxidative stress, resulting in impaired respiratory function
      f. No specific treatment other than symptomatic and supportive care is available.
  6. **Abetalipoproteinemia** characterized by low levels of low-density lipoprotein (LDL) and very-low-density lipoprotein (VLDL); defective assembly and secretion of apolipoprotein B (Apo-B)–containing lipoproteins by the intestines and the liver; mutations affect *MTP* gene
      a. Areflexia, proprioceptive dysfunction, loss of reflexes, and Babinski sign (prominent findings); by 5 to 10 years, gait disturbances and cerebellar signs seen
      b. Malabsorptive state early with steatorrhea and abdominal distension; pes cavus and scoliosis in most; pigmentary retinopathy; acanthocytosis on peripheral blood smears

(constant finding); decreased serum cholesterol; increased high-density lipoprotein (HDL) cholesterol levels; low levels of LDL, VLDL, and triglycerides
   c. High-dose vitamin E ameliorates neurologic symptoms. Give vitamins D, A, and K too.
7. **Hypobetalipoproteinemia** autosomal-dominant indistinguishable from abetalipoproteinemia; mutations affect *Apo-B* gene, which affects turnover of apolipoprotein B
   a. Progressive ataxia with other neurologic dysfunction and systemic features
   b. Varying combination of cognitive delay or decline, abnormalities of muscle tone, seizures, and movement disorders
   c. Inheritance varies; may involve defects in DNA repair
8. **Cockayne syndrome:** autosomal-dominant (CSB) and recessive (CKN1) forms; defective repair transcriptionally active DNA; fibroblasts abnormal UV sensitivity
   a. Blindness, cataracts, and pigmentary retinopathy; no increase in incidence of malignancy; microcephaly; ataxia, pyramidal, and extrapyramidal dysfunction; seizures; systemic hypertension, sexual infantilism, renal and hepatic dysfunction
   b. Calcification of basal ganglia on CT; white matter changes on MRI
   c. No treatment is available; early death in the second or third decade is usual
9. **Xeroderma pigmentosum** genetically heterogeneous; defect in DNA excision repair following UV exposure; differs from Cockayne syndrome: presence skin tumors, absence intracranial calcifications, different molecular defect; no treatment available. ataxia, chorea, and axonal polyneuropathy; cutaneous photosensitivity and multiple cancers; mental and motor retardation; microcephaly; sensorineural deafness
10. **Ataxia telangiectasia** progressive, recessively inherited ataxia; presents early childhood; more common in Amish, Mennonite, Costa Rican, Polish, British, Italian, Turkish, Iranian, and Israeli descent; defective protein (possibly phosphatidylinositol-3 kinase); mutations affect *ATM* gene locus; onset 1 to 3 years; no treatment is available
    a. Choreoathetosis; cutaneous and bulbar telangiectasia; immunodeficiency symptoms; oculomotor apraxia; progressive ataxia, slurred speech; susceptibility to leukemia, lymphoma
    b. Genetic test for 11q22.3; elevated (>10 ng/mL) serum alpha-fetoprotein in 90% to 95% of patients; breakpoints involved in translocation at the 14q11 and 14q32 sites
11. **Refsum disease** is autosomal-recessive disorder; impaired oxidation of phytanic acid; elevated phytanic acid causes neurotoxicity; onset 20s to 30s; relapsing-remitting course
    a. Cerebellar ataxia; early night blindness, pigmentary degeneration of retina; polyneuropathy; sensorineural deafness; ichthyosis and cardiac arrhythmias
    b. Elevated phytanic acid levels in the plasma and urine are diagnostic
    c. Drastic reduction in dietary phytanic acid (supplemented by plasmapheresis) at onset can ameliorate the neuropathy and possibly other clinical abnormalities
12. **Cerebrotendinous xanthomatosis** is an autosomal-recessive disorder caused by a defect in bile acid synthesis; cholestanol accumulates in tissues, nervous system; the defect is due to deficiency of hepatic sterol 27–hydroxylase, a mitochondrial enzyme
    a. Palatal myoclonus, seizures, peripheral neuropathy, progressive ataxia with mental decline, pseudobulbar palsy, tendon xanthomas, and cataracts
    b. Elevated cholestanol and apolipoprotein B in cerebrospinal fluid (CSF), low plasma cholesterol; elevated plasma cholestanol, low-to-absent chenodeoxycholic acid in the bile
    c. Lifelong oral chenodeoxycholic acid (750 mg per day) is effective if initiated early; hydroxymethylglutaryl coenzyme A (HMG-CoA) reductase inhibitor also to inhibit cholesterol biosynthesis
13. **Biotinidase deficiency:** lack of free biotin results in dysfunction of three mitochondrial carboxylases; mutations of 3p25 locus for biotinidase
    a. delayed presentation (second year of life), intermittent ataxia, sensorineural hearing loss, myoclonic seizures, developmental delay, skin rashes and alopecia
    b. May see hyperammonemia, hypoglycinemia, metabolic acidosis, lactic acidosis; possible excess excretion of hydroxyisovaleric acid, methylcrotonylglycine, hydroxypropionate, and methylcitrate in the urine
    c. Biotin 5 to 20 mg per day orally is remarkably effective in reversing neurologic and cutaneous symptoms. Hearing and visual dysfunction may be resistant to treatment.

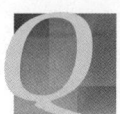# STUDY QUESTIONS FOR CHAPTER 13

Directions: Each of the numbered items or incomplete statements in this section is followed by answers or by completions of the statement. Select the ONE lettered answer or completion that is BEST in each case.

1. A 61-year-old man presents with 6 months of a rest tremor in his right hand. Which of the following additional factors makes a diagnosis of Parkinson disease most likely?

    (A) Rigidity
    (B) Bradykinesia
    (C) Postural instability
    (D) Weakness
    (E) Response to levodopa

2. A 52-year-old woman has noted progressive slowness of one year's duration. Which of the following features is most consistent with a diagnosis of multiple system atrophy?

    (A) Mild restriction of downgaze
    (B) Abnormal anal sphincter EMG
    (C) Rest tremor
    (D) Cerebellar ataxia
    (E) Autonomic insufficiency

3. A 66-year-old woman is brought to your office by her family for complaints of dementia and rigidity. On physical examination, you note generalized bradykinesia with prominent apraxia and agraphesthesia of the right hand. What is the most likely diagnosis?

    (A) Parkinson disease
    (B) Lewy-body dementia
    (C) Multisystem atrophy
    (D) Progressive supranuclear palsy
    (E) Corticobasal ganglionic degeneration

4. A 12-year-old boy is brought to your office by his mother because of unusual movements. There is a history of similar movement in his father and a paternal uncle, but not in his two older siblings. You observe sustained muscle contractions in all four limbs and his face, and classify it as dystonia. Which of the following is most likely true of this patient's condition?

    (A) It most likely began in his arms and then became generalized
    (B) It was most likely inherited as an autosomal dominant condition
    (C) Benzodiazepines are the medication of choice for this boy
    (D) The movements are likely to be similar at rest and in action
    (E) His generalized dystonia is unusual in children

5. A 14-year-old boy is brought to your office with 2 years of tics involving his face and arms and unformed vocal tics. What disorder is most likely to be present in a family member?

    (A) Bipolar disorder
    (B) Major depression
    (C) Obsessive compulsive disorder
    (D) Parkinson disease
    (E) Schizophrenia

6. A 39-year-old man comes to your office for evaluation of gradually developing ataxia. You note increased reflexes, upgoing toes, impaired extraocular movements and exophthalmos. What is the most likely diagnosis?

    (A) Abetalipoproteinemia
    (B) Dentatorubropallidoluysian atrophy
    (C) Friedreich ataxia
    (D) Hartnup disease
    (E) Machado-Joseph disease

7. A 16-year-old girl with episodic ataxia is referred for neurologic consultation. On examination, you note no ataxia, but do see continuous wriggling movements in her face and hands. What is the most likely inheritance pattern of this disorder?

    (A) Autosomal dominant
    (B) Autosomal recessive
    (C) Mitochondrial
    (D) X-linked dominant
    (E) X-linked recessive

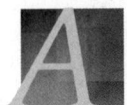# ANSWERS AND EXPLANATIONS

1. E. The cardinal features of Parkinson disease are tremor, rigidity, bradykinesia, and postural instability. In addition to asymmetric resting tremor, the factor that makes Parkinson disease a likely diagnosis is response to levodopa.

2. B. Although cerebellar ataxia and autonomic insufficiency are classical findings of multiple system atrophy, an abnormal anal sphincter EMG is the most sensitive and specific of the listed features. Restriction of downgaze is classically a feature of progressive supranuclear palsy, whereas rest tremor is seen in Parkinson disease.

3. E. Corticobasal ganglionic degeneration is characterized by parkinsonism and findings referable to the parietal lobe. These can include alien-limb phenomenon, limb apraxia, dystonia posturing, and agraphesthesia. The other choices listed are not associated with these findings.

4. B. Most inherited dystonic disorders are inherited in an autosomal dominant fashion. In children, dystonia tends to begin in the lower extremities before generalizing. Anticholinergics such as trihexyphenidyl, not benzodiazepines, are the first-line treatment for treatment of dystonia in children. Dystonia is a dynamic disorder that varies in rest and action.

5. C. The patient described in the vignette has symptoms most consistent with Tourette syndrome. This disorder is often associated with obsessive compulsive disorder and attention-deficit hyperactivity disorder in first degree relatives.

6. E. All of the disorders listed can produce ataxia, but the vignette is most consistent with Machado-Joseph disease. This disorder, also known as spinocerebellar ataxia-3 produces ataxia, pyramidal and extrapyramidal signs, amyotrophy, facial and lingual fasciculations, ophthalmoplegia, and exophthalmos. Abetalipoproteinemia and Friedreich ataxia should cause decreased reflexes. Dentatorubropallidoluysian atrophy produces ataxia, dementia, polymyoclonus, and dementia. Hartnup disease produces intermittent ataxia, neuropsychological dysfunction, and a pellagra-like rash.

7. A. The patient described in this vignette most likely has episodic ataxia 1, an autosomal dominant channelopathy involving the voltage-gated potassium gene characterized by sudden episodes of ataxia precipitated by movement, startle, or emotion and continuous myokymia in between attacks.

CHAPTER 14

Infection

I. History and Examination

A. Clinical hallmarks are fever, headache, altered mental status, and, sometimes, focal neurologic findings; these are nonspecific findings. Fever and altered mental state that remain unexplained require lumbar puncture.

B. Seizures, focal neurologic findings, papilledema or depressed consciousness mandate imaging before lumbar puncture.

C. Acute meningitis (AM)
   1. **Onset** hours to days; vomiting possible
   2. **Etiology:** bacterial, viral, systemic conditions, chemical (especially nonsteroidal anti-inflammatory drugs [NSAIDS])
   3. Often can find a **predisposing condition**
   4. **Viral:** fever, headache unrelieved by analgesics, lethargy, myalgias, nuchal rigidity

D. Subacute versus chronic
   1. **Gradual onset** over weeks to years; can appear to be serial episodes of AM
   2. **Chronic-low fever**, focal findings more common than AM
   3. **Infectious causes:** tuberculosis (TB), cryptococcosis, coccidioides, histoplasmosis, spirochetes
   4. **Noninfectious causes:** sarcoid, systemic lupus erythematosus (SLE), vasculitides, neoplasm
   5. **Always test for** cryptococcosis and syphilis; easily diagnosed and have good treatments

E. Encephalitis = cortical inflammation
   1. Mental status changes and seizures early, viral or component of systemic infection

F. Abscess: most common finding is hemicrania or generalized headache, seizures, and focal deficit; fever indicates the primary systemic source is active

G. Examination
   1. Observe for rashes over the body
   2. Nuchal rigidity
   3. Kernig and Brudzinski signs
      a. **Kernig:** passively extend knee while patient is seated and feel resistance. Most practitioners do something different, but what is the point calling the sign Kernig's if you are not doing what the originator did?
      b. **Brudzinski signs:** he actually described three signs
         i. Nape-of-the-neck sign: passive flexion of neck causes flexion of hip and knee

ii. Identical contralateral reflex sign: passive flexion of hip and knee on one side causes the same on the other side
iii. Reciprocal contralateral reflex sign: when performing (ii) contralateral leg, which has flexed, then has a spontaneous extension

II. Cerebrospinal Fluid

A. **Anatomy**
  1. Total cerebrospinal fluid (CSF) in adults is 140 mL
     a. 30 mL in subarachnoid space—why we don't aspirate CSF during lumbar puncture
     b. CSF produced at 21–22 mL per hour
        i. To reduce CSF production: acetazolamide (50%), ethacrynic acid with furosemide (25% in animals), or both (75%, again animal data); active secretion of CSF requires Na/K, ATPase pump
        ii. CSF production changes by 7% for each 1% change in osmolality (in animals)
  2. CSF resorption occurs through arachnoid villi, which are primarily located on the superior sagittal sinus.
  3. Normal pressure (adults) is <150 mm CSF, H_2O indeterminate 150 to 200, abnormal > 200; may be slightly higher in obese patients
     a. Opening pressure is measured in lateral decubitus; there is no reason not to get an opening pressure; if patient is sitting up, lay patient down when you get CSF
     b. Elevations seen in CSF during infections fluctuate considerably.
     c. Normal pressure in infancy is about 100
     d. Elevated by Valsalva, decreased by hyperventilation, no change in pregnancy; prior to measure, make certain legs are straight and patient is relaxed

B. **Lumbar puncture**
  1. Herniation
     a. Normally lumbar puncture (LP) causes a transient decrease in CSF pressure
     b. Space-occupying lesions have a relative pressure gradient
        i. LP can cause herniation through increasing this pressure gradient
        ii. If it happens, it does not usually happen immediately, rather it happens in the ensuing hours as CSF drains through the puncture hole
        iii. Risk of herniation following LP with brain abscess is about 15%
  2. Get a blood glucose immediately before the LP
  3. In absence of focal neurologic examination with normal mental state and no papilledema, perform LP immediately
  4. Start empiric treatment; do not delay as morbidity and mortality is directly related to how long patient waits before antibiotics are initiated; treat as is for bacterial meningitis

C. **CSF appearance**
  1. Color should be clear
     a. Turbid or opalescent = white blood cells (WBCs) 200/mm^3, red blood cells (RBCs) 400/mm^3
     b. Cloudy and xanthochromic or pinkish with 400 to 6,000 RBC/mm^3
     c. Bloody if > 6,000 RBC/mm^3
     d. Xanthochromia means yellowish
        i. It usually, but not always, appears 2 to 4 hours after subarachnoid hemorrhage
        ii. Caused by hemoglobin, protein >150 mg/dL, or serum bilirubin >10 mg/dL
  2. Should flow like water—can be more viscous with carcinoma, cryptococcosis, Tb

D. **How much CSF and what to order?**
  1. Medical residents rarely send enough fluid to get good results in aseptic meningitis.
  2. Tube 1: cell count (0.5 mL) with differential (0.5 to 4.5mL)

3. Tube 2: Gram staining (0.25 mL), glucose and protein (0.5 mL). Acid-fast bacillus (AFB) (0.25 mL) If your laboratory will do a acridine orange stain, then, it should always be asked for (0.25 mL). Always ask for an acridine orange stain also as it is more sensitive for finding bacteria and your laboratory will not do it unless specifically asked.
4. Tube 3: Cultures go here: bacterial culture (0.5 mL to 5 mL—the more fluid, the higher yield), aseptic meningitis: AFB smear and mycobacterial culture/India ink and fungal cultures (as much as you can get—recommended amount is 20 mL), viral culture (2 mL), polymerase chain reaction (PCR) (0.5 to 1 mL per PCR)
5. Tube 4: Special tests: VDRL (0.5 mL), Cryptococcus antigen (0.5 mL), fluorescence treponemal antibody (FTA) (0.25 mL)
6. You should expect to tap about three times in aseptic meningitis
7. The cell count is somewhat unreliable after about 30 to 60 minutes, so CSF specimen should be hand delivered/tubed to the proper laboratory tech immediately
8. Remember that the risk of postlumbar puncture headache is not correlated with amount of fluid withdrawn, so take as much as you need.

E. **Bacterial meningitis**
1. Neonate: 50% Gram-negative bacilli, 25% group B *Streptococcus*, 10% Listeria, 5% *Staphylococcus*
2. Children: 50% *Haemophilus influenzae* flu, 30% *Neisseria*, 15% *Streptococcus pneumoniae*
3. Adults (>15 years): 40% *S. pneumoniae*, 25% *Neisseria*, 10% *Staphylococcus*, 5% *Streptococcus*
4. 15,000 cases per year in United States
5. Begin treatment as soon as LP done with ceftriaxone intravenous (IV) 2 g every 12 hours (can also use cefotaxime, but have to dose more frequently and may have to adjust for creatinine clearance); all patients should get dexamethasone (DSM) IV 0.15 mg/kg every 6 hours for 4 days and 15 minutes prior to antibiotics, unless you are sure of the organism; this is not a choice, unless you wish to defend yourself in court, as DSM blocks tumor necrosis factor (TNF) production and its use is supported by convincing evidence-based medicine. Although vancomycin has erratic and low CSF penetration, all patients should receive this agent as well: 15 mg/kg (max 750 mg) every 6 hours; course should be 14 days and never switch to oral meds.
6. Some notes for specific situations:
   a. Elderly, alcoholic, or immunocompromised—add ampicillin IV 2 g every 4 hours
   b. Head trauma/postneurosurgery—use ceftazidime instead of ceftriaxone and no steroids
   c. Shunt infection (adult)—use rifampin in place of ceftriaxone and no steroids; if child, as bacterial meningitis, just don't use dexamethasone
7. Complications of meningitis include: hydrocephalus, stroke, syndrome of inappropriate antidiuretic hormone secretion (SIADH), empyema, abscess, seizures, cranial nerve dysfunction (CN VII most likely affected), disseminated intravascular coagulation (DIC) (think meningococcus); ventriculitis possible in neonates
8. CSF results (see Table 14.1)

Table 14-1: CFS Results

Condition	Opening pressure (cm H$_2$0)	Cells	Protein	Glucose as % of serum	Miscellaneous
Normal	7-18, up to 25 if obese	0-5 monos, PMN never nl 1 anything	15-45	50-66	Clear colorless
Traumatic		700 RBCs; 1 WBC	Slight increase		Subtract 1 mg/dL protein per 1,000 RBC
Subarachnoid hemorrhage	Increased	Initially RBCs, Later WBCs	50-400 50-800		Bloody RBCs replaced by xanthochromia in 2 weeks
Bacterial meningitis	Often increased	To 50,000 WBCs; mostly PMNs; monos = partially treated	100-1,000	Less than 40	Turbid lactic acid >= 3.5 mmol/L C-reactive protein 99% sensitive
Aseptic meningitis	Increased if herpes	To 450 WBCs; mostly monos; early PMNs	40-100		PCR sens/spec >90% for herpes
Fungal meningitis	Often increased	30-300 monos	100-700	Less than 30	Opalescent *Cryptococcus* + India ink
TB meningitis	Often increased	50-500 monos, lymphocytes; PMN early	60-700	20-40	Can be opalescent +AFB
Parameningeal infection	If increased then blocked	0-800 WBCs	Any		
Multiple sclerosis		5-50 monos	15-800		IgG with oligoclonal bands
Polio		Pleocytosis	40-100		Muscle pain relieved by exercise
Guillain-Barré		Normal or 10-50 monos	Anything possible		> 2.5 g/dL protein ⇒ cord compression
Sarcoid		6-200 lymphs	Usually <200		+ACE, Increased IgG
Syphilis		200-300	40-200 can include plasma cells		+VDRL +FTA 10% of taps are contaminated by blood ⇒ false +

If box empty = identical to normal tap.

ACE, angiotensin-converting enzyme; FTA, fluorescent treponemal antigen; monos, monocytes; IgE, immunoglob-

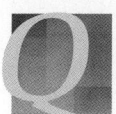 STUDY QUESTIONS FOR CHAPTER 14

Directions: *Each of the numbered items or incomplete statements in this section is followed by answers or by completions of the statement. Select the ONE lettered answer or completion that is BEST in each case.*

1. A 63-year-old man is admitted with new-onset headache and confusion. He has an emergent CT, which is negative. He has a lumbar puncture, which grows *Streptococcus pneumoniae*. After 2 days of treatment the patient is not oriented to place, but is otherwise not confused. He has a follow-up lumbar puncture that shows: RBCs 456 cells/mm^3 WBCs 1,000 cells/mm^3, neutrophils 60%, monocytes 40%. What do you do?

(A) Nothing as this is an expected finding.
(B) Nothing until sensitivity results return, but this is not an expected finding.
(C) Patient not being covered adequately by antibiotics and you would broaden coverage.
(D) This result has no meaning.

2. During a spinal surgery, when the dura is initially opened, the neurosurgeon will stop a gushing of fluid. Why?

(A) Practice
(B) Safety as subarachnoid space can transmit pressure differences
(C) Safety as subarachnoid space will be affected by rapid loss of fluid.
(D) Class 1 (randomized controlled trials) evidence-based medicine

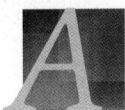

ANSWERS AND EXPLANATIONS

1. A. This LP suggests partially treated meningitis, so is expected. B. This is expected. C. There is no need to broaden coverage if patient is responding. D. Distracter.

2. B. The subarachnoid space has only 30 mL of fluid at any one time, so rapid volume loss will cause a large pressure gradient, which can be detrimental. Both A and C are true, but B is what explains the practice. D. Neurosurgery has almost no Class 1 evidence-based medicine.

CHAPTER 15

Neoplasm

I. Introduction

In 2003, the American Cancer Society (ACA) reported the diagnosis of almost 17,000 primary brain tumors, and in that same year the mortality from these tumors resulted in approximately 13,000 deaths. Primary central nervous system (CNS) tumors have surpassed acute lymphocytic leukemia as the most common pediatric cancer. In addition, the overall incidence of several major types of CNS tumors has been reported to be increasing; whether this increase is real or artifactual is a matter of debate but the trends are certainly alarming.

II. Pathophysiology

The pathophysiology of CNS tumors is unique in oncology: survival depends on local control of the primary tumor not the elimination of distant metastasis. For this reason the terms benign and malignant are not applicable to tumors of the CNS and in there place terms such as high grade and low grade are used, which are indications of a tumor's potential for growth. In addition, most histologically benign CNS tumors extensively invade normal tissues. Standard TNM tumor staging is also of little value as CNS tumors rarely metastasize out of the CNS itself. Nodal involvement is also rare, as the CNS lacks lymphatics. Generally, CNS tumors exert their effects and hence present in one of two ways, either as a result of mass effect or as a consequence of their involving critical brain structures.

A. Physiologically, tumors differ from the surrounding "normal" brain tissue in several distinct ways: first, tumors secrete angiogenic factors that stimulate neovascularization. This neovascularization is highly permeable, lacking the "normal" blood–brain barrier; in addition, these tumors are hypervascular and very edematous, consistent with local inflammatory cytokine excess. This neovascularization has several diagnostic and therapeutic implications. Diagnostically, contrast-enhanced imagining yields a highly visible enhancing lesion, and diffusion-weighted MRI techniques are capable of identifying lesions based on their edematous nature. From a therapeutic standpoint, chemotherapeutics, which do not normally cross the blood–brain barrier, may access the tumor cells. In addition, since tumors of the CNS exert their effects through or as a result of their mass, and tumors are by nature edematous and inflamed, steroid therapy typically results in significant mass reduction and reprieve from recently acquired symptomatology.

B. As noted previously, even benign-appearing CNS tumors almost always extensively infiltrate normal tissues, the implications of this make curative resection largely unachievable. Moreover, these same tumors have also been found clinically to be resistant to broad sterilizing fields of radiation and insensitive to chemotherapeutic regimens. Prognostic factors for primary CNS tumors include tumor grade, histopathologic characteristics such as high mitotic indices, neovascularization and local necrosis are all poor prognostic features; moreover, location of the lesion, patient age, performance status, extent of the patient's surgical resection, and sensitivity of tumor to radiation and chemotherapeutic modalities have all been show to be prognostic indicators. Surgical resection can in fact be curative for meningiomas and ependymomas, whereas resection is never curative for malignant glioma. Children fare better than adults with malignant glioma; conversely, adults with brainstem gliomas fare better than children.

III. Epidemiologic Considerations

CNS tumors have a male predominance, with approximately 9,500 new cases of primary CNS tumors reported by the ACA in 2003 versus 7,000 new cases among women. Primary CNS tumors are more than twice as common as Hodgkin disease and with few exceptions are largely incurable. Noteworthy is the fact that the number of primary CNS tumors is dwarfed by the number of metastatic brain and spinal lesions. It has been estimated that in excess of 100,000 people this year will have been found to have an asymptomatic metastatic brain lesion. In addition, an estimated 80,000 cases of spinal cord compression secondary to metastatic disease will occur each year. Epidemiologic evidence has only identified two known environmental risk factors for developing tumors of the CNS: exposure to ionizing radiation and immunosuppression.

IV. Genetics

Five percent of all primary CNS tumors are associated with a known hereditable syndrome.

A. In addition to the hereditary immunodeficiency syndromes like Wiskott-Aldrich syndrome, which predispose one to developing CNS lymphoma, the various heritable syndromes associated with the deletion of known tumor suppressor genes, in addition to the related systemic syndromes, often predisposes one to developing primary tumors of the CNS.
   1. As many as 15% of patients with neurofibromatosis type 1 will develop gliomas, in addition to their added predisposition to developing schwannomas, meningiomas, and ependymomas.
   2. See Table 15-1 for specific associations.

B. The tumor suppressor genes associated with primary tumors of the CNS are as diverse as the many syndromes with which they are associated and include, *p53, VHL1, RB, NF-1, TSC-1, TSC-2, NF2, MENIN, PTCH, APC, hMLH1, hMLH2, hPMS2, PTEN, hSNFS*, and *INI1*. Moreover, 7% of individuals with newly diagnosed glioma, lacking any known predisposing syndrome, have

Table 15-1 *Associations between Genetic Syndromes and Tumors*

Syndrome	Tumor
Neurofibromatosis II	Meningioma, schwannoma, ependymoma
Von Hippel Lindau	CNS hemangioblastoma
Li-Fraumeni	Many including glioma, medulloblastoma
Tuberous sclerosis	Subendymal giant cell astrocytoma, cortical tuber, and glioma
Gorlin syndrome (basal cell nevus syndrome)	Medulloblastoma
Turcot syndrome (hereditary nonpolyposis colorectal cancer syndrome)	Many including glioblastoma and medulloblastoma
Cowden syndrome	Gangliocytoma, meningioma, astrocytoma
Rhabdoid predisposition syndrome	Primitive neuroendocrine tumors, medulloblastoma, choroids plexus tumors

been found to have a first degree relative who has also been diagnosed with glioma, strongly implying the existence of other, as yet to be characterized, tumor syndromes.

V. Presentation

Presentation is the following usually the result of the tumor causing local irritation (often resulting in seizures); compression of a blood vessel and resultant ischemia, obstruction of CSF pathway resulting in hydrocephalus, or most unfortunately, with mass effect resulting in herniation.

A. New headaches are the most common presentation of patients with brain tumors and in 40% of patients this is their first symptom. Headaches secondary to brain tumors are characteristically present upon awakening; initially headache resolves within an hour and may be followed immediately by emesis. The headaches are often characteristically worse with increased intracranial pressure such as that caused by coughing or sneezing. This is in contrast to migraine headaches, which often awaken the patient and may be followed several hours later by emesis. Lateralized headaches are an accurate predictor of tumor laterality. Headache as sole symptom is rarely caused by brain neoplasm.

B. The second most common presentation of brain tumors is with seizure. Tumors presenting initially with seizure typically reside in or around the motor strip or the temporal lobe, and typically tumors presenting with seizure either compress the cortex as with meningiomas or cause local irritation.

C. Other symptoms include transient blurry vision secondary to papillary edema, depression, panic attacks, emotional changes and/or other mental status changes including apathy and irritability. In addition, in patients with episodic hemiparalysis or episodic aphasia, a CNS tumor should be suspected. Tumors of the CNS may also present with false localizing phenomena resulting from the shifting of cerebral structures and resultant nerve compression or herniation.

VI. Diagnosis of Primary CNS Tumors

Diagnosis of primary CNS tumors is strongly implied by radiographic imaging, although obtaining a biopsy to obtain a tissue diagnosis is essential in making the definitive diagnosis of cancer, a must before therapy can proceed.

A. The gold standard radiographic test to rule out a tumor of the CNS is contrast-enhanced MRI. The sensitivity of this test is exquisitely high, much higher than that of computed tomography (CT). Tumors can be placed into three broad categories: extradural, intradural, and intra- and extraaxial. These categories permit relative broad differentials to be made (Table 15-2). Tumors, with their higher water content and surrounding edema appear as hypointense lesions on T1-weighted images and as hyperintense lesions on T2-weighted images. Moreover, in the case of hemorrhage, contrast will leak from the vasculature and appear as a hyperintense lesion on T1-weighted imaging and usually as a hypointense lesion on T2-weighted images. In addition, radiographic presentation can often distinguish between metastatic lesions, low-grade gliomas, and high-grade gliomas.

B. Metastatic lesions have a regular spherical rim on imaging and often with multiple lesions, low-grade gliomas often lack surrounding edema and hence have clear well-defined nonenhancing borders; high-grade gliomas often have a contrast-enhancing rim with an irregular shape and thickness surrounding a hypointense lesion on T1-weighted imaging.

C. In the event that an MRI is not available or is contraindicated, contrast-enhanced computed tomography (CT) is the next best screening tool, CT scans do an excellent job of picking up calcification and spicules typically associated with neoplastic lesions.

Table 15-2	CNS Tumors
Tumor location	Tumors
Extradural	Metastatic neoplasm esp. Leukemia, Non-Hodgkin's Lymphoma, Multiple Myeloma, Osteosarcoma
Intradural–extraaxial	Meningioma Pituitary adenoma Acoustic neuroma Chordoma Choroid plexus papillomas Primary CNS lymphoma Metastatic neoplasm Cysts—arachnoid, dermoid, epidermoid Sarcoid
Intradural–intra-axial	Astrocytoma: includes pilocytic, giant cell, pleomorphic xanthoastrocytoma, anaplastic, glioblastoma Diffuse cerebral gliomatosis, diffuse pontine glioma Brainstem glioma Hemangioblastoma Oligodendroglioma Medulloblastoma Ependymoma Pineal germ cell tumor Colloid cyst Primary CNS lymphoma Metastatic neoplasm

D. **Following appropriate imaging**, biopsy and tissue diagnosis are necessary; the only exception is primary CNS lymphomas or leukemia, whereby a lumber puncture may yield sufficient malignant cells to make the definitive diagnosis.

VII. Following the Diagnosis

Following diagnosis treatment options need to be explored, including surgery, radiotherapy, chemotherapy, and symptomatic treatment with steroids and anticonvulsants.

A. **Following the diagnosis of a CNS tumor**, almost all symptomatic patients are started on steroids, typically dexamethasone initiated at 10 mg intravenous (IV) push, then 6 mg every 6 hours (10 mg every 6 hours for severe vasogenic edema). Steroids decrease inflammation, local edema, and support the restoration of the blood–brain barrier. Steroids decrease intracranial pressure, both by decreasing net tumor volume and decreasing flux of solute in cranium through the tumor's leaky vasculature. Patients often achieve excellent resolution of their symptoms within 1 to 2 days. Doses are typically tapered to the lowest effective dosage.

B. **Surgery remains the first-line treatment** of primary CNS tumors, providing immediate resolution of symptoms, and, although rarely curative, aggressive surgical resection improves both the quality of life and the quantity of life that remains.

C. **Typically following surgery**, or in the nonsurgical patient, radiation therapy is initiated. Although brain tumors are relatively radioresistant, radiation therapy has been shown to further extend both quality and quantity of life for the patient. Radiotherapy is typically delivered to a limited field comprised primarily of the tumor bed and its immediate surroundings, with dosages typically reaching 60 Gy divided into 30 daily fractions. Stereotactic radiosurgery may play an important role in the treatment of brain tumors in the future, but with the exception of metastatic lesions, data are still lacking.

D. Patients are placed on appropriate chemotherapy, that is, a lipophilic agent with good CNS penetration, which classically has been carmustine (BCNU), although other agents have also been used. Currently, newer agents such as temozolomide have come into favor because it is well tolerated, administered in pill form, and in limited studies has been shown to be superior to traditional chemotherapeutics in treating recurrent tumors.

E. Finally, anticonvulsant therapy is both necessary and effective in treating patients with brain tumors who have had at least one seizure. Valproate, carbamazepine, and phenytoin have all been shown to be effective; moreover, these agents may also be initiated prophylactically perioperatively to reduce the incidence of perioperative seizure.

F. The goal of therapy in the patient with a primary tumor of the CNS is usually directed toward improving the quality and quantity of life, that is, an interval of time in which the patient feels "well," as most of these lesions are not curable even with the most aggressive treatment plans.

VIII. Astrocytic Tumors

Astrocytic tumors are currently classified using a grading system devised by the World Health Organization (WHO). Pilocytic astrocytoma, astrocytoma, anaplastic astrocytoma, and glioblastoma are currently assigned WHO grades 1 through 4, respectively. This progressive grading system, based on pathologic criteria, has shown good correlation between tumor grade and prognosis. The following highlights a few features of each WHO grade.

A. WHO grade I pilocytic astrocytomas are focal tumors that typically contain Rosenthal fibers and piloid cells on tissue diagnosis

B. WHO grade II astrocytomas are diffuse tumors that typically have nuclear atypia

C. WHO grade III anaplastic astrocytomas have an increased fraction of mitotic cells

D. WHO grade IV glioblastoma is differentiated by any of florid vascular proliferation, hemorrhage, or necrosis; 5% will have pleomorphic multinucleated giant cells

E. The St. Anne/Mayo classification scheme is similar and is better at predicting mortality (Table 15-3).

F. Radiographically, low-grade tumors (WHO grades I and II) appear with T1-weighted imaging as a nonenhancing area of somewhat diffuse hyperintensity beginning immediately below the cortex, whereas high grade tumors (WHO grades III and IV tumors) typically appear as irregularly shaped, ring-enhancing lesions having irregular border thickness with surrounding edema.

Table 15-3 *St. Anne/Mayo Grading of Astrocytic Tumors*

Tumor	Grade	Criteria fulfilled
Pilocytic astrocytoma	excluded	
Astrocytoma	1	No criteria
	2	1 criterion usually nuclear atypia
Anaplastic astrocytoma	3	2 criteria usually nuclear atypia and mitosis
Glioblastoma multiforme	4	3 or 4 criteria including one or both of necrosis and endothelial proliferation

G. **High-grade diffuse astrocytic tumors** most typically present with a headache and/or mental status and personality changes; on neurologic examination focal deficits are usually present. Low-grade lesions more often present with seizure and/or other focal deficits.

H. **Differential diagnosis** includes diffuse astrocytomas; oligodendroglioma, focal astrocytotic tumors, metastasis, multiple sclerosis, cerebral infarct, and brain abscess. Of note, differentiating a high-grade astrocytoma from demyelinating disease is very difficult and may require biopsy; an incomplete ring of enhancement is one of the most distinguishing radiographic features of demyelinating disease versus a high-grade diffuse astrocytic tumor.

I. **Tissue diagnosis** is absolutely necessary and is typically achieved by open resection, although stereotactic needle biopsy is alternatively used when the diagnosis is in doubt or in the nonsurgical patient. The definitive treatment of these tumors involves complete gross resection, as determined by a postsurgical MRI, followed by radiation therapy to a limited field encompassing the tumor bed with 2 to 3 cm margins to a total dose of between 50 and 60 gray divided over 30 fractions. Within the given range, larger doses and larger margins are typically utilized for higher-grade tumors. Following radiation therapy these patients are typically started on chemotherapy, most commonly BCNU or temozolomide, although multidrug regimens are also used with equivalent efficacy. The inevitable tumor recurrence may be treated with stereotactic radiosurgery and/or an alternative chemotherapeutic agent.

J. **Prognosis for diffuse astrocytic tumors** is terminal, with an approximate median survival of 1 year for glioblastomas, 3 years for anaplastic astrocytomas, and 4 years for astrocytomas, whereas 80% with pilocytic astrocytoma achieve long-term survival.

K. **Astrocytic tumors** constitute 60% of clinically significant primary brain tumors.

IX. Oligodendrogliomas

Oligodendrogliomas represent another major group of primary CNS tumors. These tumors often appear in the young and middle aged, most commonly arising in the frontal cortex, are slow-growing in nature, and are uniquely chemo and radiosensitive, unlike their astrocytic counterparts.

A. **These tumors most commonly present** with seizures, and as is true for other tumors of the CNS, MRI is the initial test of choice.

B. **Oligodendrogliomas** may appear on MRI as a heterogeneous mass similar to astrocytomas; generally they do not enhance but their high-grade counterpart, anaplastic oligodendrogliomas, do enhance. A CT scan is often useful in differentiating from astrocytic tumors, as oligodendrogliomas often have numerous calcifications.

C. **Biopsy is necessary** to make a diagnosis; histologically there may be no definitive way to distinguish these tumors from astrocytomas, although cells with a "fried egg" appearance are characteristic of oligodendrogliomas. WHO grading of these tumors is similar to that for astrocytomas, with anaplasia and the presence of mitosis characteristic of higher-grade lesions. Definitive treatment of low-grade oligodendrogliomas is gross total resection; no further treatment is necessary. In the event of recurrence, higher-grade lesions, or subtotal resection, additional therapy consisting of radiation (as described for astrocytomas) and chemotherapy (typically a multidrug regimen consisting of vincristine, lomustine [CCNU], and procarbazine). Prognosis for patients with low-grade oligodendrogliomas is good, with mean survival of 10 years; the anaplastic variant carries a much grimmer prognosis and is comparable to glioblastoma.

X. Meningiomas

Meningiomas are the most common tumor of the meninges and account for 20% of all clinically significant primary CNS tumors.

A. These tumors have a peak incidence of 45 years of age and occur more frequently in women. The female predominance of these tumors may in part be explained by the tumor's frequent expression of the progesterone receptor. There is an association between meningioma and breast cancers.

B. In addition, the NF-2 gene has been found to be mutated in as many as 60% of all meningiomas, and multiple meningioma is highly suggestive of neurofibromatosis.

C. Meningiomas are largely benign slow-growing tumors; only 5% of all meningiomas are classified as high grade, that is, anaplastic or frankly malignant. They may undergo sarcomatous degeneration and may not recur. May also grow into venous sinus.

D. Meningiomas typically present with seizure.

E. Imaging of meningiomas iso to hypeintensity in both T1- and hypertensity in T2-weighted imaging and enhances intensely with contrast. There is typically no surrounding edema, and the presence of a dural tail that spreads from the tumor is pathognomonic for these tumors. Meningiomas are frequently calcified and induce a thickening of their overlying bony structures, called hyperostosis, identifiable even on plain films of the skull.

F. Definitive diagnosis is by biopsy.

G. Treatment may be limited to watchful waiting in a tumor the symptoms of which, typically seizures, can be controlled with antiseizure medication, as many of these tumors simply stop growing, and the risk of definitive surgical resection outweighs the risk of medical management. If definitive treatment is needed, gross total resection is indicated and, when successful, no further treatment is necessary. In the advent of subtotal resection, postoperative radiotherapy to a limited field is indicated and is highly effective at achieving local tumor control. Stereotactic radiosurgery is possibly the preferred definitive therapy for tumors <3 cm greatest dimension, having the benefit to the patient of being noninvasive.

H. Prognosis is >98% disease-specific survival 5 years following diagnosis.

XI. Benign and Spinal Tumors

A. **Pituitary adenoma** divided into micro- (<10 mm) and macroadenomas (>10 mm)
   1. They are benign epithelial tumors arising from the adenohypophysis.
   2. 75% secrete hormones—10% secrete more than one
      a. Prolactin is the most common (40%), producing amenorrhea, galactorrhea, and infertility
      b. Growth hormone (20%) produces acromegaly or giantism
      c. Adrenocorticotropic hormone (ACTH, 17%) produces Cushing disease
   3. 25% of tumors do not secrete hormones and present due to compression causing initial bitemporal superior quadrantopia and later bitemporal hemianopsia; the tumor can compress normal pituitary tissue causing panhypopituitarism, can invade the cavernous sinus, can compress the foramen of Munro, and cause pituitary hemorrhage
   4. When there is good evidence for tumor and an MRI is negative, positron emission tomographic (PET) scan will detect many missed adenomas
   5. Treatment is bromocriptine for prolactinoma or transsphenoidal resection in ACTH and macroadenomas that produce symptoms.

B. **Colloid cysts** have variable MR findings, but have an epithelial wall that can be visualized and are located in the third ventricle, making identification virtually unmistakable. May cause nonlocalized intracranial hypertension and hydrocephalus. Surgical resection is curative.

C. **Spinal tumors**
   1. Nerve sheath tumors most common spinal tumor
      a. Most frequent symptoms pain and radiculopathy
      b. Schwannoma are Schwann cells that do not envelop adjacent nerve root, so they appear as masses that project from the nerve. They often have decreased T2 in the center. Frequently arise from the eighth cranial nerve; if vestibular branch, called acoustic neuroma. The earliest symptom is hearing loss. Bilateral acoustic neuromas are pathognomonic for *NF-2*. Treatment is watchful waiting with frequent audiometry, surgical removal which means permanent deafness, or, in specialized centers, multichannel auditory brainstem implantation.
      c. Neurofibroma path fibroblasts: Schwann cells amidst nerve cells and a matrix of mucopolysaccharides that creates the characteristic swelling
      d. Malignant degeneration in 10%; malignant schwannomas don't have central decreased T2
   2. Gliomas represent some 20% of spinal tumors.
   3. Ependymomas are discussed in subsequent section (XII).
   4. Metastatic intraparenchymal or metastatic spinal leptomeningeal tumor

XII. Tumors Predominantly Affecting Children

See Table 15-4 for the most common tumors with their localization. See Table 15-5 for imaging characteristics of infratentorial tumors, which are asked about often.

Table 15-4 *Most Common Tumors of Childhood*

Fossa	Neoplasm
Infratentorial (70%)	Medulloblastoma
	Cystic cerebellar astrocytoma
	Brainstem glioma
	Ependymoma
Supratentorial (30%)	Craniopharyngioma
	Pineal tumor

Table 15-5 *Imaging of the Most Common Childhood Posterior Fossa Tumors*

Tumor	Pilocytic astrocytoma	Medulloblastoma	Ependymoma	Diffuse pontine glioma
T1	Tumor = brain, cyst = CSF	⇓	⇓ Heterogenous	=
T2	Tumor = brain, cyst = CSF	=	Heterogenous	⇑ Poor definition
Proton density	Both ⇑	⇑	⇓ Heterogenous	⇑
Enhancement	Tumor, yes	Dense	Yes, irregular	⇑⇓
Hemorrhage	Unusual	Unusual	Common	Common
Calcium	Common	Unusual	Common	Unusual

=, isointense; ⇑, hyperintense (bright); ⇓, hypointense (dark); ⇑⇓, variable.

A. **Medulloblastoma:** most common primary central nervous system malignancy among children, constituting 20% of childhood CNS tumors; medulloblastoma per WHO is an embryonal tumor of uncertain cellular lineage; arise from floor of fourth ventricle
   1. The peak incidence of these tumors occurs between the ages of 5 and 8 years, with a 2:1 male predominance; a second incidence peak occurs in young adults ages 20 to 30 years and accounts for 20% of medulloblastomas.
   2. This tumor typically presents with symptoms consistent with hydrocephalus secondary to obstruction of the fourth ventricle and include headaches, nausea, and vomiting. Because these tumors almost always arise in the vermis of the cerebellum, additional signs and symptoms include gait ataxia sparing the extremities, dizziness, vertigo, and nystagmus.
   3. MRI typically demonstrates an enhancing lesion, characteristically located in the cerebellar vermis, on T1-weighted imaging. Biopsy of the lesion shows a poorly differentiated neuroectodermal neoplastic cells, often demonstrating characteristic Homer-Wright rosettes and/or palisading tumor cells. Definitive treatment consists of gross total resection when technically feasible followed by irradiation to the entire neuronal axis, necessitated by the predilection of these tumors to spread throughout the CNS, and chemotherapy again, typically consisting of vincristine, CCNU, and procarbazine.

B. **Pilocytic astrocytoma and brainstem glioma** are detailed in the section on astrocytoma.
   1. Pilocytic astrocytomas are usually cystic, arising in the lateral cerebellar hemispheres. Symptoms usually include ipsilateral appendicular ataxia and head tilt toward lesion.
   2. Brainstem glioma usually arises in mid pons and is found predominantly in late childhood and adolescence.

C. **Ependymoma** benign, ependymal cells, original from roof of fourth ventricle
   1. Usually in childhood, intraparenchymal and in adulthood, intraspinal.
   2. Symptoms usually mental status changes and frontal lobe signs from hydrocephalus from fourth ventricular compression—most common site
   3. 10% have plastic ependymoma extension through foramina creating projections that compress tonsils and/or upper cervical cord
   4. Histology with pseudorosettes and rosettes; on imaging, nearly one half calcified
   5. Prognosis related to location and extent of surgical resection
   6. Subependymomas are benign mixed tumors containing both astrocytes and ependymal cells located intraventricularly, usually fourth ventricle, usually incidental findings at autopsy; rare in children

D. **Craniopharyngioma**
   1. Sella turcica, suprasellar cistern, third ventricle
   2. Two types
      a. Adamantinomatous usually childhood, almost always cystic, frequently calcify
         i. Arise from epithelial tissue of Rathke pouch or adenohypophysis
         ii. Pathology is clumps of wet keratin with dystrophic calcification, cholesterol crystals in the cystic fluid; often invades adjacent brain-provoking gliosis
      b. Papillary—squamous tissue, usually adult encapsulated, solid, third ventricle; originate in hypothalamus; cause hypopituitarism and initially inferior bitemporal hemianopsia; cause suprasellar calcification; are cystic
   3. Treatment for both is surgical
   4. Suprasellar region

E. **Pineal tumors**
   1. Pineal germ cell tumors
      a. Most common pineal tumor is germinoma (half of all pineal tumors) which is 90% male, typically adolescent, composed of large spherical epithelial cells, separated by reticular connective tissue
         i. Symptoms due to three mechanisms: (1) most tested is hypothalamic involvement causing growth failure and diabetes insipidus, precocious puberty possible, but the

most common symptoms are (2) hydrocephalus causing intracranial hypertension and (3) diencephalon–midbrain compression causing Parinaud syndrome
- ii. Check α-fetal protein to detect choriocarcinoma and β human chorionic gonadotropin (β-hCG) to detect either choriocarcinoma or immature (i.e., malignant) teratoma.
- iii. Exquisitely radiosensitive, so very high rates of survival even if widely metastatic
   b. Second most common pineal tumor is teratoma, with all three cell types
      - i. Usually appear during childhood, almost always cystic
2. Pineal cell tumors are neuroepithelial tumors arising from pineal gland
   a. Pineocytoma usually in adults, solid tumor, aggressiveness depends on differentiation; enhances homogenously
   b. Pineoblastoma highly cellular infiltrative similar to medulloblastoma, Flexner–Wintersteiner rosettes (lumen is surrounded by neoplastic cells with cytoplasmic extensions), disseminates early
      - i. Trilateral retinoblastoma is bilateral retinoblastoma and pineoblastoma.
3. Pineal cysts asymptomatic even if large; present in about one third of routine autopsies; must be distinguished from pineal tumors; they are round, smoothly marginated, and homogenous on MR imaging; proton-weighting can be markedly increased; do not enhance, except for residual pineal tissue; these are easily recognized by MRI

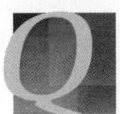 # STUDY QUESTIONS FOR CHAPTER 15

Directions: *Each of the numbered items or incomplete statements in this section is followed by answers or by completions of the statement. Select the ONE lettered answer or completion that is BEST in each case.*

1. You are asked to see a 43-year-old woman for treatment of a glioblastoma multiforme. Which of the following is true concerning the epidemiology of CNS tumors?
   (A) They are more common in men than in women.
   (B) They are equally common in men and women.
   (C) Smoking is a risk factor for development of brain tumors.
   (D) There are no known risk factors for development of brain tumors.
   (E) They are more common than metastatic disease.

2. A 47-year-old woman is referred to your care for management of meningioma. She is one of six family members to have this tumor. Which of the following genetic syndromes is associated with meningioma?
   (A) Cowden
   (B) Gorlin
   (C) Li-Fraumeni
   (D) Turcot
   (E) Von Hippel-Lindau

3. In reviewing the neuropathology of a tumor of a 54-year-old man with a glioma, the neuropathologist points out increased mitotic cells, hemorrhage, and necrosis. What is the World Health Organization (WHO) histologic grade of this tumor?
   (A) Grade I
   (B) Grade II
   (C) Grade III
   (D) Grade IV

4. A 7-year-old boy is under your treatment for medulloblastoma. Which of the following is true concerning this tumor?
   (A) The peak incidence is in children younger than 5 years
   (B) There is a second peak in patients in their 50s
   (C) There is a 2:1 male-to-female predominance ratio
   (D) It is the most common posterior fossa tumor in children after hemangioblastoma
   (E) It most commonly arises in the cerebellar hemispheres

5. A 71-year-old woman comes to your clinic because she is concerned that she has a brain tumor. She has developed persistent frontal headaches over the last 3 months. Which of the following is the most common presentation of brain tumor in adults?
   (A) Headache
   (B) Hemiparesis
   (C) Increased intracranial pressure
   (D) Seizures
   (E) Weight loss

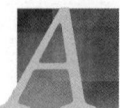# ANSWERS AND EXPLANATIONS

1. A. Central nervous system tumors are slightly more common in men than in women. Risk factors for developing tumors of the CNS are exposure to ionizing radiation and immunosuppression. Smoking is not a recognized risk factor. There are approximately 180,000 metastatic CNS tumors per year, compared to about 16,000 primary tumors.

2. A. Cowden syndrome is associated with gangliocytomas, meningiomas, and astrocytomas. Gorlin syndrome is basal cell nevus syndrome in association with medulloblastoma. Li-Fraumeni is associated with an increased risk of gliomas and medulloblastomas. Turcot syndrome is hereditary nonpolyposis colorectal cancer syndrome associated with glioblastoma and medulloblastoma. Von Hippel-Lindau syndrome is associated with hemangioblastoma of the CNS.

3. D. The presence of hemorrhage and necrosis qualifies this tumor as WHO grade IV. Grades I, II, and III do not have necrosis. Enhanced mitotic activity distinguishes anaplastic (grade III) from grade II.

4. C. Medulloblastoma is about twice as common in boys as in girls. Its peak incidence is in children between ages 5 and 8 years, with a second peak in young adults ages 20 to 30 years. Medulloblastoma is the most common posterior fossa tumor in children and usually arises from the vermis rather than from the cerebellar hemispheres.

5. A. Headache is the most common presentation of brain tumor in adults, but it is accompanied by other meurological dysfunction. This is followed by seizures. The other causes listed are less common presentations.

CHAPTER 16

Headache and Pain

I. Headache Epidemiology

Headache occurs in more than 90% of the population at some time in their life.

A. Migraine and chronic headaches are common causes of morbidity and disability; disruption of relationships and comorbidity (psychiatric, neurologic, and pain) are common; tension headaches: frontal ⇒ sinus, temporal ⇒ TMJ, neck ⇒ cervical.

B. Misdiagnosis of migraine occurs frequently and causes delay in treatment. Most common misdiagnoses are tension-type headache and sinus headache due to prominent neck and facial pain, respectively. If patient misses work or school, most likely migraine.

II. International Headache Society Classification/Diagnosis

A. Developed to standardize headache diagnosis for research studies

B. Used in clinical practice as guideline. The following represents selected useful points.

C. Primary headache categories
  1. **Migraine without aura:** at least five attacks; headache attacks last 4 to 72 hours (untreated or unsuccessfully treated); includes at least two of the following: unilateral location, pulsating quality, moderate or severe pain intensity, aggravation by or causing avoidance of routine physical activity (e.g., walking or climbing stairs); during headache at least one of following: nausea and/or vomiting, photophobia, phonophobia; features headache worsened by exercise, relieved by sleep
     a. Migraine without aura is most common (85%).
     b. Migraine without aura often has a menstrual relationship (thought to be due to the fall in estrogen).
     c. Triad of nausea, incapacitation, photophobia (any two) has best correlation with migraine diagnosis.
     d. If migraines occur >15 days per month for >3 months it is chronic migraine; often daily headache loses associated symptoms and resembles tension-type headache with migraine exacerbations.
     e. Transforms to chronic migraine with medication overuse, trauma (physical, emotional), or infection.
     f. Note: Patients often have facial or neck pain with migraine, which has posed diagnostic confusion in the past but is now recognized as a common symptom.

2. **Migraine with aura:** at least two attacks; aura consisting of at least one of the following, but no motor weakness: fully reversible visual symptoms including positive features (e.g., flickering lights, spots, or lines) and/or negative features (i.e., loss of vision), fully reversible sensory symptoms including positive features (i.e., pins and needles) and/or negative features (i.e., numbness), fully reversible dysphasic speech disturbance; at least two of the following: homonymous visual symptoms and/or unilateral sensory symptoms, at least one aura symptom develops gradually over 5 minutes and/or different aura symptoms occur in succession over 5 minutes, each symptom lasts > 5 and < 60 minutes; foral seizure progression is seconds to minute; migraine occurs about 20 minutes
    a. **Differential diagnosis:** carotid dissection, arteriovenous malformation (AVM), and seizure; careful history usually identifies aura
    b. **Visual aura most common:** fortification spectrum, scintillating scotoma ("teichopsia"), stars ("photopsia")
3. **Migraine variants**
    a. Typical aura with nonmigraine headache (does not fulfill preceding criteria)
    b. Typical aura without headache ("acephalgic" migraine, retinal migraine)
    c. Familial hemiplegic migraine; migraine with aura including motor weakness and at least one first- or second-degree relative has migraine aura including motor weakness
    d. Status migrainosus (debilitating migraine attack lasting for more than 72 hours)
4. **Tension-type headache:** At least 10 episodes; headache lasting 30 minutes to 7 days; headache has at least two of the following characteristics: bilateral location, pressing/tightening (nonpulsating) quality, mild or moderate intensity, not aggravated by routine physical activity such as walking or climbing stairs; both of the following: no nausea or vomiting (anorexia may occur), no more than one of photophobia or phonophobia; note: history and physical/neurologic examination do not suggest other pathology
5. **Cluster headache:** at least five attacks; severe or very severe unilateral orbital, supraorbital, and/or temporal pain lasting 15 to 180 minutes if untreated; includes at least one of the following: ipsilateral conjunctival injection and/or lacrimation, ipsilateral nasal congestion and/or rhinorrhea, ipsilateral eyelid edema, ipsilateral forehead and facial sweating, ipsilateral miosis and/or ptosis, a sense of restlessness or agitation; attacks have a frequency from one every other day to 8 per day
6. **Short-lasting unilateral neuralgiform headache attacks with conjunctival injection and tearing (SUNCT):** attacks last 5 to 240 seconds, occur from 3 to 200 times per day, are associated with prominent autonomic features (see preceding text)
7. **Other primary headaches:** paroxysmal hemicrania, stabbing headache, cough headache, exertional headache (may be confused with subarachnoid hemorrhage, but headache goes away when exertion stops), headache associated with sexual activity, hypnic headache (nocturnal with autonomic features), primary thunderclap headache (subarachnoid hemorrhage ruled out), hemicrania continua, new daily-persistent headache

D. **Secondary headache categories**
1. Headache attributed to head and/or neck trauma, cranial or cervical vascular disorder, nonvascular intracranial disorder, a substance or its withdrawal, infection or disorder of homeostasis
2. Headache or facial pain attributed to disorder of cranium, neck, eyes, ears, nose, sinuses, teeth, mouth, or other facial or cranial structures
3. Headache attributed to psychiatric disorder

E. **Cranial neuralgias, central and primary facial pain**
1. **Trigeminal neuralgia:** paroxysmal attacks of pain lasting from a fraction of a second to 2 minutes; can affect one or more divisions of the trigeminal nerve; the pain is intense, sharp, superficial or stabbing; precipitated from trigger areas or by trigger factors; no clinically evident neurologic deficit; there may be baseline aching pain in addition to sharp brief lancinating pain

2. **Glossopharyngeal neuralgia:** paroxysmal attacks of pain lasting from a fraction of a second to 2 minutes; the pain is unilateral, sharp, stabbing, and severe; distribution within the posterior part of the tongue, tonsillar fossa, pharynx, or beneath the angle of the lower jaw and/or in the ear; precipitated by swallowing, chewing, talking, coughing, and/or yawning
3. **Occipital neuralgia:** paroxysmal stabbing pain, with or without persistent aching between paroxysms, in the distribution of the greater, lesser, and/or third occipital nerves; tenderness over the affected nerve; pain is eased temporarily by local anesthetic block of the nerve.

III. Pathophysiology

A. **Tension-type headache** (TTH)
   1. Episodic TTH is not as well understood—the "common cold" of the headache world.
   2. Chronic TTH is caused by prolonged painful input from pericranial myofascial tissues, like tender points.
   3. Central sensitization of pain pathways may be caused by or associated with the activation of neuronal nitric oxide synthase and the generation of nitric oxide.
   4. Short latency responses recorded in tonically active sternocleidomastoid muscle after stimulation of the infraorbital branch of the trigeminal nerve (trigeminocervical reflex) is abnormal in chronic TTH.

B. **Migraine**
   1. Lower threshold for migraine attacks autosomally dominant inherited trait with variable penetrance
   2. The nervous system more sensitive to the environment including endogenous and exogenous triggers (hormonal shifts, changes in sleep/eating/stress levels, bright light, noise, weather changes, and foods and drink ingested)
   3. Biobehavioral changes may be noticed by the patient as prodromal symptoms, possibly related to hypothalamic changes: irritability, euphoria, cravings, increased sensitivity to surroundings, yawning, nausea
   4. Cortex experiences a wave of excitation followed by depression of metabolic activity moving from occipital to frontal lobes at a rate of about 3 mm per minute (spreading cortical depression); when clinically expressed, aura is experienced
   5. Corresponding blood flow changes occur matching the neuronal demands of the cortex
   6. Brainstem and trigeminal nerve activation cause neurogenic inflammation of meningeal vessels with vasodilation, increased permeability, probably associated with dysfunction of 5-HT inhibitory receptors
   7. Peripheral sensitization of trigeminal nerve endings causes pain within the meningeal artery, pulsations and movement of the head (causing traction on the meninges)
   8. Sensory relays travel back to the trigeminal nucleus caudalis, and pain signals are sent to the thalamus and to the cortex and brainstem structures
   9. Central sensitization occurs with hyperexcitability in the trigeminal nerve distribution and allodynia in the scalp, face, neck, and traveling to other body parts, and prolongation of the headache phase
   10. After-effects due to slow recovery of cortical neurons (hangover cognitive slowing), allodynia of head

C. **Cluster**
   1. Hypothalamic dysfunction/activity on PET scans (possible explanation for cyclical nature of attacks)
   2. Increased parasympathetic activity causes ipsilateral autonomic changes of the face
   3. Some meningeal inflammation may be present as this headache is responsive to 5-HT agonists acutely

IV. Nonpharmacologic Management

A. **Goal setting:** migraine, other primary headaches are not "curable"; therefore, the goal of treatment is maintenance of function, quality of life, understanding reasonable goals will aid in a successful outcome

B. **Education:** patient will benefit from understanding that primary headaches are a neurologic disorder; healthy lifestyle changes can limit disability: diet/nutrition, exercise, sleep hygiene, and stress management

C. **Psychophysiologic management**
   1. **Biofeedback:** learning to control parts of the body utilizing feedback from a machine relating to blood pressure, pulse, surface electromyogram (EMG), galvanic skin response, and temperature
   2. **Autogenic exercises:** practicing control of autonomic nervous system function through relaxation, thereby warming the finger temperature (aided by a small finger thermometer)
   3. **Progressive muscle relaxation:** systematically concentrating on relaxing muscle groups one at a time in a contiguous fashion ultimately ending in the whole body being very relaxed
   4. **Cognitive behavioral therapy** for stress management and comorbid psychiatric symptoms

V. Pharmacologic Management

A. Acute treatment
   1. **Migraine selective** (also used in cluster headache)
      a. **Triptans:** seven exist with minimally variable bioavailability, lipophilicity, and half-lives. They are **5HT 1 B/D agonists:** they are excitatory at the 5-HT receptor in three areas restoring normal function
         i. Meningeal blood vessel: vasodilation is normalized and capillary permeability lessened
         ii. Trigeminal nerve endings on the meningeal blood vessels: inhibition of release of inflammatory peptides such as calcitonin gene-related peptide
         iii. Trigeminal nucleus caudalis: decreases pain impulse generation
      b. **Ergotamine:** less selective for the 5-HT 1 receptor; therefore, it has more side effects (nausea/vomiting and nonmeningeal vasoconstriction)
      c. **Dihydroergotamine (DHE-45):** a parenteral form of ergot with fewer side effects than parenteral ergotamine; used most often for intractable migraine or status migrainosus
   2. **Nonselective**
      a. **Nonsteroidal anti-inflammatory drugs** (NSAIDs)
         i. Nonselective—high-dose naproxen, ibuprofen, indomethacin, salicylates
         ii. Cyclooxygenase (COX-2) inhibitors—caution: relative hypercoagulability with cardio/cerebrovascular history
      b. **Caffeine:** alone or combined with simple analgesics
      c. **Metoclopramide:** found to be more effective than placebo especially with aspirin
      d. **Chlorpromazine** or prochlorperazine
      e. **Butalbital, caffeine, and aspirin or acetaminophen combinations:** caution due to the prolonged receptor activity of butalbital predisposing to chronic headache; has never been studied in migraine
      f. **Dichloralphenazone, isometheptene mucate, acetaminophen combination:** effective in mild to moderate headache
      g. **Opioid analgesics** provide humane rescue therapy in severe attacks
      h. **Dexamethasone**

B. **Preventive treatment:** attention to physical and psychiatric comorbidity important
   1. **US Food and Drug Administration (FDA) approved** (i.e., can be marketed as such): β-blocking agents—propranolol and timolol; anticonvulsants—divalproex sodium, topiramate, and neurontin

2. **Non-FDA approved** (i.e., clinicians have to use their knowledge): calcium channel blocker—verapamil, tricyclic antidepressants—amitriptyline, imipramine, doxepin, other antidepressants—selective serotonin reuptake inhibitors (SSRIs) help in coping skills, comorbid depression, serotonin and norepinephrine reuptake inhibitors (SNRIs) (venlafaxine, mirtazapine) may be slightly more effective for headache, other anticonvulsants—gabapentin, NSAIDs—COX-2, naproxen, indomethacin

VI. Pediatric Headache

Individual episodes tend to be shorter: 2 hours on average

A. **Migraine with aura** is slightly more prominent in patients younger than age 20.

B. **Migraine equivalents** may occur in the patient with an immature nervous system: Episodic vertigo, episodic vomiting ("abdominal migraine"), confusional migraine, tendency toward motion sickness is commonly associated with later development of migraine

VII. Headache in the Elderly

A. **Postmenopausal women** have decreasing prevalence of migraine with each decade of life

B. **Hormone replacement therapy** (HRT) can be an issue but is generally best decided upon using factors other than headache

C. **Giant cell arteritis**
 1. May produce pain in the temple, periauricular area, jaw, or lateral neck
 2. Chewing or other jaw movements may exacerbate the pain
 3. Polymyalgia rheumatica symptoms often occur in tandem: polyarthralgias, jaw claudication, rash, weight loss
 4. 70% will have a significantly raised erythrocyte sedimentation rate (>50)
 5. Treatment can be initiated prior to temporal artery biopsy
 6. Stroke in the ophthalmic artery causing blindness or other cerebral vessel is a preventable sequela
 7. Tapering steroid therapy starting at 60 to 100 mg/day for at least six to twelve months is the appropriate treatment

VIII. Headache Emergencies and Other Pathology in Which Headache is Prominent

A. **Sudden onset headache**
 1. **Subarachnoid hemorrhage:** computed tomography (CT) and lumbar puncture (LP) with centrifugation of CSF
 2. **Acute meningitis:** CT (to rule out hemorrhage) and LP with stains and cultures
 3. **Thunderclap headache** (peak onset occurs within 1 minute but no pathology is found): conventional angiography to rule out an occult aneurysm is controversial; usually caused by SAH or ICP but may be related to migraine

B. **Indolent headache**
 1. **Bacterial or viral meningitis:** meningismus, fever, high white blood cell (WBCs) count, change in mental status, seizures
 2. **Sinusitis:** especially suspect sphenoid sinusitis, which may need MRI or coronal CT
 3. **Neoplasm:** usually focal neurologic deficit; symptoms or papilledema will be present

4. **Subdural hemorrhage:** trauma overlooked in elderly, more predisposed to stretching of bridging veins

C. **Posttraumatic headache**
  1. Headache may take any form (tension-type, migraine, cluster, nonspecific)
  2. Intensity of the headache is usually in direct opposition to the force/severity of the trauma (patients who survived prolonged coma rarely complain of headache).
  3. Neuroimaging abnormalities are almost never present.
  4. Headache usually resolves by 6 to 12 weeks; longer than 6 months likelihood of full recovery is poor

IX. Pain: Definition and Clarifications

A. **International Association for the Study of Pain (IASP) definition of pain:** "An unpleasant sensory and emotional experience associated with actual or potential tissue damage, or described in terms of such damage"

B. **Pain is subjective.** One *learns* application of the word through experiences related to injury in early life.

C. **Pain is an experience we associate with actual or potential tissue damage.** It is unquestionably a sensation in a part or parts of the body, but it is also *always unpleasant* and therefore also an emotional experience.

D. **Pain has a significant emotional component.**

E. **Neuralgia:** pain in the distribution of a nerve or nerves

F. **Neuropathic pain:** pain initiated or caused by a primary lesion or dysfunction in the nervous system

G. **Dysesthesia:** an unpleasant abnormal sensation, whether spontaneous or evoked, and includes
  1. **Hyperalgesia:** an increased response to a stimulus that is normally painful
  2. **Allodynia:** pain due to a stimulus that does not normally provoke pain

H. **Hyperpathia:** A painful syndrome characterized by an abnormally painful reaction to a stimulus, especially a repetitive stimulus, as well as an increased threshold.

I. **Analgesia:** absence of pain in response to stimulation that would normally be painful

J. **Anesthesia: absence of sensation**

K. **Placebo effect:** psychological factors influence magnitude of analgesia; conditioning, suggestion, and endogenous opioid systems are critical factors in placebo analgesia

X. Neurophysiology of Prolonged or Chronic Pain

A. **Peripheral (nociceptor) sensitization and central sensitization**

B. **Wind-up** occurs in spinal cord wide dynamic range (WDR) neurons.
  1. Neurons are hyperexcitable and sensitized to further nociceptive input.
  2. Occurs in response to ongoing, untreated, uninterrupted peripheral nociception
  3. WDR neurons continue to fire faster and faster; independent of any input.

C. **Allodynia:** pain due to a stimulus that does not normally provoke pain (touch, warmth)
   1. Nociceptors respond to normally innocuous stimuli via bradykinin or histamine sensitization.
   2. Central nociceptive neurons become responsive or more responsive to tactile stimuli
   3. Central inhibition is reduced, allowing nociceptive central neurons to respond more to tactile stimuli
   4. Dorsal horn rewiring: tactile afferent fibers synapse *directly* onto nociceptive central neurons

D. **Kindling**
   1. There is an episode of a biological neuronal dysfunction such as depression, seizure, or migraine in response to a trigger or series of events.
   2. The episodes occur more consistently or quicker in reaction to the trigger or similar event.
   3. Finally, the episodes may occur spontaneously without a trigger or event.
   4. The episodes then may occur so frequently that they are almost continuous or chronic.
   5. Note the similarity between kindling (higher centers) and wind-up (spinal cord) in neuronal behavior.

XI. Adaptive versus Maladaptive Pain

A. **Adaptive pain** is usually acute or post-surgical, allows us to protect ourselves
   1. Inflammatory/nociceptive; responsive to opioid treatment and opioid/serotonergic/GABAergic and dopaminergic endogenous pain modulation

B. **Chronic pain** by definition is pain that lasts >3 months

C. **Maladaptive pain** lasts after the injury has healed, has no biologic purpose, is a disease in and of itself, is neuropathic pain, not associated with activation of nociceptors, often not responsive to opioid treatment

D. **Neuropathic pain is most likely due to peripheral or central sensitization of nociceptive neurons.**

E. **Complex regional pain syndrome (CRPS)**
   1. **Symptoms:** disproportionate extremity pain, swelling, and autonomic (sympathetic) and motor symptoms; upper extremities slightly more commonly affected than lower.
      a. Type 1: "reflex sympathetic dystrophy (RSD)" occurs after injury other than direct nerve trauma
      b. Type 2: "causalgia" occurs after nerve trauma
   2. **Pathophysiology:** unknown changes in the peripheral and central somatosensory, autonomic, and motor processing and a pathologic interaction of sympathetic and afferent systems are described; treatment is mobilization of the limb by aggressive physical therapy and sympathetic nerve block; diagnosis is usually established by triple phase bone scan examining limb for autonomic dysfunction.

F. **Fibromyalgia:** history of widespread pain of right and left sides of the body, above and below the waist, along the axial skeleton, duration of pain is constant, lasting more than 3 months; to meet the diagnostic criteria, pain must occur in 11 of 18 paired tender points

XII. Evaluation of the Patient in Pain

A. **History:** location may be misleading due to referred pain
   1. **Quality:** neuropathic pain is burning, stabbing, or shocklike; neuromuscular pain is more often aching, throbbing; note: there is a lot of crossover in pain quality in clinical practice

B. **Physical**
  1. Trigger points (neuromuscular bulges, causes a painful muscle twitch when palpated)
  2. Pain upon light touch (allodynia, CRPS, peripheral neuropathy)
  3. Pain upon even slight passive movement (CRPS, acute injury)
  4. Evidence of sensory loss (anesthesia dolorosa, radiculopathy, compressive or peripheral neuropathy)

C. **Laboratory:** Important to rule out known/treatable causes of peripheral neuropathy, compressive neuropathy, metabolic peripheral neuropathy, radiculopathy, headache, neck and back pain, vasculitis, temporal arteritis, just to name a few. The physical exam will lead the examiner in the appropriate work-up.

D. **Psychological pain** impacts upon the patient's social sphere including spouse, children, family, friends, and work relationships, often to an extreme and deleterious way; in the extreme it commonly leads to divorce, isolation, and unemployment.

E. **Pain does not equal pain behavior** except in infants, where no other way to assess pain.

XIII. Pain Management

A. **Acute pain:** opioids are highly effective in this setting; simulates endogenous opiates at the opiate receptor
  1. NSAIDs, salicylates, and acetaminophen decrease prostaglandin synthesis.
  2. **Anesthetics:** lidocaine and other amide local anesthetics slow down the depolarization of the nerve cell membrane; this effect is based on the interaction with a specific receptor site in the sodium channel

B. **Chronic pain management**
  1. **Pharmacologic**
     a. **Nonopiate:** anti-inflammatories, antidepressants (mainly tricyclic), and phenothiazines can be very effective but have risks of hypotension and dyskinesia; benzodiazepines can be problematic due to addiction and withdrawal seizures; muscle relaxants, both peripherally acting such as tizanidine, and centrally acting such as baclofen; anticonvulsants stabilize neuronal membranes and decrease depolarization
     b. **Chronic long-acting opioids—principles of treatment:** the patient should consult with another physician for second opinion; a clear-cut diagnosis must be established (this does not mean any test results need to show the pathology, however); previous nonopioid treatment must have been tried and must have failed; use of the opioid must help the patient function better than he or she would without the opioid

C. **Procedural** with blocks and **surgical** with a variety of procedures

D. **Psychological/behavioral**
  1. **Psychophysiologic:** biofeedback, autogenics
  2. **Cognitive:** coping skills
  3. **Supportive:** individual and group therapy

XIV. Addiction and Detoxification

A. **Pseudo-addiction:** patient behaviors that may occur when pain is undertreated; patients with unrelieved pain may become focused on obtaining medications, may "clock watch," and may otherwise seem inappropriately "drug seeking"; even such behaviors as illicit drug use and deception can occur in the patient's efforts to obtain relief; pseudo-addiction can be distinguished from true addiction in that the behaviors resolve when pain is effectively treated

B. Detoxification: involves abruptly or slowly withdrawing opioid medication and/or other substances (benzodiazepines, alcohol, etc.), providing support for their greatest comfort during the process
1. **Clonidine** can help with withdrawal symptoms.
2. **Diphenhydramine or quetiapine** can help promote restful nighttime sleep.
3. **Dicyclomine and loperamide** help with gastrointestinal overactivity.
4. **Anti-inflammatories and muscle relaxants** may help with pain, muscle tension.
5. **Dopamine agonists** may help with restlessness.
6. **Neuromodulators/anticonvulsants** may help stabilize and promote endogenous pain modulation.
7. **Psychosocial support** in outpatient or inpatient setting is essential.

STUDY QUESTIONS FOR CHAPTER 16

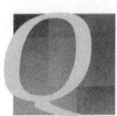

Directions: *Each of the numbered items or incomplete statements in this section is followed by answers or by completions of the statement. Select the ONE lettered answer or completion that is BEST in each case.*

1. A 56-year-old man has had a dozen nighttime attacks of severe right-sided head pain of 30-minutes duration associated with conjunctival injection and tearing. What is the most likely diagnosis?
   (A) Cluster headache
   (B) Migraine headache
   (C) Sudden-onset unilateral neuralgiform headache attacks with conjunctival injection and tearing (SUNCT)
   (D) Tension headache
   (E) Trigeminal neuralgia

2. A 36-year-old woman has very brief paroxysmal attacks of pain involving the back of her tongue and throat. These attacks are precipitated by chewing and swallowing, and she has lost 10 pounds as a result. What is her most likely diagnosis?
   (A) Trigeminal neuralgia
   (B) Glossopharyngeal neuralgia
   (C) Occipital neuralgia
   (D) SUNCT
   (E) Migraine headache

3. A 71-year-old man has had multiple episodes of left temporal headache exacerbated by chewing. He also describes recurrent blurry vision in his left eye and chronic shoulder and hip aches. What is the most appropriate treatment for this patient?
   (A) Dihydroergotamine
   (B) Ibuprofen
   (C) Muscle relaxants
   (D) Oxygen inhalation
   (E) Prednisone

4. A 25-year-old woman has five to 10 migraine headaches per month and misses at least one day of work as a result of these headaches. Which of the following anticonvulsants is the most effective treatment for migraine headache?
   (A) Carbamazepine
   (B) Gabapentin
   (C) Lamotrigine
   (D) Phenytoin
   (E) Topiramate

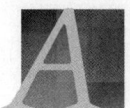 ANSWERS AND EXPLANATIONS

1. A. Cluster headache is characterized by severe unilateral orbital, supraorbital, or temporal pain that lasts between 15 minutes and 3 hours. It includes ipsilateral conjunctival injection and/or lacrimation, ipsilateral nasal congestion and/or rhinorrhea, ipsilateral eyelid edema, ipsilateral forehead, and facial sweating. Migraine and tension headaches are not typically associated with the autonomic findings noted in this patient. SUNCT is of shorter duration (typically 5 to 250 seconds), but shares many of the same features as cluster headache. Trigeminal neuralgia pain lasts for seconds at a time.

2. B. Glossopharyngeal neuralgia consists of brief paroxysmal attacks of pain that characteristically affect the posterior part of the tongue, tonsillar fossa, pharynx, beneath the angle of the jaw, or ear. Trigeminal neuralgia affects the face in the distribution of the trigeminal nerve and is precipitated by touch. Occipital neuralgia affects the back of the head. SUNCT is a sudden-onset headache that is usually orbital, supraorbital, or temporal. Very brief paroxysmal attacks are not characteristic of migraine.

3. E. This man's clinical history is most consistent with giant cell arteritis, a headache disorder of the elderly characterized by pain in the temple, periauricular area, jaw, or lateral neck. Jaw claudication, scalp tenderness, and polymyalgia rheumatica are frequently associated. To prevent loss of vision, prednisone should be administered urgently. Dihydroergotamine is effective for migraines but not for giant cell arteritis. Ibuprofen can be used to treat multiple headaches. Muscle relaxants are most appropriate for tension headaches. Oxygen inhalation is an effective treatment for cluster headaches.

4. E. Of the listed anticonvulsants, topiramate is the most effective migraine prophylactic agent. The number needed to treat for a 50% reduction in headache frequency is 3.3–3.5 for both gabapentin and topiramate, but the gabapentin studies have methodologic limitations.

CHAPTER 17

Epilepsy

I. Definitions

A. **Seizures** are divided into generalized and partial types
   1. **Generalized:** tonic-clonic, tonic, clonic, myoclonic, absence, atypical absence, atonic
   2. **Partial:** simple and complex partial

B. **Epilepsies**, conversely, are divided into four categories: generalized onset versus focal, and symptomatic versus "idiopathic" or genetic (Table 17-1)
   1. **Generalized** epilepsies are treated with valproic acid (VPA), topiramate (TPM), lamotrigine (LTG), zonisamide (ZNS), levetiracetam (LEV). **Focal** are treated with any antiepileptic (Table 17-2).

II. Generalized Idiopathic Seizures

Generalized idiopathic seizures are bilateral without focal onset—patients always lose consciousness during event); these represent electrophysiologic not structural brain diseases; no aura

A. **Convulsive types**
   1. **Tonic clonic** (grand mal in older terminology): initial drug of choice is VPA
      a. Important to distinguish from focal onset with secondary generalization, for which initial drug of choice is probably tegretol
      b. Some people experience signs that the seizure is about to occur, feeling of dread (prodrome).
      c. Initial loss of consciousness, falling to ground, trunk flexion, opening of eyes and mouth, upward deviation of eyes; followed by 10 to 20 seconds of extension (tonic phase); electroencephalogram (EEG) shows spike/spike waves followed by 10 seconds of 10-Hz spikes
      d. Followed (by clonic phase) with 4- to 8-Hz flexor spasms; EEG shows spikes mixed with slow waves becoming polywave and spike pattern
      e. Postictus variable expression ranging from confusion to obtundation to undirected violence; EEG is initially slowed followed by resumption of normal activity; patient should have careful neurologic examination while postictal, as transient unilateral hemiparesis, called Todd paralysis, suggests focal brain lesion, rather than generalized condition
      f. If patient does not wake up before next attack or seizure lasts for more than 5 minutes, patient is in status epilepticus: treat aggressively to prevent brain injury
      g. Tonic-clonic seizures in a newborn appear as migratory jerking movements that seem to haphazardly migrate among the limbs and can affect the face; EEG can be diagnostic
   2. **Purely clonic, purely tonic, or clonic-tonic-clonic** types also exist.

B. **Nonconvulsive types**
1. **Absence** (petit mal in older terminology): drugs of choice: LTG, VPA, or ethosuximide, but individual practices may prefer one over another due to lack of high quality trials
   a. The patient stares and briefly stops responding; patients do not lose muscle tension and fall and can continue to perform complex activities; 90% will have a 3-Hz clonus of fingers, face, or eyelids; EEG shows 2.5- to 3.5-Hz spike and wave; patient quickly resumes consciousness with no postictal state
   b. Can be induced by 30 to 120 seconds of hyperventilation
   c. Usually begin after age 4 and are frequent
   d. Can last for hours; this is called absence status
   e. 50% of patients subsequently develop major motor seizures
2. **Atypical or complex absence:** drug of choice is VPA
   a. EEG rates 2 up to 6, myoclonus, less complete loss of consciousness possible
   b. EEG: runs of slow spike and wave without alteration of consciousness possible
3. **Lennox-Gastaut syndrome**
   a. Falling attacks with peak onset of 3 to 6 years, followed by other seizure activity as well as atypical absence; 20% had West syndrome (see infantile spasms below); more than 90% are mentally challenged by age 5
   b. Tonic seizures EEG shows 1.5- to 2-Hz paroxysmal fast activity and no postictal depression; atypical absence show 2 to 2.5-Hz spike and wave
   c. Check skin carefully for neurocutaneous syndrome and obtain MRI to evaluate structural abnormality, including cortical maldevelopment
   d. Very difficult to treat; start with VPA or clonazepam; may utilize a ketogenic diet if medications fail to control seizures; vigabatrin is utilized but not available in the United States due to potential for retinal hamartomas and 30% chance of visual field constriction

C. **Myoclonic seizures:** drug of choice is VPA for men, for women TPM, ZNS, LEV
1. **Benign myoclonus of infancy:** myoclonus with normal EEG and neurologically intact; need not be treated

Table 17-1 *Categories of Epilepsy*

	Generalized onset	Focal onset
Symptomatic	West syndrome	Temporal lobe epilepsy
	Lennox-Gastaut	Frontal lobe epilepsy
"Idiopathic" or genetic	Absence	Benign rolandic
	Juvenile myoclonic	Benign occipital

Table 17-2 *Treatment of Epilepsy*

Spectrum of action	Medication
Any seizures	Valproate, topiramate, lamotrigine, levetiracetam, zonisamide. Felbamate as last resort (rare fatal aplastic anemia and liver failure)
Simple/complex partial seizures, secondarily generalized, and tonic-clonic seizures	Carbamazepine, oxcarbazepine, phenobarbital, phenytoin, primidone, tiagabine
Special cases	Ethosuximide for absence Acetazolamide for absence as a second agent ACTH for infantile spasms Valium and others for status

2. **Benign myoclonic epilepsy:** onset 4 months to 2 years; one third have family members affected; brief myoclonus with head to chest, eyes upward, and arms upward and outward, legs flex; EEG shows 3-Hz spike and wave; treat with TPM, LTG
3. **Severe myoclonic epilepsy:** healthy infant has a febrile, usually prolonged and sometimes focal, generalized seizure and then has intellectual decline to mental retardation; after one year of age will begin to have generalized myoclonic seizures; resistant to therapy; avoid carbamazepine as it increases seizure frequency
4. **Infantile spasms:** onset 4 to 7 months, always before age one; series of rapid flexor spasms of arms, neck, and truck; extensor spasms where head moves back and arms spread outward; 20% have tuberous sclerosis; many have underlying brain abnormalities; EEG while awake or light sleep shows chaotic high voltage with random spikes and slow waves; this is called hypsarrthymia and is diagnostic; treat with adrenocorticotropic hormone (ACTH), which stops the seizures but does not affect prognosis of those with brain abnormalities
5. **Disseminated myoclonus:** search should begin for drug intoxication, aseptic meningitis, or subacute sclerosing panencephalitis; if it occurs in adulthood with dementia consider Creutzfeldt-Jacob; epileptologists would not call this a syndrome
6. **Juvenile myoclonic epilepsy (JME):** two different syndromes; triad of disorders
   a. **JME with absence:** the first manifestation (affects about one third) at ages 6 to 14 is absence seizures, the second during adolescence is myoclonus, and the third (affects most) also while to teen is tonic-clonic seizures in morning; JME is the latter two manifestations; myoclonus is characterized by brief, bilateral but not necessarily symmetric upper extremity flexor jerks; EEG shows bilateral spike/polyspike and wave at 3.5- to 6-Hz, often maximally frontocentral; treat with valproate if male, or female LTG, ZNS, LEV

III. Partial = Focal Seizures

Drug of choice: LTG, oxcarbazepine for infants; this is due to structural brain dysfunction; if macroscopic visualized by CT and if microscopic by MRI; usually CT/MRI negative; often begins with aura and may have post-event neurologic dysfunction (Todd paralysis)

A. **Simple partial = without altered consciousness**
   1. Frontal lobe = contralateral frontal
      a. Most common type is a turning of head and eyes away from seizure; can occur with an ipsilateral tonic contraction, which occurs in the supplementary motor cortex
      b. Jacksonian = tonic contraction of hand/foot/limb/face; can march = spread to ipsilateral muscles; high incidence of starting in face, hands is likely due to large cortical representation; motor cortex = clonic contractions; premotor = tonic contractions; Brodmann 8 = flailing movements; amygdala/operculum = ictal aphasia if left or vocal arrest
      c. Somatosensory can be well localized to postrolandic cortex; if there is a visual component or temporary blindness, there is a occipital localization; if it is lateral occipital, the visual symptom can begin as twinkling lights; complex hallucinations are likely due to temporal–occipital junction; a feeling of vertigo suggests parietotemporal junction or posterior superior temporal; olfactory suggests parahippocampus or uncus origin

B. **Complex partial = with impairment of consciousness**
   1. The initial event of the seizure can be aura, which can be any number of visual, emotional experiences, autonomic disturbance (feeling in abdomen or chest), or bad taste or smell.
   2. This is followed by an alteration of consciousness after which the person is amnesic for this alteration. This usually includes some kind of motor automatisms, during which time the person is clearly not responsive. If the patient is partially responsive, this usually localizes their seizure to the right temporal lobe. Although violence during this period is possible (about 2%), that someone could commit murder as portrayed in the movies is extremely rare, as violence in these cases is resistive and nongoal directed.

3. Two-thirds have or have had generalized tonic clonic seizures.
4. The classic finding is medial temporal sclerosis.
5. Postictus is usually evident on EEG as generalized slowing.
6. A rare syndrome is the transient epileptic amnesia, which is the only manifestation of temporal lobe epilepsy; the mechanism of transient global amnesia is rarely epilepsy
7. Although the data are limited, nearly one third have depressive disorder, another one third have anxiety disorder, and fully one tenth are psychotic.
8. There is a personality disorder associated with temporal lobe seizures: rigid thinking, verbose, preoccupied with naive and often religious ideas, emotional outbursts are common, hypergraphia

IV. Special Syndromes

A. **Febrile seizures**, two major types
   1. **Simple febrile seizures** ages 6 months to 5 years, single generalized tonic-clonic seizure, EEG normal, do not treat; in general, if there are no abnormalities on neurologic exam or family history of seizure, most child neurologists would not order an EEG (this is *not* a guideline); risk for seizure disorder in later life about 2%
   2. **Complicated febrile seizures:** acute encephalopathy presents as prolonged focal or generalized seizures or repeated seizures; risk for seizures in later life at least 8%.
   3. Consider lumbar puncture if any chance of infection, as one fourth of meningitis in children presents with a seizure; a key defining feature is that children generally do not wake up after a seizure if it is meningitis

B. **Rolandic epilepsy**, for example, benign rolandic epilepsy of childhood
   1. Seizure wakes child from sleep, with ipsilateral twitching that spreads; can become a tonic-clonic seizure; lasts 1 to 2 minutes with preservation of consciousness; EEG shows uni/bilateral spikes in central/central and temporal regions; MRI if atypical features, hard to control; treatment not needed if seizures infrequent, consider for family
   2. Age of onset 3 to 13 years; seizures stop by age 16 treated or not

C. **Reflex epilepsy** occurs uncommonly with epileptic individuals having provoked seizures with a specific stimulus; the most common is hot water, but there are also visual, auditory, somatosensory, and other rarer types

D. **Epilepsia partialis continua** is persistent clonus in one muscle group that may continue for up to months; EEG shows slow waves or sharp wave/spike in contralateral hemisphere; there is always an underlying cerebral lesion. Epilepsia partialis continua is a risk factor for Rasmussen encephalitis, which features continuous focal seizures and progressive hemiparesis

V. Syndromes Mimicking Seizures Dependent on Age

A. **Jitteriness** (newborns particularly with perinatal asphyxia or addicted mothers)
   1. Low Hz, high-amplitude limb shaking often with jaw involvement in response to touch, noise, or other stimulation; do not expect change in respiratory pattern or abnormal eye movements; this is overreaction to stimulation; can need sedation for feeding if results from drug use in addicted mother; usually, reduced stimulation is all that is needed

B. **Cyanotic syncope** (<2 years old); breath-holding spells with loss of consciousness affects 5% of infants; usually provoked by something; if lasts longer than a few seconds, can see tonic posturing and eyes rolling upward; EEG shows flattening
   1. Treatment is no medication except perhaps a caution not to hold infant upright during times of decreased cerebral perfusion; children do not die; drug not available in the United States, unless you are an astronaut on the International Space Station, can be used (piracetam).

C. Pallid syncope (≤ 2 years old)
  1. In response to unexpected painful event, the infant becomes pale and limp and loses consciousness; the body can then stiffen with clonic movements; it results from reflex asystole; infants do not die from this even though it can be very scary; no need to treat

D. Benign nocturnal myoclonus (all ages): repeated flexion of upper extremity in early stages of sleep; don't treat or it will become worse; EEG normal

E. Psychogenic seizures (also referred to as hysterical seizures or pseudoseizures): prolactin and creatinine kinase levels normal, tend to occur in front of other people; unlikely to include incontinence, tongue biting, or have postictal phase; consider conversion reaction; question patient for history of prior physical or sexual abuse

VI. Convulsive Status

A. **Act quickly**—this is an emergency

B. **Diagnosis:** 2+ convulsions without recovery of consciousness or any seizure lasting longer than 5 minutes; formal definition is 20 minutes, but risk of going into status skyrockets at 5 minutes

C. Immediately, just as in-hospital administer **Advanced Trauma Life Support (ATLS):** begin primary survey with a modified ABCDE that takes no more than 10 minutes; most hospitals require staff to be paged
  1. **Airway**—determine airway patency, place on O_2 and obtain pulse oximetry
  2. **Breathing**—intubate first and ask questions later if any sign of respiratory depression
  3. **Circulation**—vital signs every 5 minutes, continuous electrocardiogram (ECG), intravenous (IV) line with normal saline (NS)
  4. **Disability**—blood sugar level, get blood for STAT toxin screen, chem-7, and coagulation panels, AED levels (if appropriate); empirically give thiamine 250 mg IV followed by 1 amp dextrose 50 grams (D50) in an alcoholic; do not routinely give D50 as this likely worsens outcome
  5. **Exposure/environment**—ensure that patient is in a safe region to continue seizing

D. **Break the seizure.**
  1. IV lorazepam 0.1 mg/kg at 2 mg/minute every 5 minutes up to 9 mg; for a child, give 0.05 to 0.1 mg/kg IV up to 5 mg; if IV route is not available, give same dose rectally using Diastat or could try 10 mg midazolam in 2 mL buccally if you are prepared to intubate by yourself; IV lorazepam should terminate about 90% of status; IV diazepam is slightly less effective at about 75% and is shorter acting with more respiratory or cardiovascular activity
  2. After two doses of lorazepam or alternatively as soon as given lorazepam, start phenytoin load; use whatever is available to you locally—equivalent preparations:
     a. Phenobarbitone 10 mg/kg at 100 mg/minute (available in United Kingdom) or phosphenytoin 15 mg (elderly) to 20 mg (adults) PE/kg at 150 mg PE/minute (children 3 mg PE/kg/minute) (PE = phenytoin equivalent)
     b. Many epileptologists swear by Depacon (IV VPA) 20 mg/kg up to 200 mg/minute or 3 mg/kg/minute, because it is safer.
     c. If in children, can try phenobarbital immediately after benzodiazepines as long as the child is intubated first
  3. Refractory status: If you don't have a second IV by now, get it. If you continue to give benzodiazepines, will likely cause cardiovascular collapse. In any case, have dopamine ready. If you need a pressor, start it at 5 mg/kg/minute and titrate up if this occurs.

4. Intensive care unit (ICU) transfer at 30 minutes; get an arterial line for pressor support and continuous EEG is helpful; in children, if you are trained or can get a neurosurgeon to help, put in an intracranial pressure (ICP) bolt to ensure sustained increased ICP does not occur; if you haven't intubated, you should do so now; can try VPA IV especially if partial status epilepticus, if you want; otherwise, go for an anesthetic coma using midazolam 0.2 mg/kg then 0.2 mg/kg/hour titrated, or propofol 2 mg/kg IV push, then 2 mg/kg/hour titrated; if these fail, can consider pentobarbital coma; load this correctly: 15 mg/kg at 25 mg/minute, maintenance 2.5 mg/kg/hour titrated to burst suppression

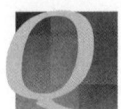

STUDY QUESTIONS FOR CHAPTER 17

Directions: *Each of the numbered items or incomplete statements in this section is followed by answers or by completions of the statement. Select the ONE lettered answer or completion that is BEST in each case.*

1. A 3-year-old child with seizures shows a chaotic pattern of multifocal spikes mixed with slow waves. What do you treat this with?

   (A) ZNG
   (B) VPA
   (C) Phenobarbital
   (D) ACTH

2. A man describes smelling burnt rubber and then losing consciousness. His wife mentions that he then walks in circles. What do you order for studies?

   (A) EEG
   (B) MRI
   (C) EEG and MRI
   (D) EEG, MRI/MRA

3. A 45-year-old man is brought to the emergency room after a seizure, and while his initial history is being obtained, he has a generalized tonic-clonic seizure that persists for 10 minutes. When you arrive at the bedside, he is still seizing. What is the most initial appropriate course of action?

   (A) 2 mg intravenous lorazepam
   (B) Load with phenytoin 50 mg/kg
   (C) Load with VPA 20 mg/kg
   (D) Portable EEG
   (E) Intubation

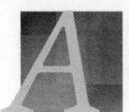# ANSWERS AND EXPLANATIONS

1. D. This is hypsarhythmia, which is treated with ACTH. (A), (B) are good agents for generalized epilepsies. (D) Phenobarbital is generally only used when the newer agents fail, as it has many side effects.

2. C. This is temporal lobe seizures until proven otherwise. Patients are always evaluated with EEG and MRI as they have a very high incidence of tumors. (A), (B) would be an incomplete evaluation. (D) MRA is not needed. MRA is used to evaluate for aneurysms, not in this case.

3. E. The first priority in treating a patient with status epilepticus is to ensure airway patency and to perform basic life support measures. A patient with a generalized tonic-clonic seizure lasting at least 10 minutes should be intubated. Although lorazepam, phenytoin, and valproic acid are all appropriate medications for status epilepticus, the first priority is airway protection. A portable EEG is unlikely to add anything to the clinic diagnosis of convulsive status epilepticus, and is not emergently indicated.

CHAPTER 18

Cognitive and Emotional Alteration

I. Delirium

A. First and foremost **dementia must be differentiated from delirium**.
 1. **Delirium** has four primary features according to *Diagnostic and Statistical Manual of Mental Disorders,* Fourth Edition (DSM-IV).
    a. Reduced ability to focus or shift attention causing disturbance in consciousness
    b. Develops over hours to days and often fluctuates during the day
    c. Change in perception or cognition not accounted for by a preexisting dementia
    d. Evidence that the condition is caused by an underlying medical condition, drug/substance effect
 2. **Dementia** has three cardinal features.
    a. Impairment of cognition, especially memory
    b. Behavioral disturbance
    c. Interference with activities of daily living and functional independence

B. For every patient meeting criteria for dementia there should be a search for potentially **reversible causes**.
 1. **A potentially reversible cause** is found in about 20% of patients with dementia. The most common causes appear to be depression (6% of all patients), drugs (4%), hydrocephalus (3%), alcohol (2%), and metabolic causes (2%).
 2. **All patients with a dementia should get the following:** complete blood count, chemistry panel, thyroid function tests, a vitamin B_{12} level, and brain imaging study (CT or MRI).
 3. **Consider, depending on the circumstances:** erythrocyte sedimentation rate (ESR), urine analysis (U/A), chest x-ray (CXR), blood cultures, urine drug screen, heavy metal screen, HIV test, Venereal Disease Research Laboratory (VDRL) test, cerebrospinal fluid (CSF) analysis, electroencephalogram (EEG), positron emission tomography (PET)/single-photon emission computed tomography (SPECT) if computed tomography (CT)/magnetic resonance imaging (MRI) normal
 4. **Normal pressure hydrocephalus** classically is the triad of gait disturbance, cognitive dysfunction, and urinary incontinence.
    a. Gait disturbance is variable, but most often unsteadiness/imbalance that causes greatest difficulty with stairs
    b. Cognitive dysfunction and unconcern for this
    c. Urinary symptoms seem to occur in three stages: first is urgency/frequency, then urgency associated with incontinence, finally indifference to incontinence
    d. Diagnosis with the Miller Fisher test: objective gait assessment before and after withdrawal of about 30 mL spinal fluid, and isotope cisternogram (isotope remains in ventricles); CT/MRI shows enlarged ventricles (especially temporal horns) out of proportion to size of sulcal CSF spaces
 5. **Alcoholic dementia:** status is somewhat ambiguous, but it is a term that is commonly used; global cognitive decline (not just of memory as this is Korsakoff syndrome), often

with dilated ventricles, accompanied by loss of control and emotional lability; often at autopsy, the dementia is explained by another etiology, especially trauma or Wernicke-Korsakoff syndrome
6. **Paretic neurosyphilis:** a form of tertiary syphilis with gradual development of cognitive decline often with odd behavior, disinterest in grooming, and irritability, occasionally with megalomania; this is followed by progressive unsteadiness, hand/facial tremulousness, dysarthria, hurried speech, continued cognitive decline leading to a bedridden state (hence paresis), and eventual aphasia/agnosia/apraxia
7. **Late, chronic meningitis:** can lead to hydrocephalus with dementia, stupor, and paralysis or a tabes dorsalislike condition
8. **Tumors:** early symptoms lack of spontaneity, forgetfulness, faulty insight, fatigue, loss of interest in normal activities, or apathy make it easily confused with depression; cognitive dysfunction is the presenting complaint in one third of patients with metastatic intracranial tumor; this is followed by slowed reaction time and mental slowing, eventually manifesting as long pauses after questions are asked but when answers are made they are often unusually intelligent for what might be expected from a typical delirious patient who also may have long pauses; or, it can be outright dementia

II. Mild Cognitive Impairment (MCI)

A. **Definition**
   1. **Objective memory impairment for age**, with this as primary complaint for visit, preferably confirmed by informant
      a. Normal aging and MCI can often be differentiated by asking about missed appointments; patients with memory impairment as part of normal aging will not typically miss these, whereas patients with MCI will, assuming that the patient did not miss them normally previously
   2. **Otherwise normal cognition and activities of daily living** (ADLs); patient is not demented by AD criteria
   3. **Specialized neuropsychologic testing** is pretty good at getting a definite diagnosis.
      a. This testing is also effective for differentiating from dementia and pseudodementia of depression

B. **Subtypes**
   1. Amnestic MCI is what we just described. Rate of progression to AD is 10% to 15% per year.
      a. About 60% of these patients will be diagnosed with AD in 5 years, with about a 10% a year conversion to dementia. Those apolipoprotein E4 allele carriers are likely to progress more rapidly to AD.
      b. Hippocampal atrophy measured by volume by MRI is predictive of AD conversion.
   2. Multiple domain MCI: more than one domain of cognition, but none sufficiently severe to be dementia; likely etiologies include AD, vascular cognitive impairment, and normal aging
   3. Single nonmemory domain: the likely etiologies include AD, Lewy body dementia (LBD), primary progressive aphasia, and frontotemporal dementia

III. Alzheimer Disease (AD)

A. **Epidemiology:** affects about 4 million in the United States at a cost of about $100 billion per year; accounts for between one half and three quarters of all dementias
   1. Affects 2% of individuals ages 65 to 69 years and the incidence doubles every 5 years until age 90
   2. Familial AD affects <5% of AD, but is autosomal dominant

3. Apolipoprotein E is involved in cholesterol transport and has three different alleles: ε2, ε3, and ε4; homozygous ε4: >90% chance for AD by age 85; genotyping is not recommended, as there is no treatment for this condition at this time; not all patients with homozygous pattern become demented
4. Risk factors of lesser importance: female, <8 grades in school, history of head trauma causing unconsciousness, or myocardial infarction
5. Family history of AD in first-degree relative increases risk of developing AD by 4 times.
6. Median survival is slightly <6 years.

B. **Pathology**
1. **Gross:** marked atrophy, especially of amygdala and hippocampus with relative sparing of the occipital pole
2. **Micro:** synaptic loss, neuritic plaques (NPs) and neurofibrillary tangles (NTs) not unique to AD
    a. Plaques and tangles
        i. NP = sphere with core of amyloid surrounded by degenerating nerve endings
        ii. Diffuse plaque = poorly defined amyloid
        iii. Burnt-out plaques = isolated dense amyloid core
        iv. This amyloid is really amyloid precursor protein that has been abnormally processed into fragments called amyloid beta; these are toxic and insoluble in the brain
        v. Need sufficient number of NPs and NTs for diagnosis at necropsy, as small numbers may be seen in nondemented individuals
    b. Amyloid angiopathy may cause ischemia or lobar hemorrhage.
    c. Overall decline in cholinergic activity; also decreases in corticotropin-releasing factors, glutamate, norepinephrine, serotonin, and somatostatin

C. **Symptoms**
1. Memory loss interfering with ADLs is most common presenting complaint.
    a. Initially difficulty recalling information, later includes remote memory
2. Language initially decreased conversation, then mild loss of fluency and naming, and with progression loss of fluency
3. Visual tasks—initially misplacing objects and driving problems then getting lost where patient was before familiar and finally unable to do even basic things
4. Behavioral includes delusions, depression, and insomnia
5. Neurologic signs includes agraphesthesia, positive face-hand test, and frontal release signs; gait problems late in the disease course; be cognizant that patients show cognitive impairment without other neurologic signs; the presence of early neurologic signs should suggest alternative diagnosis

D. **Diagnosis-two criteria:** DSM-IV and National Institute of Neurological and Communicative Disorders and Stroke–Alzheimer's Disease and Related Disorders Association (NINCDS-ARDRA)
1. **DSM-IV:** delirium ruled out, no other cause identified, gradual onset of cognitive decline with impairment of recent memory and disturbance of one of: language, word-finding, praxis, visual processing, construction, executive function, or visual agnosia
2. **NINCDS-ARDRA**
    a. Probable AD: deficits in two or more areas of cognition, no disturbance of consciousness, onset ages 40 to 90, progression, absence of other conditions that could explain dementia; it also has supporting and consistent features; not sudden onset, focal neurologic findings; no seizures/gait problems early in its time course
    b. Possible AD: probable AD with atypical onset, presentation, etc., or presence of second brain disorder that could cause dementia but is not believed to be the cause
    c. Definite AD: probable AD with tissue confirmation

E. **Treatment**
1. **Cholinesterase inhibitors** for mild to moderate AD
    a. Donezipil 5 to 10 mg, galantamine 8 to 24 mg, rivastigmine 3 to 12 mg, Namenda 5 mg and NMDA receptor effect; may use with other medication for enhanced effect

b. Rivastigmine is not hepatically metabolized, the other two agents are
c. They have mild but measurable increases in functioning and likely delay institutionalization of the patient.
2. **Memantine** for moderate to severe AD, possibly disease modifying
   a. Memantine and donepezil were more effective than donepezil alone
3. **Vitamin E** 1,000 IU orally b.i.d. has been shown to slow the progression of AD
   a. Selegiline 5 mg orally b.i.d. can be considered if the vitamin E can not be taken, as it is no more effective than vitamin E alone, and there are no additive benefits
   b. High dose vitamin E (400 IU/day) is probably associated with increased all-cause mortality, as well as increased risk of congestive heart failure, so probably should only be recommended for patients with AD and those with at least one family member affected if they do not have cardiovascular disease
4. **Nonsteroidal anti-inflammatory drugs** (NSAIDs) have no role in the treatment of AD. They have probably been shown to have neuroprotective effect on development of AD but also increase cardiovascular mortality. There is no convincing evidence that risk of use outweighs benefit.
5. **Behavioral problems** are expected occurrences with AD and can be alleviated with pharmacologic intervention. Depression is especially common in early AD, and treatment can enhance quality of life.

IV. Dementia with Lewy Bodies (DLBs)

A. **Epidemiology:** accounts for 15% to 25% of irreversible cases of dementia

B. **Variable time course of disease features**
   1. **Cognitive impairment:** fluctuations are a defining feature of DLB, with times of near normal cognition
   2. **Psychiatry:** visual hallucinations, illusions, and delusions are common. Depression and anxiety are both very common; occasional Capgras syndrome (spouse replaced by identical appearing imposter) and late course aggression.
   3. **Motor:** Spontaneous parkinsonism is a common hallmark of the disease. Can include myoclonus, which can be confused for Creutzfeldt-Jacob.
   4. **Sleep:** rapid eye movement sleep behavior disorder; patients act out dreams physically while sleeping. Dreams are often described as a chase or violent actions. This often starts years before dementia begins. Often causes excessive daytime sleepiness.
   5. **Autonomic problems** like orthostatic hypotension, urinary incontinence, constipation, or impotence.

C. **Diagnosis** (McKeith criterion)
   1. **Core features:** progressive cognitive decline interfering with normal functioning, objective testing deficits, prominent/persistent memory impairment (may be absent early)
   2. **Fluctuating consciousness/alertness**, recurrent visual hallucinations, spontaneous features of parkinsonism
      a. Two features for clinically probable DLB, one feature for clinically possible

D. **Treatment:** cholinesterase inhibitors—dramatic improvement in cognitive impairment
   1. Can try carbidopa/levodopa, dopamine agonists, or psychostimulants
   2. Classic: arguments with self in mirror—cover the mirror
   3. Emotional lability/depression treat as though depression

V. Frontotemporal Lobar Dementia (Formerly Called Pick Disease)

A. **Affects 5% to 7%** of those affected by dementia

B. **Really three different forms** (rule in by Neary criterion)
   1. **Frontal lobe dementia**
      a. Core features: include gradual progression, insidious onset, and early impairment of social conduct, regulation of personal conduct, insight, and emotional blunting
   2. **Progressive nonfluent aphasia** primarily affecting the dominant (left) hemisphere
      a. Core features: gradual progression, insidious onset, nonfluent spontaneous speech with at least one of agrammatism, phonemic paraphasias, anomia
   3. **Progressive fluent aphasia/semantic dementia** predominantly affecting the dominant (left) anterior temporal lobe
      a. Core features: insidious onset, gradual progression, loss of word meaning, semantic paraphasias
   4. **Prosopagnosia** when the right temporal lobe is affected more than other areas; this is a subset of semantic dementia with cardinal features of: insidious onset, gradual progression, and either prosopagnosia (impaired facial recognition) or associative agnosia (impaired recognition of object identity)
   5. **Diagnostic exclusions:** abrupt onset with ictus, head trauma related to onset, early amnesia, spatial disorientation, logoclonic, festinant speech, myoclonus, corticospinal weakness, cerebellar ataxia, choreoathetosis; also imaging and laboratory testing must not show another obvious cause for the abnormality

C. **Other syndromes**
   1. **Primary progressive aphasia:** language difficulty with at least one of word-finding difficulties, abnormal speech, decreased comprehension, and impaired spelling; these language findings should be only feature for at least 2 years before other parts of brain become affected; syndrome will affect frontal, temporal, and parietal regions of brain
   2. **Frontotemporal dementia with parkinsonism:** autosomal dominant syndrome linked to chromosome 17q21–22, which codes for microtubule associated tau protein
   3. **Frontotemporal dementia with motor neuron disease**: course is faster due to dysphagia and/or respiratory failure
   4. **Corticobasal degeneration:** asymmetric rigidity, apraxia, and alien limb phenomena

D. **Treatment:** Anticholinesterase inhibitors have met with anecdotal success. Safety is main issue with removal of firearms, power tools, and periodic driving examinations.

VI. Vascular Cognitive Impairment

A. **Generally diagnosed when patient has** cerebrovascular disease, vascular risk factors, and dementing illness. There are usually multiple infarcts, but critical area like thalamus, single large infarct, or intracranial hemorrhage can cause this.
   1. National Institute of Neurological and Disorders and Stroke–Association Internationale pour la Recherche et l'Enseignement en Neurosciences (NINDS-AIREN) criteria include: cognitive decline with impairment of memory and two other areas, both neurologic examination and imaging consistent with stroke, temporal relationship of stroke to cognitive decline with a duration of no more than 3 months

B. **Symptomatology** depends on location of strokes.

C. **Treatment is cholinesterase inhibitors/memantine and risk factors**

D. **Risk reduction with antihypertensives suggest a relative risk reduction of about 12%.**

VII. Fatigue

Fatigue is weakness/exhaustion from physical/mental exertion.

A. Approach: assess neurosis/depression, recent/ongoing infections, anemia/azotemia, endocrine survey, current/recent medications; physical overwork
  1. If decreased strength, abnormal reflexes, fasciculation/atrophy consider neuromuscular disease

B. Causes: psychiatric illness fatigue without medical disease (note: anxiety-depressive illness present commonly as fatigue)
  1. **Presentation:** increased fatigue in morning, early morning wakening/insomnia, increased with specific activities/situations, patient status post stress/grief situation, lack of concentration on menial tasks, easily worried, multiple/dramatic medical complaints
  2. **Diagnosis:** Peak muscle test shows no physical weakness
  3. **Treatment:** specific to psychiatric disorder

C. Medical illness
  1. **Myopathic fatigue:** fatigue secondary to weakness in muscles; found in many myopathies
  2. **Neurologic:** overwork fatigue (loss of muscle fibers leads to increased work for remaining muscle fibers)
      a. Common in amyotrophic lateral sclerosis (ALS), post polio syndrome, Guillain Barré, chronic polyneuropathy, paralysis
      b. Also occurs in patients with incessant muscle activity (i.e., Parkinson disease, Huntington disease)
      c. Multiple sclerosis—exact cause of fatigue unknown, possibly related to CSF interleukins
  3. **Systemic disease:** many including acute/chronic infection, metabolic/endocrine disease, carcinoma, nutritional deficiency/pregnancy, sleep apnea, medications (β-blockers, anticonvulsants, anxiolytics, antidepressants, antipsychotics, chemotherapy/radiation therapy)
  4. **Postviral/chronic fatigue:** unknown etiology; may occur months/years after viral illness; female > male; age onset 20 to 40s; Centers for Disease Control and Prevention (CDC) criteria include persistent/disabling fatigue for at least 6 months with more than four of following: impaired concentration/memory, sore throat, tender lymph nodes, muscle pain, multi-joint pain, headaches, unrefreshing sleep, postexertional malaise >24 hours
      a. **Diagnosis:** exclusion (normal laboratory test results, electromyogram [EMG], nerve conduction study [NCS])
      b. **Treatment:** nonspecific; exercise, antidepressants

VIII. Anxiety

Anxiety is an intermittent or sustained emotional state characterized by feelings of nervousness, irritability, uneasy anticipation, apprehension; usually accompanied by physiologic features; mediated by autonomic nervous system (ANS), thyroid, adrenal

A. Panic attacks
  1. **Presentation/diagnosis:** overwhelming fear/apprehension with series of sympathetic-mediated physiologic reactions (shortness of breath [SOB], dizziness, sweating, trembling, chest pain, abdominal pain, diarrhea, palpitations, feeling that one is about to die); usually occur during calm/nonthreatening situation; escalate over minutes to hours; abate over 20 to 30 minutes; followed by tiredness; sometimes associated with depression/new-onset schizophrenia
  2. **Treatment:** Rx SSRI and benzodiazepam, psychoanalysis
  3. **Must distinguish from temporal lobe seizures** (no loss of consciousness [LOC] in panic attack) and dizziness secondary to vertebrobasilar ischemia, labyrinthine dysfunction; should also rule out somatic disease such as thyrotoxicosis, Cushing, pheochromocytoma, hypoglycemia, and menopause
  4. **Agorophobia:** fear about having a panic attack in places/situations where can't get help, typically restricting what they can do

B. **Anxiety neurosis**
   1. **Presentation/diagnosis:** episodic or sustained anxiety without mood disorder; may include phobic neurosis
   2. **Treatment:** antidepressants/anxiolytics, psychoanalysis

C. **Stress syndrome**
   1. **Presentation/diagnosis:** change in behavior/physiology secondary to environmental challenges that overwhelm adaptive capacity; differs from anxiety in that stressor is external versus internal
   2. **Treatment:** antidepressants/anxiolytics, psychoanalysis

D. **Irritability/irritable aggression:** normal reaction but can be intensified; excessive in patients with depression/mania, sociopathy, premenstrual syndrome (PMS)/postnatal, Alzheimer/dementia, temporal/frontal lobe trauma

IX. Limbic System and Emotion

A. **Hallucinations/delusions:** can be caused by
   1. **Abnormality in perception/thinking:** florid delirium from any cause
   2. **Abnormality in cognition:** common in manic/schizophrenic episodes
   3. **Severe acute pain:** patients have brief attention span followed by groaning and anger

B. **Emotional lability:** easy vacillation from one emotional state to another; response is usually appropriate to stimulus, but excessive; common with diffuse cerebral disease (AD) and frontal lobe damage

C. **Pathologic laughing and crying:** disordered emotional expression with outbursts of involuntary, uncontrollable laughing/crying; usually after very minor stimulus and characterized as having no real feeling or displayed emotion; *causes:* local are lacunar vascular disease, ALS, MS; diffuse are hypoxic-hypotensive encephalopathy, encephalitis, cerebral trauma; medication (rare): imipramine and fluoxetine
   1. **Pseudobulbar palsy:** loss of voluntary movements of muscles innervated by motor nuclei of lower pons and medulla (facial) where reflective pontomedullary activities are preserved (yawning, coughing, crying, and spasmodic laughing), caused by injury (usually vascular or demyelinating) to corticobulbar tract

D. **Rage:** minor provocation leading to blindly impulsive violence and destruction; response out of proportion to stimulus; further stimuli increases violence; impressive physical strength; loss of contact with reality
   1. **Neurologic disease:** usually secondary to severe trauma to medial or anterior temporal lobes; also herpes simplex encephalitis, lobar hemorrhage, hemorrhagic leukoencephalitis
   2. **Acute toxic-metabolic encephalopathy:** patient's attention cannot be obtained; "flailing limbs"; found with phencyclidine (PCP)/cocaine and hypoglycemic reactions
   3. **Temporal seizure:** rare cause; may have prodrome of increased excitability with aggressive behavior/rage in ictal/postictal state; brief; poorly directed
   4. **Episodic reaction without neurologic abnormality:** less understood, some people just like that; alcohol or drug use; *treatment*: lorazepam or haloperidol for acute management

E. **Placidity and apathy:** patients with cerebral disease frequently display quantitative reduction in all activity, not just motor; may be caused by acute lesions to nondominant parietal lobe; common presentation is patient status post infarction who is indifferent to his paralysis, unconcerned with personal relationships/family's sadness, generally inattentive; also found with AD, normal pressure hydrocephalus, corpus callosum tumors

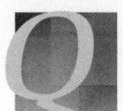 STUDY QUESTIONS FOR CHAPTER 18

Directions: *Each of the numbered items or incomplete statements in this section is followed by answers or by completions of the statement. Select the ONE lettered answer or completion that is BEST in each case.*

1. A patient comes to you with gait apraxia, severe cognitive impairment, and urinary incontinence. What are the two most useful two tests to diagnose the condition?

I. CT, II. MRI, III. SPECT, IV. LP, Removal of CSF, V. VP shunt

(A) I, II
(B) I, IV
(C) II, IV
(D) III, V

2. A patient comes to your attention brought in by his wife who complains that her husband has been using the word "thing" for common objects like a pot or watch. On the neuroimaging that you order to evaluate this condition, what do you expect?

(A) Left anterior temporal
(B) Right anterior temporal
(C) Left posterior temporal
(D) Right posterior temporal

3. A 77-year-old woman with a history of a left capsular infarction develops a dense left hemiparesis. During recovery, she is noted to have unexpected emotional outbursts or laughter and crying. What is the most appropriate treatment for this condition?

(A) Carbamazepine
(B) Fluoxetine
(C) Lorazepam
(D) Quetiapine
(E) Valproic acid

4. A 74-year-old man is brought to your office for difficulties with his memory and performance of his activities of daily living. In order to evaluate his dementia, his primary care physician has already ordered an MRI, TSH, VDRL, and vitamin B_{12} level. What is the likelihood of finding a reversible cause of dementia?

(A) 1% to 2%
(B) 5% to 10%
(C) 10% to 20%
(D) 20% to 30%
(E) 30% to 40%

5. A 63-year-old woman has been having problems with her memory. She relates examples of forgetting her keys around the house and forgetting to pick up certain items at the grocery store. She otherwise has no impairment of her activities of daily living. Other than mild impairments of 5-minute recall, her neurologic examination is normal. What is the most likely diagnosis?

(A) Alzheimer disease
(B) Frontotemporal dementia
(C) Lewy body dementia
(D) Mild cognitive impairment
(E) Vascular dementia

6. A 79-year-old woman is brought to your office for abnormal speech. For the last 2 years, her family has noted the gradual development of word-finding difficulties, decreased comprehension, and poor spelling. More recently, she has been having problems with memory. On your examination, you note prominent abnormalities in language and memory. What is the most likely diagnosis?

(A) Alzheimer disease
(B) Frontotemporal dementia
(C) Lewy body dementia
(D) Primary progressive aphasia
(E) Vascular dementia

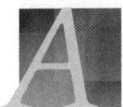 # ANSWERS AND EXPLANATIONS

1. B. CT and LP removal of 20 to 30 mL CSF with objective improvement of gait.

2. A. Lesion in the left anterior temporal lobe.

3. B. This patient is demonstrating pathologic laughter and crying. Common causes include bilateral cerebrovascular disease, ALS, and MS. The most appropriate treatment is fluoxetine.

4. C. In 10% to 20% of cases, a reversible cause of dementia can be found.

5. D. This patient has impairments in memory by history and physical examination, but no other abnormalities suggestive of Alzheimer disease. This makes a diagnosis of mild cognitive impairment the most likely of the options listed. People with Alzheimer disease commonly have broader impairments of their activities of daily living. Frontotemporal dementia classically affects personal and social conduct before memory. Lewy body dementia features cognitive fluctuations and visual hallucinations as early symptoms, rather than memory impairments. Vascular dementia is characterized by episodic accumulation of deficits and is usually accompanied by an abnormal neurologic examination.

6. D. Although she has difficulty with memory, the prominent language problems preceding her memory problems are most consistent with primary progressive aphasia. In Alzheimer disease, language deficits can also be seen, but the memory difficulties are usually earlier and more prominent. Frontotemporal dementia classically affects personal and social conduct before memory. Lewy body dementia features cognitive fluctuations and visual hallucinations as early symptoms, rather than memory impairments. Vascular dementia is characterized by episodic accumulation of deficits and is usually accompanied by an abnormal neurologic examination.

CHAPTER 19

Pediatrics

I. Altered States of Consciousness

A. **Hypoxia**
  1. **Chronic:** associated with a variety of cardiac and pulmonary conditions in patients who become depressed or undergo personality change, seen with PaO_2 < 60 mm Hg, focal neurologic findings if < 40 mm Hg; associated with progressive, irreversible mental decline; following cardiac surgery, hemichorea may develop as a complication
  2. **Acute:** absence of papillary reaction on presentation = will not recover enough to be independent; unconsciousness for 2 months = no language skills or ability to walk
     a. Delayed postanoxic encephalopathy 1 to 2 weeks after recovery, progressive decline
     b. Postanoxic action myoclonus: voluntary motor activity includes myoclonus
  3. **Persistent vegetative state (PVS):** eyes open, sleep–wake cycles but no consciousness; ethically okay to remove all medical treatment/feeding in collaboration with family; 3 months of PVS and will never regain functionality

B. **Infection**
  1. **Herpes simplex virus (HSV)** accounts for about 15% of encephalitis cases; 80% with focal abnormalities, 20% with behavioral changes or seizures; look for T2 hyperintensity in the temporal and inferior frontal lobes; electroencephalogram (EEG) may show periodic lateralized epileptiform discharges (PLEDs). CSF lymphocytic pleocytosis in 97%; red blood cells (RBCs) 0–500/mL; protein elevated and glucose normal; 25% will not follow this pattern. Treat with acyclovir if there is any question that HSV is cause.
  2. **Aseptic meningitis:** usual etiologic agent is enterovirus; one fourth with antecedent illness
     a. **Typical signs:** abrupt onset fever, headache, stiff neck (absent in infants), irritability, lethargy; seizures and coma possible for infants; CSF WBCs (polymorphonuclear cells [PMNs] early, lymphs later) 10 to 200/mL, protein 50 to 100 mg/dL, glucose normal except can be decreased with mumps; treat as bacterial meningitis until cultures come back negative
  3. **Septic meningitis** relatively common in neonates
     a. **Neonatal**
        i. Onset within first 5 days of life: almost always *Escherichia coli* or group B streptococci; mortality ranges up to 50%; symptoms hypo/hyperthermia, vomiting, and lethargy
        ii. After first 5 days of life also includes *Listeria monocytogenes* and other enterococci and enterobacilli; mortality 10%; symptoms lethargy, disturbed feeding, followed by hyperthermia, respiratory distress, seizures, children often have bulging fontanel
        iii. CSF is not the same for preterm and term babies as with adults; as CSF is a frequently tested concept, knowing the norms might be helpful; normal during neonatal period is WBCs 0 to 22/mL^3, protein 20 to 160 mg/dL, glucose 34 to 110

mg/dL; normal for premature neonates is WBCs 0 to 25/mL^3, protein 65 to 150 mg/dL, glucose 25 to 60 mg/dL; infected CSF WBCs (leukocytes) >1,000/mL, protein 30 to 1,500 mg/dL; treatment: ampicillin and gentamicin through 2 weeks after CSF culture is negative

   b. **Children** (≤ age 13, but this definition not universally accepted): most likely culprits are *Streptococcus pneumoniae* and *Neisseria*; other sources include *Haemophilus influenzae;* the child appears sick and does not want to be touched or moved, and has fever, headache, lethargy, and neck stiffness; seizures occur often and consciousness declines; treatment: immediate blood cultures, ampicillin, cephalosporin, and dexamethasone; obtain lumbar puncture (LP) as soon as possible; the evidence for getting a computed tomography before LP in children is marginal

      i. Afterwards, 10% will have bilateral or unilateral hearing loss, 5% will have neurologic deficit, so all patients get their hearing tested after hospitalization

   c. **Tuberculosis** 5% of bacterial meningitis, most common in patients 6 months to 2 years old; suspected patients should get a purified protein derivative (PPD) in emergency department; if untreated, child will likely die within a month; associated with syndrome of inappropriate antidiuretic hormone secretion (SIADH) causing hyponatremia and hypochloremia; treatment: if PPD is positive, give isoniazid (INH); start RIPE early, as mortality ranges up to 20% even with early appropriate treatment (RIPE is rifampin, isoniazid, pyrazinamide, and ethambutol)

4. **Arboviral** account for 10% of cases of meningitis; no treatment for most of them, geographic location is very important; CSF typically shows aseptic meningitis; diagnosis by titer

   a. **La Crosse** is the most common arboviral source of meningitis in the United States; La Crosse located in Wisconsin and New York State: 2 to 3 days of flulike symptoms followed by headache, rapidly followed by seizures

   b. **St. Louis** most common viral source of epidemic meningitis in the United States; the disease has a range of severity with progression of symptoms over 1 to 2 weeks including weakness and tremor; no seizures; children without residual impairment, adults not so lucky

   c. **Japanese B** is most important worldwide, for nonimmunized travelers during the rainy season in Asia; vaccination protects >90%; 2 to 3 days of headache and fever then delirium and later hypotonia and masklike face

   d. **Eastern equine** onset rapid with headache and fever followed by seizure/coma; focal lesions present on magnetic resonance imaging (MRI) in basal ganglia and thalamus

   e. **Western equine** in the Midwest particularly, California and North and South Dakotas, behavioral change followed by drowsiness and coma; EEG abnormal in one temporal lobe, so easily confused with herpes

5. **Fungal infections:** most infections occur in immunocompetent children

   a. *Cryptococcus neoformans* is uncommon before age 10. Chronic, waxing and waning headache that eventually becomes continuous; low grade fever and uncharacteristic mood swings are common symptoms; test for CSF antigen and India ink smear

   b. *Coccidioides immitis* should be considered in any child who develops chronic headache after an upper respiratory infection and who lives in the Southwest or San Joaquin Valley in California; frequently see eosinophils in CSF; test CSF with antibodies and culture

6. **Reye syndrome** is still seen in small epidemics concurrent with influenza/chicken pox epidemics when children are given aspirin; typically there is progression of vomiting followed by vomiting with lethargy over a day or so followed by delirium; diagnosis is suggested by the quartet of hypoglycemia, hyperammonemia, increased LFTs, and normal bilirubin; as this syndrome is deadly, all children should be admitted to the pediatric intensive care unit (PICU) with hypertonic glucose and head elevation; early intubation and mannitol is recommended for increased intracranial pressure with compromise.

C. **Immunosuppressive therapy**
   1. Steroid doses of 0.5 to 1 mg/kg/day can produce hyperactivity and anxiety, doses of 2 mg/kg/day can produce a delirium with schizophrenic features
   2. Cyclosporine causes confusion, fatigue, cortical blindness with visual hallucinations about 5% of the time
   3. OKT3 use—about 25% develop sterile febrile meningitis by the first 5 days, which resolves in a few weeks without discontinuing the drug

D. **Migraine variants**
   1. **Transient global amnesia:** no other signs but retrograde amnesia after attacks; EEG can show background slowing in one temporal lobe; probably a form of migraine
   2. **Confusional migraine:** child becomes rapidly delirious with impaired consciousness and combativeness, lasts 2 to 20 hours, then child falls into a deep sleep; expect a family history of migraine and EEG to show slowing, either occipitally or temporally

II. Headache and Increased Intracranial Pressure (ICP)

A. **Common sense about childhood headaches**
   1. 75% is due to migraine; 10% of children have migraines; children want to go to bed
      a. Intermittent headaches in child who looks sick and recovers completely are migraines
      b. Likely two kinds of headaches—constant mild due to analgesic rebound and migraine
   2. Chronic low intensity headache is not likely serious disease; new onset, serious headache that the child does not recover from likely is due to serious medical or neurological illness
   3. Intense pain lasting a few seconds in an otherwise normal child will probably never be explained unless it is an adolescent with pain on the top of the head that drops the child to the floor and is repeated over days; this is "ice pick" headache, a migraine equivalent

B. **Migraines**
   1. **Prophylaxis:** may still use propanolol at 1 mg/kg/day titrated to 2 mg/kg/day, as it should have no cardiovascular effect on children with normal cardiovascular systems; avoid in asthma; warn about depression and fatigue as the most frequent side effect causing discontinuation
   2. **Treatment:** sleep is best; try promethazine to relieve nausea/vomiting and cause them to fall asleep; triptans are safe in children
   3. **Visual hallucinations** with migraine may be associated with time/body distortions called "Alice in Wonderland" syndrome
   4. **Migraine with aura:** can end by vomiting; migraine without aura vomiting may be more prominent than the headache; neither should be maximal in intensity at outset
   5. **Benign exertional headache:** seen in sports and during sex, migraine variant; headache relieved when activity stops

C. **Headaches with particular attention to childhood features**
   1. **Cluster headaches:** onset >10, headache often begins during sleep, lasts 30 to 90 minutes and happens two to six times per day; the child will pace; treatment; 100% oxygen or lithium for chronic cluster headaches that never seem to go away
      a. **Chronic paroxysmal hemicrania:** shorter and more frequent than cluster headache, try indomethacin first, acetazolamide is second line
      b. **Hemicrania continua:** continuous cluster headache for days to weeks; diagnosis of exclusion when other possible causes have been eliminated; treatment: indomethacin
   2. **Headache mimics**
      a. Sinusitis is the most common misdiagnosis, may be given in the history; patient awakens with headache and after being up and about, it goes away

b. Seizures can rarely be manifested by headaches that are clearly not migraines, can consider getting an EEG in such cases
c. Caffeine can cause dull frontal headache when addicted
d. Monosodium glutamate (MSG) and nitrites can cause throbbing headaches in sensitive children
e. An adolescent who complains of chronic mild headaches should be asked about possible chronic marijuana use irrespective of age
f. 10% of children with lupus have severe headaches; treat with analgesics

D. **Increased intracranial pressure**
  1. Symptoms in children usually includes headache, but can include diplopia, personality changes, and nausea and vomiting, particularly on waking in the morning
  2. Symptoms in infants include failure to thrive, increased head size, and high pitched cry; also impaired upward gaze, sixth nerve palsy, and bulging anterior fontanel; of note is that papilledema is uncommon
  3. **Hemorrhage**
     a. **Shaking injuries/retinal hemorrhages:** look for healing fractures in the posterior rib cage; order a skeletal survey; if the parents ask to sign the child out against medical advice (AMA), it is your duty to refuse; CT shows characteristic subdural blood collections; treatment: bilateral subdural taps, which can be done daily to remove as much fluid as possible; despite treatment outcome is poor
     b. **Preterm peri- or intraventricular hemorrhage (IVH):** very common, found in 20% who weigh less than 1.5 kg at birth; ultrasonography is the standard of care for all with birthweight < 1.8 kg; treatment is primarily monitoring for posthemorrhagic hydrocephalus with ultrasonography that occurs in 10% after IVH; may be asked about grades of hemorrhage grade I—isolated to subependymal, grade II—IVH, grade III–IVH with ventricular dilation, grade IV—IVH with ventricular dilation and extension into the brain parenchyma
        i. Full-term infants less commonly get IVH. Typical scenario is difficult birth with resuscitation at birth, with seizures on the second day of life; treat same as preemies.
  4. **Pseudotumor cerebri:** headaches, vomiting, diplopia, with papilledema and sixth nerve palsy; all get imaging to exclude tumor or hydrocephalus; get basic labs to exclude secondary causes like iron deficiency anemia, hyperthyroidism (primary or secondary), hypoparathyroidism, adrenal insufficiency (primary or secondary), pregnancy; ask about diet and supplements, as vitamins A and D deficiency or vitamin A excess can cause condition; drug-related causes: oral contraceptives, tetracycline, and nalidixic acid; treat with lumbar puncture with drainage of CSF until pressure is one half of the opening pressure; can in addition give acetazolamide; treatment is necessary to reduce the risk of visual loss; formal visual fields should be monitored to check for inferior nasal quadrant defect and enlarging blind spot

III. Developmental Delay

A. **Screening tests:** it is crucial for residents to understand appropriate screening tests for developmental delay; DQ = age that child scored/chronological age; DQ < 70% defines delay; always do a screening neurologic examination; always refer for specialized testing except established mental retardation (MR) diagnosis unless you have a specific chromosomal abnormality diagnosed
  1. **Up to age 3**, use the Denver II or CAT (clinical adaptive test)/CLAMS (clinical linguistic and auditory milestone scale), loss of primitive reflexes
  2. **From age 3 to 5**, Denver II is okay, but Goodenough-Harris draws a figure and Gesell figures should also be included in the evaluation
  3. **After age 5**, it is harder to test, but Goodenough-Harris "draw a figure" and Gesell figures continue to be useful

B. **Speech**
   1. **Normal development:** by 6 months, babies articulate the consonants M, D, and B, but these do not mean anything to the child and can be heard even from deaf children; it is not until about a year that mama/dada mean anything
   2. **Hearing impairment:** the major cause of isolated speech delay is hearing loss and all children with isolated speech delay should receive audiometry
   3. **Autism:** failure of language development, impairment of relationships, restricted activities, and onset before age 3

C. **Motor development:** usually manifestation of ataxia, plegia, or movement disorder, which are covered in individual sections

D. **Global delay:** screen with MRI to detect malformation or perinatal disease; if you recognize a syndrome that is chromosomally based, it is worthwhile to investigate it, as it can be helpful in giving advice to parents and children who may carry the gene; classic chromosomal abnormalities where infant is likely to survive past first year:
   1. **Down syndrome trisomy 21:** incidence 1 in 660, number 1 genetic cause of delay
      a. 6/10 features in neonate suggests diagnosis: hypotonia, poor Moro reflex, hyperflexibility, excess skin on back of neck, flat facies, anomalous auricles, slanted palpebral fissures, pelvic dysplasia, single transverse palmar crease, mid phalanx dysplasia of the fifth finger
      b. Testing—karyotype for diagnosis, echocardiogram, thyroid stimulating hormone (TSH) (yearly), complete blood count (CBC), liver function test (LFT); adult survivors are at a high risk for lymphoma and early onset Alzheimer disease
         i. Meiosis nondisjunction (94%)—incidence rises with maternal age in general; if have one child due to nondisjunction, risk for another child is 1 in 200 if maternal age <35 and double age-specific risk if >35
         ii. Robertsonian translocation (5%)—if mother is carrier, 15% risk of recurrence, 2.5% if father is the carrier, 100% if the translocation is 21:21, <1% if neither
         iii. Mosaicism (1%)—nondisjunction during mitosis after zygote is formed.
   2. **Fragile X syndrome:** incidence 1:1,500 males; trinucleotide repeat CGG in Xq27.3, with number of repeats correlating with severity of disease, normal <50 copies, disease > 200 copies; number 2 genetic cause of delay
      a. Most noticeable feature is long face and large everted ears; autism very common (60%), macrocephalic, postpubertal macroorchidism, tall
      b. X-linked: all mothers of affected males are carriers
      c. Females will generally only have learning disabilities
      d. Testing—karyotype of lymphocytes cultured in folate-deficient medium
   3. **Neurocutaneous syndromes**
      a. Neurofibromatosis (NF) AD clinical manifestations highly variable; NF-1 1:3,000 peripheral type, NF-2 central type; diagnosis by two of the following: at least six café au lait spots, two+ neurofibromas, axillary/inguinal freckles, at least 2 Lisch (iris hamartoma) nodules, first-degree relative with NF-1, osseous dysplasia. NF-2 classically has bilateral acoustic neuromas; also optic gliomas
      b. Tuberous sclerosis (TS) AD, again variable expression even in same family; TS-1 9q34, TS-2 16p13.3, although both appear to have the same symptoms; developmental delay and hard to control seizures are the rule; if survive to childhood, may develop a Shagreen patch (raised plaque over back), facial adenoma sebaceum, retinal tumors, rhabdomyoma of the heart, renal cysts and tumors; mental regression is progressive as cortical hamartomas form; routine MRI is necessary every 2 years because subependymal giant cell astrocytomas (WHO grade I astrocytoma) can form
      c. Chediak-Higashi patients have strangely shaped areas of skin depigmentation with anemia and neutrophil dysfunction causing frequent infections; developmental regression, seizures, and peripheral neuropathy appear within the first 2 years; death usually occurs before age 10

E. **Loss of milestones**
  1. **Homocystinuria** autosomal recessive (AR)
     a. Screen for methionine in urine and/or blood; diagnose with cultured fibroblasts showing a deficiency of cystathionine synthase
     b. Intelligence declines progressively in untreated children; associated features include ataxia, dystonia, aphasia, pseudobulbar palsy, and seizures
     c. Hyperhomocysteinemia causes blood vessel intimal thickening with ensuing thromboembolic disease, a rather unsettling but frequent presentation; another presentation is lens dislocation; all children with either should be screened
     d. One third are pyridoxine responsive and treat with 0.5 to 1 g per day pyridoxine and folate; one third are somewhat responsive; diet of methionine restriction is unpalatable and most do not tolerate and require betaine 6 to 9 g per day, which recycles homocysteine to methionine
  2. **Maple syrup urine disease:** three forms of disease associated with deficiency of branched chain keto-acid dehydrogenase; AR recessive 19q13.1-2
     a. **Classic form:** almost no enzyme; normal newborns develop seizures by second week that become progressively more frequent and severe
     b. **Intermittent form:** small amount of enzyme; episodic ataxia and lethargy with protein or stress due to infection; can die during an attack from metabolic acidosis; treat with thiamine 100–1,000 mg per day; no delay expected between attacks
     c. **Intermediate form:** moderate delay is expected unless there is early intervention; screen with ferric chloride test on urine and diagnose with branched chain amino and ketoacids (quantitative); protein restricted diet is treatment
  3. **Phenylketonuria:** AR 12q24.1 deficiency of phenylalanine hydroxylase, compulsory screening for the musty odored urine; phenylalanine restricted diet in all newborns with phenylalanine concentration of 20 mg/dL or greater; requires referral as diet therapy is complicated; almost no patients continue the diet into adulthood; quitting after age 12, causes about a 7 point IQ drop compared to parents, whereas with continuation of the diet, IQ is not different from that of parents; more importantly, many parents who stop the diet have been resistant to change their diets back for their children, with disastrous effects
  4. **GM1 gangliosidosis:** AR 3p deficiency of β-galactosidase; onset between 6 months and age 1 1/2 with weakness, incoordination, and slowed development followed by spasticity, seizures, and loss of milestones; cherry red macula and coarse facial features may be present; death by 7 years
  5. **Tay Sachs disease or infantile GM2 gangliosidosis:** AR deficiency of hexosaminidase A; 10 time more prevalent in Ashkenazi Jews than the rest of the population; most have an abnormal Moro reflex and a cherry red macula by 3 to 6 months; rapid loss of milestones occurs as the child becomes spastic, unresponsive, and severely retarded by age 1; prenatal diagnosis by amniocentesis
  6. **Sandhoff disease:** AR deficiency of both hexosaminidase A and B
     a. Exactly like Tay Sachs but can affect other organs; to be suspected in every Tay Sachs presentation that does not affect a Jewish child; prenatal diagnosis by amniocentesis of N-acetylglucosaminyl oligosaccharides (usually have to specifically request this)
  7. **Gaucher disease:** AR 1q21 deficiency of glucocerebrosidase; three types: type I does not affect nervous system, type II onset before 6 months of age, type III onset during childhood; type II presents with motor milestone regression and cranial nerve palsies, followed by splenomegaly and hypotonia then spasticity; death by first 2 years; type III is treated by modified β-glucosidase and does not progress rapidly
  8. **Krabbe disease** (globoid cell leukodystrophy): AR deficiency of galactosylceramide β-galactosidase; onset 1 to 7 months with enhanced startle, progressive hypertonicity, peripheral neuropathy, and often chronic fever; within 2 to 4 months the infant is in permanent opisthotonos; almost all die or are in a chronic vegetative state by age 1

a. Also has late-onset form with developmental regression, cortical blindness, and spasticity; it is called juvenile Krabbe disease even though it presents age 2 to 6+
9. **I-cell disease:** AR 4q21–23 deficiency/dysfunction of *N*-acetylglucosamine phosphotransferase is similar to Hurler syndrome with striking gum hypertrophy; consider for all infants with Hurler symptoms but negative for mucopolysacchariduria
10. **Mucopolysaccharidoses** (MPSs) all are AR except II, which is X; all are treated with bone marrow transplantation; screen by testing for mucopolysacchariduria; definitive diagnosis by testing for specific enzyme deficiency in cultured fibroblasts
    a. MPS I (Hurler); 4p16.3 deficiency of lysosomal hydrolase α-L-iduronidase; development is normal in first year, and delayed in the second with corneal clouding, facial feature coarsening, hepatosplenomegaly, and dwarfism; radiographs show specific abnormalities including bony hypoplasia, enlarged sella turcica, and shallow orbits
    b. MPS II (Hunter) Xq28 deficiency of iduronate sulfatase similar to Hurler without corneal clouding; watch for nerve entrapment and hydrocephalus; progression is variable
    c. MPS III (Sanfilippo); slow, progressive mental deterioration age 2 with coarsened features, hepatosplenomegaly; often presents with hyperactivity and sleep disorder
11. **Niemann-Pick disease:** AR deficiency of sphingomyelinase
    a. Type A presents in first months of life with feeding difficulty and hepatomegaly; a cherry red macula may be present; progressive blindness, emaciation, and hyperactive reflexes develop; screen for vacuolated leukocytes
    b. Type C 18q11–12; similar to type A, but presents later after age 2 and slowed progression; look for cerebellar ataxia or dystonia; there is also an adolescent form
12. **Mitochondrial diseases:** mitochondria are transmitted maternally
    a. Alexander disease: 11q13 NADH-ubiqone oxoreductase flavoprotein-1; presents with megalencephaly, spasticity, and seizures; MRI shows leukodystrophy of deep white matter but sparing the periventricular region; presents any time from birth to childhood, and death occurs within 2 years of presentation
    b. Leigh disease (subacute necrotizing encephalomyelopathy): AR and X-linked forms, deficiency of enzyme of energy metabolism, most common form is cytochrome C oxidase deficiency; usually presents in first 2 years with respiratory problems, variable ocular dysmotility and hearing problems, and hypotonia; if survives to childhood will have very thin legs called stork legs; symptoms worsened by a high carbohydrate meal; MRI reveals T2 hyperintensity of the bilateral basal ganglia, thalamus, and dorsal brainstem; treatment: restrict carbohydrates, high dose thiamine helpful in some, acetazolamide helpful if X-linked form
    c. Menkes kinky hair syndrome Xq13: at about 3 months infant becomes lethargic and less reactive, with myoclonic seizures provoked by stimulation, with progressive developmental regression; look for high-arched palate, full cheeks, and wiry hair that breaks easily; most die by age 18 months; copper supplementation is somewhat helpful
13. **Lesch-Nyhan disease Xq26–27:** deficiency of hypoxanthine guanine phosphorylase; children develop motor delay by 3 months, followed by rigidity and cervical dystonia, facial grimacing, involuntary movements by age 2, and finally compulsive self-mutilation by biting fingers, lips, and cheeks, aggression, and mental retardation; although can treat some symptoms, the neurologic deterioration is relentless
14. **Rett syndrome:** Xq28 1:10,000, occurs only in females; developmental arrest at some point between 5 and 18 months, hypotonia, lack of interest in the environment followed by rapid loss of developmental milestones and stereotyped hand movements with complete loss of interest in the environment
15. **Adrenoleukodystrophy:** X-linked deficiency of peroxisomal acetyl coenzyme A synthetase; about one half will have a relentless neurologic deterioration that starts with a behavioral change, which progresses to include gait and coordination apraxias, then seizures, and finally chronic vegetative state or death; treatment is bone marrow transplantation if presents early enough

IV. Hypotonic Infant

A. **Testing**
  1. **Phasic tone** = deep tendon reflexes that respond by rapid contraction
  2. **Postural tone** = prolonged anti-gravity contraction
  3. **Diagnosis** by testing three maneuvers:
     a. **Traction response:** lift baby to sitting position by hands and should see the end lifting up immediately with lifting the body; cannot elicit if <33 weeks gestation
     b. **Vertical suspension:** lift baby in axillae without grasping thorax; baby should press down on shoulders to maintain self and should keep head up
     c. **Horizontal suspension:** suspend baby horizontally by stomach; baby should be able to intermittently keep back straight, keep head up, and limbs flexed

B. **Cerebral hypotonia**
  1. **Diagnostic clues:** dysmorphic features, abnormalities of organs or brain function, tightly fisted hand with thumb enclosed (fisting), legs crossed under vertical suspension (scissoring)
  2. **Prader-Willi syndrome:** maternal disomy of chromosome 15, and Angelman syndrome, paternal disomy of chromosome 15
     a. Prader-Willi: hypogonadism/cryptorchidism, short stature, hypotonic, deep tendon reflexes (DTRs) depressed or absent, feeding difficulties; hypotonia and feeding difficulties persist to about 10 months of age and are replaced by mental retardation and insatiable hunger; diagnosis by chromosome analysis and advise that chromosome 15 is likely the one affected
  3. **Chronic nonprogressive encephalopathy:** many causes, basically hypotonia is only symptom and gets better over time; if coupled with any other abnormality, get MRI
  4. **Riley-Day syndrome** (see subsequent section on autonomic problems)
  5. **Oculocerebrorenal syndrome** = Lowe syndrome; Xq26 recessive; hypotonic and hyporeflexive, often with glaucoma/cataracts; mental retardation and progressively worsening renal function with proteinuria and metabolic acidosis appear later; special diet may be helpful, most require bicarbonate
  6. **Cerebrohepatorenal syndrome** = Zellweger syndrome; disease of mitochondria; therefore, transmitted maternally; several gene loci; newborns identified by their dysmorphic features: pear-shaped head with wide cheeks, widened sutures, micrognathia, hypertelorism with flat nose bridge, flexion deformities of knees and ankles; associated with biliary cirrhosis, polycystic kidneys, retinal degeneration, and migration disorders of cerebral formation; seizures usually begin shortly after birth and are difficult to control; most affected infants pass by 1 year
     a. Neonatal leukodystrophy and infantile Refsum disease are milder variants

C. **Spinal cord**
  1. **Hypoxic-ischemic myelopathy with gray matter necrosis:** hypotonic, areflexic
  2. **Spinal cord injury during vaginal delivery**
     a. **Breech presentation:** 70% have injuries if head is hyperextended, can occur at any spinal level; find level by viewing where stops sweating
     b. **Cephalic presentation:** trunk fails to twist with the head fracturing odontoid process; most are unconscious at birth

D. **Motor**
  1. Get a **creatine kinase (CK) level** and an **electromyogram (EMG)** after CK level; muscle biopsy is only useful sometimes
  2. **Spinal muscle atrophy** (SMA), two forms both AR—diagnosis readily established by demonstrating gene abnormality on 5q13; SMA 3 occurs later
     a. **SMA 1**—onset birth to 6 months proximal > distal weakness, hypotonia, and areflexia; relentless progression of weakness; when gag is lost, will die due to aspiration
     b. **SMA 2**—normal at birth with delayed motor development often with fine hand tremor—usually can sit but never stand unsupported.

3. **Infantile neuronal degeneration:** AR caused by enzyme deficiency; appears as SMA but includes degeneration of cerebellum, thalamus, and sensory nerves; can be differentiated from SMA by EMG (nerve conduction velocity [NCV] decreased, sensory nerve action potentials [SNAPs] absent) and diagnosed by sending for urine sialoglycopeptides; death is nearly universal

V. Ataxia

A. **Acute or recurrent ataxia**
   1. **Reversible causes:** brain tumors usually present as subacute chronic ataxia, but may rarely bleed, cause hydrocephalus, or most commonly parents do not observe early signs until there is an obvious gait ataxia; for this reason, imaging should be performed on almost everyone; in addition, drug intoxication with phenytoin, antihistamines, or most psychoactive drugs are frequent causes, and so all should have a drug screen
      a. Myoclonic encephalopathy can be due to occult neuroblastoma; onset—birth to 4 years with chaotic eye movements, myotonic ataxia (constant rapid muscular contractions causing ataxia), and personality change that waxes over a week; screen with chest/abdomen MRI, urine homovanillic acid; treat with ACTH or steroids
   2. **Genetics**
      a. Episodic ataxia—1 autosomal dominant (AD) 12p mutation of potassium channel; at age 4 to 7, child feels sudden onset spreading stiffness and most sit down followed by ataxia lasting up to 6 hours; attacks usually start when the child is startled; treat with acetazolamide, or if that fails with phenytoin
      b. Episodic ataxia—2 AD 19p mutation of calcium channel; onset sometime during childhood with vertigo, jerk nystagmus, and ataxia lasting for up to a day; child can be affected by only one or two of the symptoms; usually becomes milder with age; almost all patients respond to acetazolamide, or if cannot be tolerated with flunarizine; anticonvulsants are not helpful, unlike for episodic ataxia-1
      c. Hartnup disease—AR defect of amino acid absorption; hallmark is severe rash that appears with sunlight exposure; stress triggers ataxia, nystagmus, emotional instability, and/or decreased consciousness; can have rash alone or neurologic attacks alone; treat with nicotinamide and high protein diet
      d. Pyruvate dehydrogenase E1 deficiency X-linked; episodic ataxia, dysarthria, dysarthria, and lactic acidosis; the lactic acidosis can be sufficiently severe to cause death; treatment prevents attacks but not progression of ataxia
   3. **Postinfectious causes** particularly varicella infection/vaccine
      a. **Acute cerebellar ataxia:** ataxia that is maximal at outset with nystagmus and clear sensorium; gets better in a few days, and complete recovery occurs in most by 6 months; one of the few cases for which brain imaging is not mandatory; no treatment
      b. **Miller Fisher syndrome:** ataxia, ophthalmoplegia, and areflexia; recovery within 6 months; no treatment
      c. **Multiple sclerosis:** 5% of cases occur in children younger than 5; similar to adult form, but usually presents with ataxia and fever; give steroids for acute exacerbations; adult MS drugs have not been tested in children
      d. Check an antibody titer

B. **Chronic ataxia**
   1. **Tumors should be considered with any ataxia accompanied by headache**; the following are all the major childhood posterior fossa tumors, but all supratentorial tumors may have ataxia with progression of the tumor; get an MRI
      a. **Cerebellar astrocytoma:** presents with headache and nausea in children >5 years, ataxia if <5 years, headache is not usually the classic increased ICP headache; get an MRI and attempt to remove surgically; with partial resection, give radiation

- b. **Brainstem glioma:** expect this to present with bilateral (facial, abducens) cranial nerve dysfunction, especially facial and abducens, although ataxia is often a feature with progression as well as hemiplegia and dysphagia; median survival is 10 months
- c. **Medulloblastoma:** most common brain tumor of infancy; vomiting, headache, refusal to stand or walk, and torticollis are most common symptoms; if reflexes are hyperactive, child may have hydrocephalus; treat with gross total resection, craniospinal radiation, and chemotherapy
- d. **Ependymoma:** slowly waxing and waning increased intracranial pressure with ataxia, intermittent nature due to temporary fourth ventricular obstruction; treat with surgery and posterior fossa radiation
2. **Malformations** all are diagnosed with MRI
   - a. **Basilar impression** = posterior displacement of the odontoid, which compresses the spinal cord or possibly the brainstem; minor trauma to the head or neck precipitates neck stiffness, headache, ataxia, and nystagmus; treat surgically
     - i. Klippel-Feil syndrome—three types: low posterior hairline, short neck, limited neck movement, and vertebral fusions (type I thoracic and cervical, type II atlantooccipital, type III cervical and lower thoracic or lumbar), associated with deafness, scapula deformity, hydrocephalus, and basilar impression
   - b. **Hypoplasia of the cerebellum** presents with developmental delay and hypotonia. Head tremor (called titubation) as well as at least one of ataxia, dysmetria, or intention tremor is always present. Look for nystagmus and expect mental retardation.
   - c. **Hypoplasia/aplasia of the vermis** can be partial or complete so has a range of presentations from asymptomatic to head tremor with truncal ataxia.
     - i. Dandy-Walker syndrome can be trisomy 9 or X-linked aplasia of the vermis, cystic dilation of the fourth ventricle, and hydrocephalus, which does not have to be present at birth; presents with ataxia or macrocephaly often with occipital bulging; treat surgically
     - ii. Joubert syndrome; AR aplasia of the vermis with oculomotor apraxia and episodic hyperpnea possibly followed by apnea when a neonate; the so-called molar tooth sign is pathognomonic: deep interpeduncular fossa, thick and straight cerebellar peduncles, hypoplastic vermis; look for anteverted nostrils and triangular-shaped mouth when open
   - d. **Chiari malformation type I** is cerebellar ectropion II; also includes downward displacement of the medulla; presentation is often during teenage years with headache, weakness, ataxia, and lower cranial nerve dysfunction; treat with surgical decompression
3. **Genetics**
   - a. **Friedreich ataxia:** AR 9q13 triplet repeat disorder most common inherited ataxia; onset between 2 and 18 years with ataxia, clumsiness, or scoliosis; ataxia and dysarthria are progressive; most patients have absent tendon reflexes and extensor plantar responses; many develop scoliosis so severe that it requires surgical stabilization; hypertrophic cardiomyopathy develops in close to half and requires close monitoring with chest x-rays and ECGs; diabetes can develop; treat symptoms, no treatment for underlying disorder
   - b. **Hypobetalipoproteinemia:** AD; unexplained progressive ataxia with high triglyceride, low high density lipoproteins (HDL), and low low density lipoproteins (LDL); give high dose vitamin E
   - c. **Abetalipoproteinemia:** AR 4q22-24; defective microsomal triglyceride transport protein causes fat malabsorption with vomiting and loose stool at birth; if left untreated, there is posterior spinal column demyelination and progressive limb ataxia; symptom progression is halted with fat restriction and high dose vitamin E
   - d. **Ataxia-telangiectasia:** AR 11q22-23; causes ataxia, chronic sinus/pulmonary infections, and oculomotor apraxia; with age, telangiectasias develop; screen by checking for acanthocytes on smear; do not use radiation to scan if at all possible, as gene defect does not allow DNA repair and affected individuals are very prone to develop neoplasia from radiation doses that would have no effect on normal children

e. **Ramsay Hunt syndrome:** AR; cerebellar ataxia and myoclonus develop due to progressive deterioration of the dentate nucleus and superior cerebellar peduncle; seizures affect most but occur infrequently; treat with anticonvulsants and valproic acid for myoclonus

VI. The Plegias

A. **Monoplegia**
  1. **Plexitis:** treat with range of motion, often uses MRI to exclude other causes
     a. **Brachial:** prior immunization by tetanus toxoid in all infants; severe arm or shoulder pain abrupt in appearance and lasting up to 3 weeks, as pain decreases, it is replaced by weakness; 90% recover in 3 years; EMG and clinical diagnosis
     b. **Lumbar:** fever then abrupt leg pain in 3 to 7 days; and about a week later by weakness
     c. **Hereditary brachial plexopathy:** AD chromosome 17; two different types; 17q25 similar to brachial plexitis with family history and the attacks recur usually about one every 3 years; 17p11.2, called hereditary neuropathy with liability to pressure palsy, have a painless monoplegia that develops after trivial trauma and has complete recovery
     d. **Neonatal brachial neuropathy:** vaginal birth trauma, occurs in 1:1,000 live births, abducted and internally rotated arm, elbow extension and lack of Moro; spontaneous recovery in more than half; consider reconstructive surgery if no recovery at 6 months
  2. **Osteomyelitis–neuritis:** infantile disease where arm is flaccid, but there is pain in shoulder caused by osteomyelitis of the humerus; aspirate shoulder joint and treat with antibiotics; consider with any infant who has brachial plexitis
  3. **Hopkins syndrome** = asthmatic amyotrophy; clinical diagnosis of sudden flaccid monoplegia during recovery of asthmatic attack; recovery is incomplete; all have been vaccinated with the polio vaccine
  4. **Injuries**
     a. Brachial plexus—mild injuries: range of motion (ROM) exercises, severe: rest limb for one month
     b. Lumbar plexus—almost always associated with pelvic fractures/dislocations

B. **Cerebral palsy (Hypoxic-ischemic encephalopathy)**
  1. **Description:** chronic motor disability affecting 2:1,000 live births, most of the time idiopathic, about one fourth will have mental retardation
  2. **Hemiplegic:** affects one side, imaging studies useful, clinical diagnosis established with hemiplegia, hand dominance formed in the first year, and no other diagnoses
  3. **Spastic diplegia:** affects legs > arms, usually caused by premature birth–induced periventricular leukomalacia; scissoring, increased deep tendon reflexes, hip dislocation, adductor response, ankle clonus, and extensor plantar response can be seen; this is a clinical diagnosis; therapy is multidisciplinary
     a. Spastic paraplegia is diplegia in which the only symptoms in the upper extremity are increased deep tendon reflexes
  4. **Spastic quadriplegia:** profound developmental delay from intrauterine disease or hypoxic ischemic encephalopathy; classic posture—head/neck retracted, hands clenched with elbow flexion, legs extended; infantile reflexes do not disappear; MRI of brain is normally checked for brain malformations

C. **Acute hemiplegia**
  1. **Cerebrovascular disease:** stroke is considered for any new onset hemiplegia; incidence is 2.5:100,000 per year; typical initial studies: CT head looking for hemorrhage
     a. Hemorrhagic sources: arteriovenous malformation (AVM), brain tumor, cocaine use (can also be ischemic)
     b. Internal carotid artery occlusion with chronic tonsillitis, cat-scratch disease, mycoplasma pneumonia; diagnose with arteriography, treat with aggressive targeted antibiotics

i. Fibromuscular dysplasia acts in many ways like internal carotid artery occlusion except that arteriography shows segmental narrowing like a string of beads.
  c. Sinus venous thrombosis
    i. In infants with heart disease; dehydrated and polycythemic; consider with any case of infant hemiplegia with seizures and decreased consciousness
    ii. In children, most likely cause is hypercoagulable states; expect increased intracranial hemorrhage and hemiplegia; treat with rehydration and decreasing anticoagulation; determine specific coagulation abnormality; search for: valvular PFD, heart disease, endocarditis
  d. Embolic arterial occlusion primarily mitral valve prolapse, also other heart abnormalities; cardiac echo is mandatory; aspirin is advised
  e. Sickle cell anemia—seizure can be initial presentation, which when ended have hemiplegia or other deficits present; manage with oxygen, fluids, and packed red blood cells; strokes can be avoided if hemoglobin S is below 30%
  f. Moyamoya—recurrent transient ischemic attacks (TIAs) or sudden hemiplegia are most common manifestations; diagnose with angiography, which appears hazy ("puff of smoke" appearance) in the affected area; often there is an underlying vasculopathy or coagulopathy, which should be looked for, and MRI shows characteristic lesions in basal ganglia

D. **Todd paralysis** = postictal hemiparesis; hemiparesis may be a seizure manifestation

E. **Diabetes mellitus:** children can get acute incidents of hemiplegia; usual manifestation is waking up with headache and hemiparesis with face/arm > leg; aphasia may be present. It lasts up to a day. Recovery is complete, but recurrences are common

F. **Chronic hemiplegia: consider brain tumor, abscess, AVM, demyelinating disease**
  1. **Sturge-Weber syndrome:** cutaneous angioma of the face with ipsilateral intracranial angioma; seizures in more than three fourths, usual onset before end of first year, usual type focal motor; most of those who develop seizures will be developmentally delayed; about half will develop hemiplegia contralateral to the cutaneous angioma; treat with hemispherectomy if seizures begin in infancy

VII. Sensation

A. **Hereditary sensory and autonomic neuropathies** (HSANs): most have no treatment
  1. **HSAN I sensory 9q AD variable penetrance (VP):** after first decade, lancinating pain in legs and feet with ulcerations; feet affected more than hands; lose pain/temperature sensation before touch/pressure; diagnose by AD and sensory loss in feet; evoked potential (EP) shows decreased conduction velocity (CV), no sensory nerve action potentials (SNAPs); sural nerve biopsy reveals greatly decreased myelinated fibers and decreased small myelinated fibers
    a. Familial amyloid polyneuropathy similar presentation, but also often includes urinary incontinence, impotence, and postural hypotension
  2. **HSAN II AR:** diffuse loss of sensation beginning at birth, loss of reflexes, often includes decreases in hearing, taste, smell; no SNAPs; motor CV normal
  3. **HSAN III** = Riley Day syndrome AR 9q: Hypotonia, feeding difficulties, poor control of autonomic functions, meconium aspiration; sucking and swallowing separately normal, but cannot be coordinated; absent fungiform papillae; diagnose by miosis with pilocarpine or methacholine drops, corneal insensitivity, and absence of tears; treatment: bethanechol orally 1 to 2 mg/kg/day
  4. **HSAN IV AR:** congenital insensitivity to pain, anhidrosis, mental retardation; often presents with repeated fevers, which can include seizures during the summer
    a. Anhidrotic ectodermal dysplasia presents similarly, but has normal pain sensation.

5. **HSAN with spastic paraplegia:** stiff-legged gait from spasticity and delayed motor milestones; sensory neuropathy with insensitivity to pain that becomes progressively worse; usually appears later; mentation is normal; diagnose when neuropathy is so bad that ulcers have begun to appear on feet

B. **Hereditary metabolic neuropathies**
   1. **Acute intermittent porphyruria:** AD 11q23.3; deficiency of porphobilinogen deaminase; most are asymptomatic, those patients that have symptoms get them during hormonal changes or when taking certain drugs like barbiturates; symptoms include abdominal pain, proximal > distal motor neuropathy (arms > legs); about one half will get psychiatric symptoms or seizures; some have depression or anxiety between attacks; screen by urinary γ-aminolevulinic acid; diagnose by red blood cell porphobilinogen deaminase level activity; treat with IV glucose and avoid triggers
   2. **Hereditary tyrosinemia:** AR deficiency of fumarylacetoacetate; presentation at age 1 with attacks of with abdominal and leg pain with limb hypertonicity; weakness may be so severe as to require ventilatory support; attacks may also include seizures of self mutilation; screening same as acute intermittent porphyria; diagnose with increased tyrosine and decreased fumarylacetoacetate hydrolase; treat with NTBC, which stands for (2-(2-nitro-4-trifluoromethylbenzoyl)-1,3-cyclohexanedione)

C. **Syringomyelia:** a fluid-filled cavity or syrinx is present in the gray matter of the spinal cord; must distinguish this condition from cystic astrocytoma, which would show solid enhancing tumor nodule on MRI, but this is done with an MRI; usually affects pain and temperature transmission first; often presents during teens; if the syrinx is in the cervical area, sensation is lost in the cape area; progression is insidious with enlargement into the ventral horn with weakness and atrophy in the hands; finally, there is loss of touch and vibratory sense; treat with shunt or excision

STUDY QUESTIONS FOR CHAPTER 19

Directions: Each of the numbered items or incomplete statements in this section is followed by answers or by completions of the statement. Select the ONE lettered answer or completion that is BEST in each case.

1. A 3-day old boy has a fever to 104°F, vomiting, and lethargy. A lumbar puncture shows 1,400 WBCs/mL with a protein of 350 mg/dL and glucose of 10 mg/dL. What is the most likely etiology of his meningitis?

   (A) *Escherichia coli*
   (B) *Listeria monocytogenes*
   (C) *Streptococcus pneumoniae*
   (D) *Neisseria meningitidis*
   (E) *Haemophilus influenzae*

2. A neonate recovers after treatment for bacterial meningitis. Which cranial nerve is most likely to be compromised as a long-term consequence of this process?

   (A) CN III
   (B) CN V
   (C) CN VI
   (D) CN VII
   (E) CN VIII

3. A 4-year-old girl with tuberous sclerosis is brought to your clinic by her parents. They would like to obtain an MRI of her head. Which tumor of the central nervous system is most frequently seen in tuberous sclerosis?

   (A) Acoustic neuroma
   (B) Hemangioblastoma
   (C) Oligodendroglioma
   (D) Optic glioma
   (E) Subependymal giant cell astrocytoma

4. During routine newborn screening, a neonate is found to have a phenylalanine concentration of 48 mg/dL. Which of the following is true concerning phenylalanine restriction?

   (A) It is not necessary, as this is a normal value for phenylalanine
   (B) It will likely preserve this newborn's intellect into adulthood
   (C) Although it may benefit the newborn through infancy, mental retardation is certain
   (D) If discontinued in the teens, the patient's intellect will likely be preserved relative to his parents
   (E) It will be of no benefit to this patient

5. At age 4 months, a baby girl develops enhanced startle, progressive hypertonicity, and chronic fever. Three months later, she is in a permanent state of opisthotonos. Among other studies, she has an EMG that demonstrates diffuse slowing of her nerve conduction velocities. Which enzyme is likely to be deficient in this baby?

   (A) Hexosaminidase A
   (B) Glucocerebrosidase
   (C) Galactosylceramide beta-galactosidase
   (D) Iduronate sulfatase
   (E) Sphingomyelinase

6. A 3-month old infant becomes lethargic and less reactive with myoclonic seizures provoked by stimulation. Over the ensuing months, progressive developmental regression is noted. Physical examination discloses a high-arched palate, full cheeks, and wiry hair that breaks easily. What is the most likely pattern of inheritance of this disorder?

   (A) Autosomal dominant
   (B) Autosomal recessive
   (C) Mitochondrial
   (D) X-linked dominant
   (E) X-linked recessive

7. You are asked to see a newborn with difficult-to-control seizures. When you arrive, you are struck by several dysmorphic features including a pear-shaped head with wide cheeks, widened sutures, micrognathia, hypertelorism, and flexion deformities of the knees and ankles. What is the most likely diagnosis?

   (A) Adrenoleukodystrophy
   (B) Homocystinuria
   (C) Hurler syndrome
   (D) Metachromatic leukodystrophy
   (E) Zellweger syndrome

8. A 3-year old girl is brought to your office for 2 months of chaotic eye movements and ataxia. A chest CT demonstrates neuroblastoma. What is the most appropriate treatment for this child?

   (A) Acetazolamide
   (B) ACTH
   (C) Carbamazepine
   (D) Haloperidol
   (E) Trihexyphenidyl

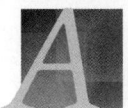# ANSWERS AND EXPLANATIONS

1. A. In neonates, the most common causes of meningitis are *Escherichia coli* and group B streptococcus. Listeria is also a common cause, but is less common than *E. coli*. The other choices listed are common causes of meningitis in older patients.

2. E. After meningitis, approximately 10% of neonates will develop bilateral or unilateral hearing loss.

3. E. Tuberous sclerosis is associated with subependymal giant cell astrocytoma. Acoustic neuroma is associated with neurofibromatosis type 2. Hemangioblastoma is seen in Von Hippel-Lindau syndrome. Oligodendroglioma is not classically associated with any of the neurocutaneous disorders. Optic gliomas are found in patients with neurofibromatosis type 1.

4. B. A normal serum phenylalanine concentration is less than 20 mg/dL. Phenylalanine restriction will likely preserve the newborn's intellect into adulthood. Teens who discontinue phenylalanine restriction will likely have a lower IQ than their parents.

5. C. The baby in the vignette has a history most consistent with Krabbe disease, which is an autosomal recessive disorder associated with deficiency of galactosylceramide β-galactosidase. Hexosaminidase A deficiency produces Tay-Sachs disease. Lack of glucocerebrosidase is the cause of Gaucher disease. Iduronate sulfatase deficiency produces Hunter syndrome. Sphingomyelinase deficiency is the cause of Niemann-Pick disease.

6. E. The infant in the vignette has a clinical history most consistent with Menkes kinky hair syndrome. This disorder is inherited in an X-linked recessive fashion.

7. E. The pattern of dysmorphic features is most consistent with Zellweger syndrome. The dysmorphisms listed are not associated with the other syndromes.

8. B. The child described in the vignette has opsoclonus-myoclonus associated with neuroblastoma. The most appropriate treatment for this condition is ACTH or corticosteroids.

CHAPTER 20

Neuroradiology

I. Our Approach

We will review modern imaging modalities and their uses. In addition, the chapter contains multiple image-based questions that explore topics often included on the Neurology board examination.

A. During neuroradiology rounds, try to be as formal as possible with every image; that is, "This is axial/coronal/sagittal, etc. T2-weighed magnetic resonance imaging (MRI), which shows a hyperintensity (hyperdensity for computed tomography [CT]) in the putamen." Precisely specify the anatomic area as well as possible. Do this for each image presented. Then say, the differential diagnosis of this type of lesion is ... If additional imaging is needed to determine the lesion from the differential diagnosis, specify it. This is excellent practice for being able to evaluate images on the boards.

II. Imaging Modalities

A. Shadow radiography (i.e. plain films)
  1. Generally only useful for cervical spine fractures, spondylolysis, flexion-extension views for spinal instability, or to show implants/wires. Shows distribution of ionized calcium.
  2. C-Spine clearance. Normally done by the trauma team in the emergency department (ED), but is fair game during the test. Order lateral C-spine plain film. Many will include a view of the dens through the mouth, called the odontoid view. Visualize C1 to C8 and the C8–T1 junction. If you cannot, get a Swimmer view (alternatively called Fletcher view). Clear the C-spine if no tenderness, neurologically intact, the patient is not intoxicated and coherent, and C-spine normal. If any subluxation <3.5 mm, get flexion-extension views, to diagnose ligamentous injury. If no movement, clear the C-spine.
  3. Skull radiogram is of limited utility except for classic findings like multiple myeloma and Paget disease; can be helpful in evaluating extraaxial skull tumors that invade outside the skull: meningioma and metastatic, especially gastrointestinal (GI) and prostate, aneurysmal bone cyst (usually occipital), and hyperostosis frontalis interna (thickened frontal bone sparing the midline). Bone scan is superior to show osteolytic and osteoblastic lesion.

B. Computerized tomography (CT)
  1. **The CT scanner** was developed directly from x-ray technology and measures the density of tissues being studied. The terms hyperdense and hypodense are used to refer to brighter and darker areas, respectively, on CT scans. Image density is often expressed in Hounsfield units (HU) (Table 20-1).

Table 20-1	Hounsfield Units for Commonly Imaged Tissues
Tissue	HU
Air	−1000 to −600
Fat	−100 to −60
Water	0
CSF	8–18
White matter	30–34
Gray matter	37–41
Fresh congealed blood	50–100
Bone	600–2000

2. **Computerized tomography** has several advantages over other imaging modalities. It is cheaper, more widely available, and faster than the other modalities that will be described. CT is the image modality of choice for head trauma, skull fracture, and acute hemorrhage. In addition, CT can be used with patients who are claustrophobic, or have metallic fragments or implanted devices.
3. **CT is clearly the superior choice in the following instances:** central nervous system (CNS) tumors with calcifications like craniopharyngioma, oligodendroglioma, retinoblastoma, or meningioma; temporal bone; fractures; or bony or chondral lesions. Some clinicians prefer it for spinal stenosis, trauma, or hardware.
4. **Dye can cause contrast-induced nephropathy.** Any creatinine level >1.4 mg/dL is at risk, and you can expect a discussion to be required with the radiologist. Either give four doses of 600 mg acetylcysteine with fluids (two the day of procedure and two the day after) or give normal saline with bicarbonate, 154 mEq/L one hour before and 6 hours after at a rate of 3 mL/kg/hour.

C. **Magnetic resonance imaging** (MRI)
   1. **MRI** has transformed diagnostic imaging with its high-resolution high-contrast images. The image propagation of MRI involves the manipulation of hydrogen atom protons within a strong magnetic field. MRI allows for multiple image acquisition techniques that allow for improved identification of tissue type and chronicity of lesions. Examining proton relaxation times (T1 and T2) among different axes to the magnetic field allows the scanner to differentiate tissue type based upon their proton composition. T1-weighted images are useful in identifying anatomy. T1 hyperintensity (bright) areas are normally fat or blood. T2-weighted images are better for identifying pathology. In T2 imaging, water is bright (Table 20-2; we suggest that this table be memorized). The mnemonic **Iddy biddy baby dada** can be helpful—for blood hyperacute is T1 **I**sointense, T2 **d**ark (iddy), acute T1 **b**right, T2 **d**ark (biddy), then subacute T1, 2 bright and chronic T1, 2 dark. (See Figures 20-3 and 20-8 left as examples of T1 and compare to Figure 20-8 right and Figure 20-16 right.) Proton density is between T1 and T2 and is excellent for showing the differentiation of white from gray matter, and is the preferred imaging modality for diffuse axonal injury. Cerebrospinal fluid (CSF) is bright and white matter is dark. Of note, the effect of MRI on a fetus is unknown, so avoid in early pregnancy. Gadolinium should be used any time that it is possible that there has been breakdown of the blood–brain barrier. (See Figure 20-6 lower left.) Gadolinium images are T1 images. They can be easily seen from T1 by examining the nasal mucosa, which will be bright with gadolinium. Gadolinium also has some more arcane uses such as detecting neurotoxicity of acyclovir.
   2. **Diffusion-weighted imaging** (DWI) can identify cellular injury within minutes of the insult and is therefore extremely useful in identifying acute ischemic strokes. When the blood supply to the brain is reduced to 20% of normal, adenosine triphosphate levels diminish, the sodium-potassium pump fails, and intracellular swelling or cytotoxic edema of the cells develops. Diffusion-weighted imaging is able to depict these areas within the brain.

Table 20-2 MRI Signal Intensities

	T1	T2	Flair	Diffusion	T1/contrast	Comments
CSF	Dark	Bright	Dark	Dark		
Gray/white	W Brighter	G Brighter	Isodense	Isodense	___	
Muscle	Isodense	Dark	Isodense	Isodense	___	
Bone	Dark	Dark	Dark			
Bone marrow	Bright	Bright	Bright			
Tumor	Dark	Bright	Bright	Less bright	Enhanced*	Depends on vascularity*
Infarct, acute	Dark	Bright	Bright	Bright	May enhance	
Infarct, old	Dark	Bright	Dark	Dark	___	
Cyst	Dark	Bright	Dark			
Fresh blood*	Dark	Dark	Dark	Isodense	___	Parenchymal*
Subacute blood*	Bright	Bright	Bright	Bright	___	Parenchymal*
Old blood*	Dark	Dark	Dark	Dark	___	Parenchymal*
Fat	Bright	Low intensity	Dark	Dark	___	
Air	Dark	Dark	Dark			
MS plaque	Dark	Bright	Bright	May enhance		
Abscess	Dark/mixed	Bright	Mixed	Bright	May enhance*	Capsule*
Vasogenic edema	Dark	Bright	Bright	Dark		
Cytotoxic edema	Bright	Bright	Bright	Bright		
Radionecrosis	Dark	Bright	Bright	Isodense	Enhanced	

Conventional MRI techniques are not able to demonstrate an acute ischemic infarction for 8 to 12 hours after onset. Diffusion-weighted MRI can show regions of ischemia within minutes of onset. (See Figure 20-7 right.)

   a. Apparent diffusion coefficient (ADC) mapping is an algorithm derived from DWI that shows additional information and is easily calculated at most neuroradiology workstations. Hyperintensity on DWI may not be a stroke, it could be an artifact from the T2-derived image called "T2 shine through" and ADC does not change for T2 shine through. In addition, it can differentiate old strokes (hypointensity) from new ones (hyperintensity) as well as differentiate vasogenic from cytotoxic edema.

3. **Fluid-Attenuated Inversion Recovery (FLAIR)** is a rapid scan technique that generates T2-weighted images and produces no appreciable signal from the cerebrospinal fluid in the ventricles or subarachnoid space. As a result, lesions in the periventricular and cortical surface regions of the brain are more distinguishable. FLAIR imaging can detect processes in these regions (e.g., meningeal disease, subarachnoid hemorrhage) that would go unrecognized with other techniques. (See Figure 20-6 lower right, and Figure 20-12 both images.)

4. **Perfusion MRI** involves introducing a tracer into the circulation and monitoring its concentration in a tissue over time using MRI. With this technique, one can determine the rate of tracer delivery and hence blood flow to a tissue. In acute infarction, the perfusion defect is generally larger than the diffusion abnormality. The difference between the two defects represents the area of the brain that is at risk for further ischemia (the ischemic penumbra). In the future, perfusion-weighted imaging used in conjunction with diffusion-weighted MRI may play a major role in the optimization of therapy for individual patients with ischemic stroke.

5. **Magnetic resonance angiography** (MRA) is a three-dimensional computer modeled image that can be rotated on an axis to visualize vessels from multiple views. MRI is mainly used to detect regions of decreased or absent blood flow caused by dissection, thrombus, or

arthrosclerotic narrowing. MRA can also be used to detect some aneurysms and vascular abnormalities. (See Figure 20-7 left.)
6. **Magnetic resonance venography (MRV)** is used to examine pathology of he venous system, namely venous sinus thrombosis. (Please see Figure 20-11).
7. **Functional MRI (fMRI)** shows areas of brain activation due to conversion of oxyhemoglobin to deoxyhemoglobin; useful for surgical planning and research
8. **MR spectroscopy (MRS)** attempts to determine the chemical environment of the brain. It can be very helpful in certain circumstances when attempting to differentiate between two things that look very similar: toxoplasmosis from CNS lymphoma, radiation necrosis from recurrent neoplasms, seizure foci, some metabolic/white matter abnormalities. It can also be used to determine if lead or carbon monoxide toxicity has affected the brain.
9. **MRI tricks of the trade** (these may prove helpful for the oral portion of examination; in actual practice, you may not have the software, but you will not know until you ask)
    a. Want to remove susceptibility distortions in DWI? Ask for line-scan diffusion imaging. This is particularly helpful when looking at DWI of the spine.
    b. Spin echo, fast spin echo (FSE), and gradient echo image details
        i. Ever had an uncooperative semi-unstable patient who moved about? Well, order a single shot FSE with high bandwidth and long echo train. The images will be artifact free and done in less than a minute for an entire brain. They won't be the highest quality, but will show obvious abnormalities.
        ii. Order FSE imaging for highly detailed orbit, labyrinth, or when worried about arachnoiditis. Do not order FSE for small/remote hemorrhages; use gradient echo instead.
        iii. Spin echo images have moderate fat suppression for T2 images.
        iv. With Gradient echo, call T2 images "T2*."
    c. Short tau inversion recovery (STIR) images remove fat from T1 images and are particularly helpful in coronal orbital images or looking for cystic lesions like giant cell tumors of the spine.
    d. What do you do if spin echo images are normal but you think something should be there? Repeat the scan using short flip angle and long TE for hemorrhage, child abuse, seizure, to follow head trauma progression or regression
    e. Cannot tell what kind of image you are looking at? All MRI images will have TE (echo delay time) and TR (repetition time) values given. Short TE is 10 to 25 msec, long TE is 60 to 100+msec, short TR is 100 to 900 msec, long TR is 1800+ msec.
        i. T1-weighted images will be short TR and short TE
        ii. Proton density images will be long TR and short TE
        iii. T2-weighted images will be long TR and long TE
    f. Not sure that your chemotherapy has been effective on the tumors and want to know quickly? Can try 31P MRS, but use it judiciously.
    g. Want to see STIR image post contrast? Ask for SPIR (spectral inversion recovery) on Philips scanners, which is a spectrally selective version of a STIR image, or SPECIAL on GE scanners.

C. Doppler ultrasound/transcranial Doppler: beneficial in measuring vessel lumen diameter, patency, and flow direction. This modality is limited in its ability to examine small vessels, aneurysms, and vascular abnormalities. Everyone who has a stroke or transient ischemic attack (TIA) should have a carotid duplex scan before they leave the hospital. TCD is essential in following patients with SAH for possible development of vasospasm.

D. Conventional angiogram is used to define aneurysms, fistulas, embolization of very bloody tumors (particularly meningiomas or arteriovenous malformations [AVMs]); it allows coiling of many aneurysms avoiding an open procedure; complication rate is about 5% and stroke rate is about 0.5%; anatomy is good on angiograms, so be prepared for them (Figures 20-1, 20-5).

E. Post myelogram CT: injected dye into the intrathecal sack and is of value in spine imaging; typically used when MRI can not be performed or to confirm equivocal MRI findings

F. Nuclear scanning: positron emission tomography (PET) measures emission of positrons from special radioactive compounds; it also has relatively poor resolution; used to differentiate radiation necrosis from neoplasm and show effectiveness of neuropsychiatric drug treatments.

G. Nota Bene: single proton emission spectroscopy (SPECT) is okay at differentiating radiation necrosis from neoplasm; it detects subclinical ischemia and is helpful in dementia; is used for information about perfusion, rather than metabolism
   1. EEG—see Chapter 4
   2. EMG-NCV—see Chapter 4

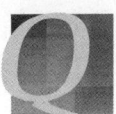
STUDY QUESTIONS FOR CHAPTER 20

Directions: *Each of the numbered items or incomplete statements in this section is followed by answers or by completions of the statement. Select the ONE lettered answer or completion that is BEST in each case.*

1. Choose the lettered item that corresponds with the numbered structure (Figure 20-1).
   (A) Anterior cerebral artery (A1 segment)
   (B) Middle cerebral artery (M1 segment)
   (C) Internal carotid artery
   (D) Berry aneurysm

2. What is the most common location for berry aneurysms?
   (A) Internal carotid artery
   (B) Anterior communicating artery
   (C) Basilar artery
   (D) Middle cerebral artery

3. In this CT image of a pediatric patient (Figure 20-2), what is the most likely etiology for the findings?
   (A) Gunshot wound to the head
   (B) Shaken baby syndrome
   (C) Dandy-Walker malformation
   (D) Schizencephaly

4. Identify the lesion at the tip of the arrow in Figure 20-3.
   (A) Hemorrhage
   (B) Meningioma
   (C) Calcified falx
   (D) Artifact

5. Identify the malformation in Figure 20-4.
   (A) Arnold-Chiari type I malformation
   (B) Arnold-Chiari type II malformation
   (C) Dandy-Walker malformation
   (D) Polymicrogyria

6. Identify the pathology in this set of images in Figure 20-5.
   (A) Aneurysm rupture
   (B) Penetrating trauma
   (C) Hypertensive intracerebral hemorrhage
   (D) Arteriovenous malformation

7. Which of the following studies should not be ordered at this time to identify the lesion in Figure 20-6.
   (A) Single photon emission computed tomography (SPECT)
   (B) Proton emission tomography (PET)
   (C) Tissue biopsy
   (D) Lumbar puncture

8. This patient has undergone a thrombotic stroke. Identify the thrombosed vessel in Figure 20-7.
   (A) ICA
   (B) MCA
   (C) Basilar artery
   (D) PCA

9. Identify the malformation in Figure 20-8.
   (A) Arnold-Chiari type I malformation
   (B) Arnold-Chiari type II malformation
   (C) Dandy-Walker malformation
   (D) Polymicrogyria

10. Describe the changes on neuropsychiatric testing that are *not* likely to have occurred in this patient with a gunshot wound to the head, seen in Figure 20-9.
    (A) Disinhibited
    (B) Impulsive behavior (pseudopsychopathic)
    (C) Inappropriate jocular affect, euphoria
    (D) Confabulation
    (E) Emotional lability

11. Identify the most likely etiology of the lesion seen in Figure 20-10.
    (A) Meningioma
    (B) Lymphoma
    (C) Intracranial hemorrhage
    (D) Sarcoidosis

12. Identify the anatomy and pathology seen in Figure 20-11.
    (A) Confluence of sinuses
    (B) Straight sinus
    (C) Superior sagittal sinus
    (D) Transverse sinus
    (E) Sigmoid sinus.

229

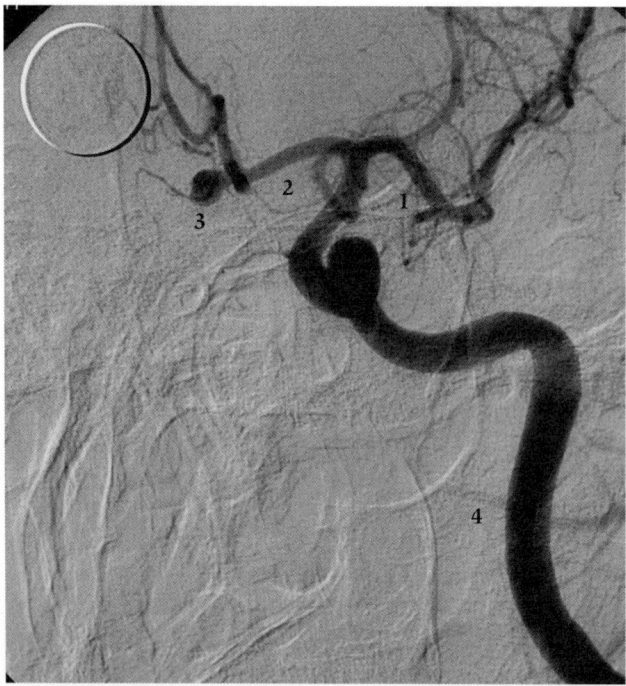

Figure 20-1 This is a carotid angiogram of the anterior circulation. It is an anteroposterior (AP) image of an internal carotid injection. The disc in the upper right corner is a dime, which is often used for measuring features like the aneurysm identified in the image as a dime is 17.9 mm. **(1)** M1 segment of middle cerebral artery; **(2)** A1 segment of anterior cerebral artery; **(3)** Aneurysm; **(4)** Internal carotid artery.

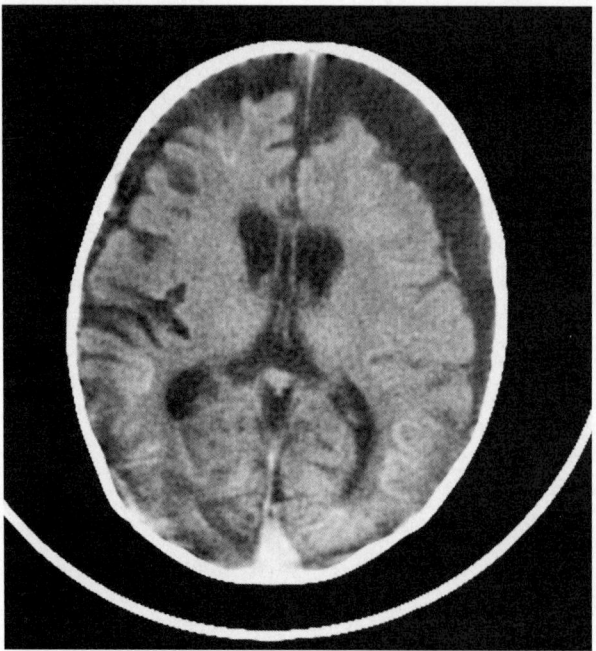

Figure 20-2 Axial CT shows bilateral hygromas and multiple petechial hemorrhages posteriorly. This is consistent with shaken baby syndrome.

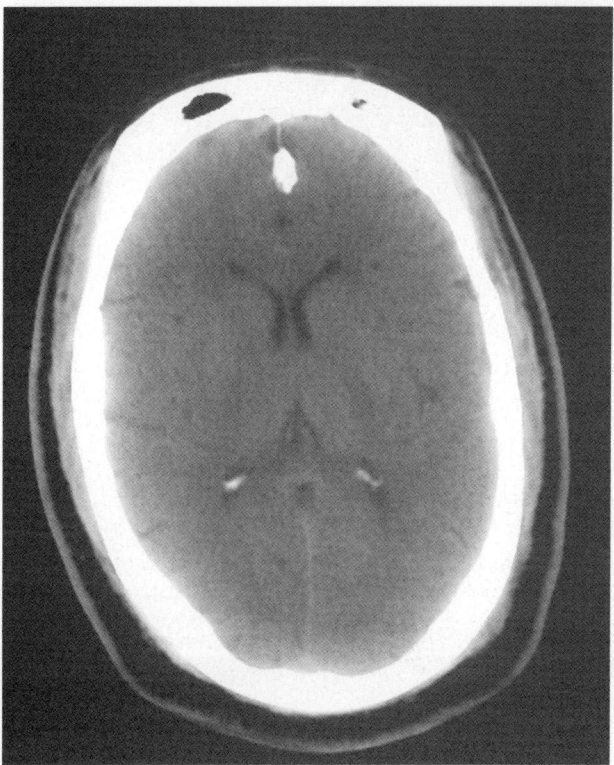

Figure 20-3 Axial T1-weighted MRI shows a hyperintensity on the falx, the same intensity as bone. This is consistent with calcified falx and possible meningioma.

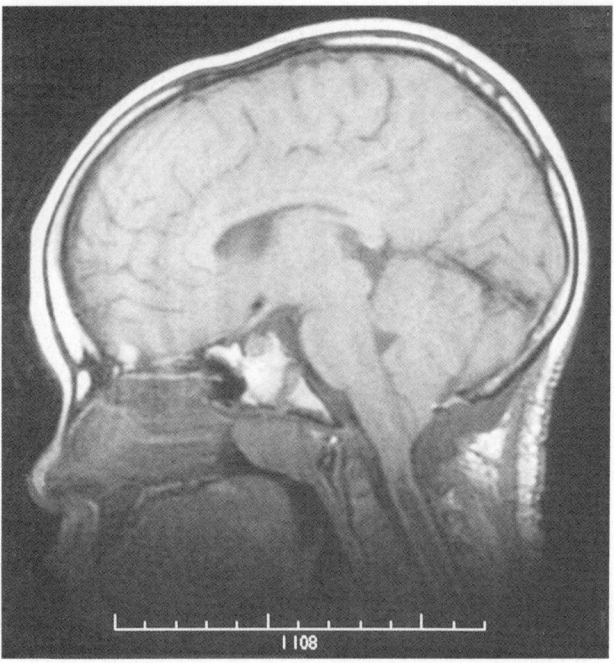

Figure 20-4 Sagittal T1 MRI showing syringomyelia and cerebellar herniation, consistent with Arnold-Chiari type I.

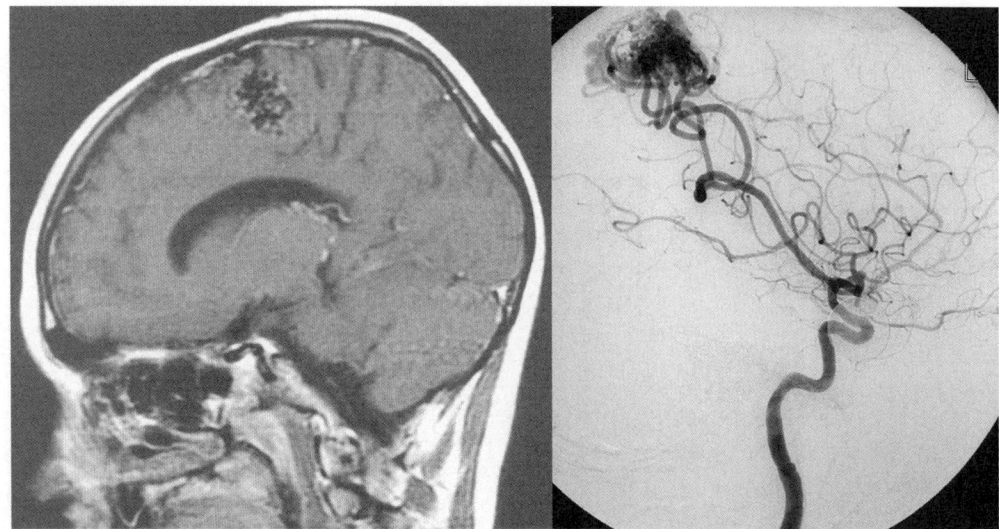

Figure 20-5 Sagittal MRI shows a heterogeneous mass with at least three clearly defined flow voids. Carotid angiogram shows a diffuse mass with vessels that appear to go into and out of the mass. This is an AVM.

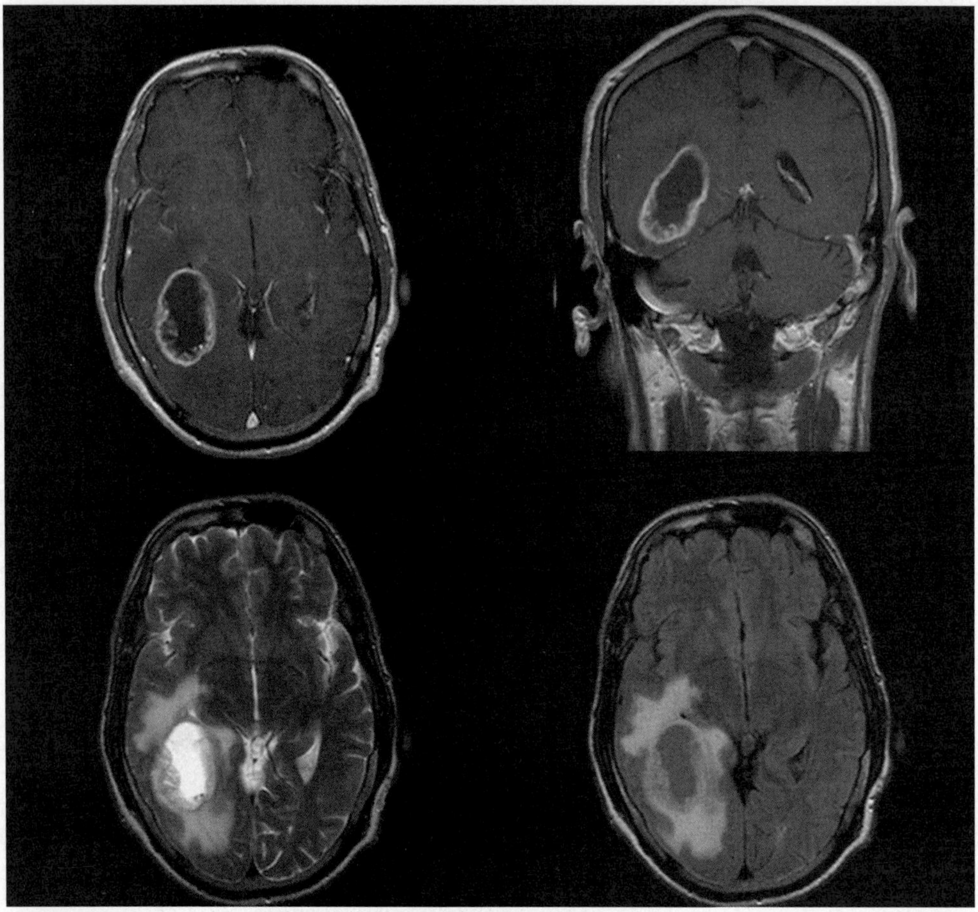

Figure 20-6 There are four MRI views: clockwise from upper left—T1 axial, T1 coronal, T1 post-gadolinium, and FLAIR images. The mass is well circumscribed with edema and enhancement.

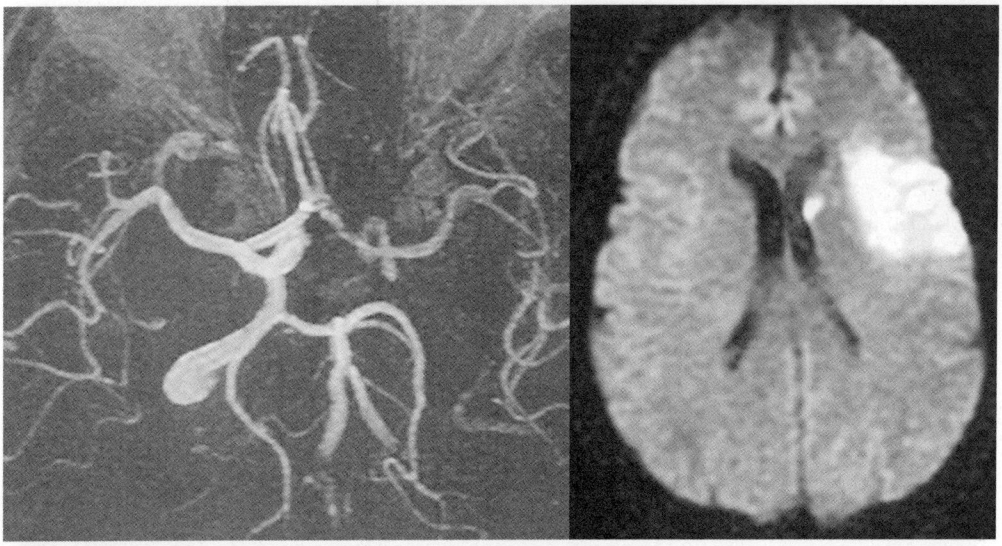

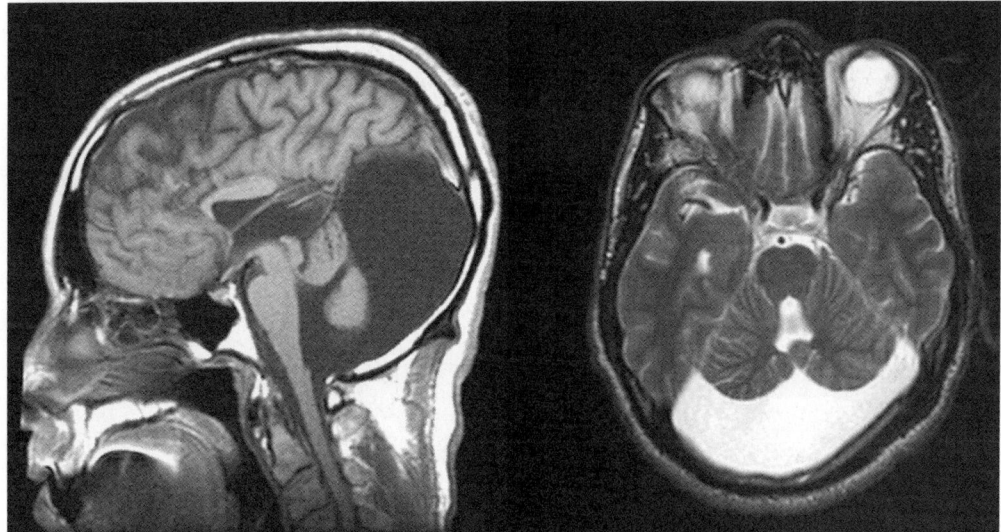

Figure 20-7 On the **left** is an MRA showing a clear cut-off of the left ICA. On the **right** is an axial diffusion-weighted MRI image showing a left hyperintense lesion, denoting a recent ischemic event.

Figure 20-8 On the **left** is a axial T1-weighted MRI showing an enlarged posterior fossa and dilation of the fourth ventricle. There is also loss of cerebellum, but without further images in the series it is difficult to localize the part(s) affected. This information is provided by the axial T2 MRI image on the **right**, which shows that defect affects the vermis. These findings constitute a Dandy-Walker malformation.

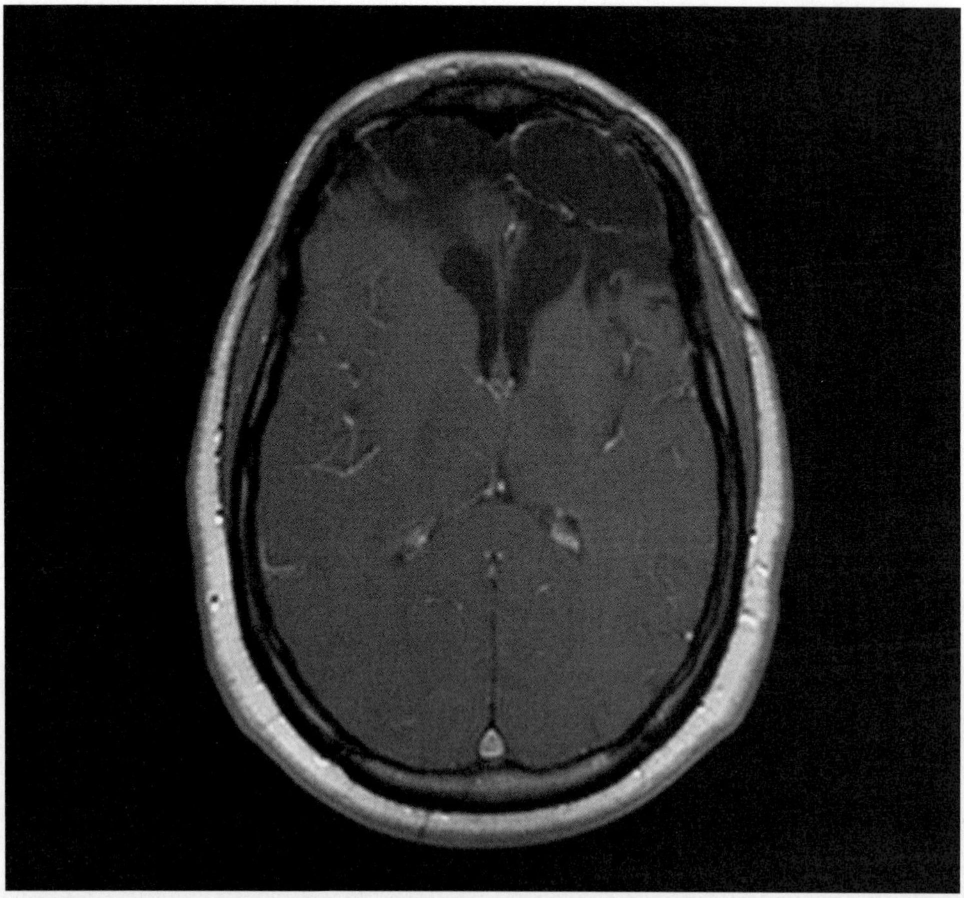

Figure 20-9 This axial T1 postcontrast MRI shows marked hypointensity in the orbitofrontal region. It was a follow-up MRI from a gunshot.

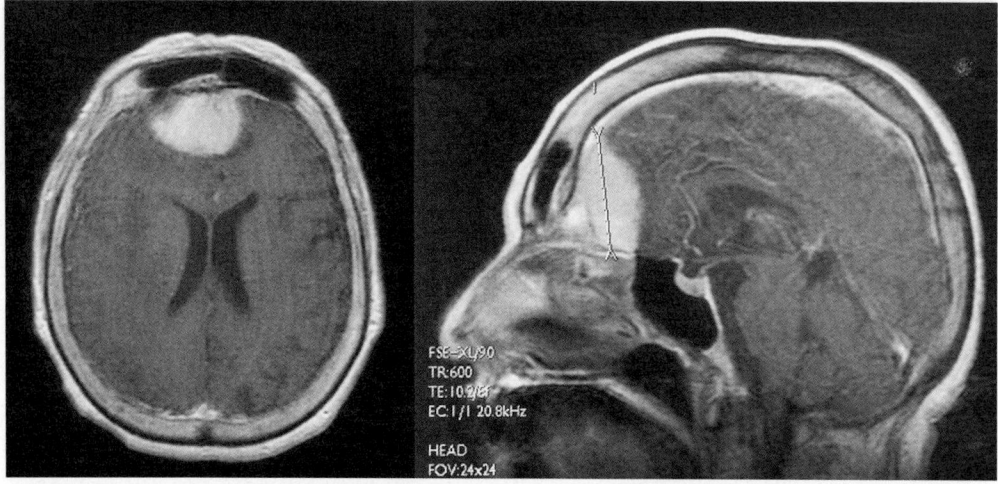

Figure 20-10 Axial **(left)** and sagittal **(right)** T1 postcontrast MRI. The axial image shows a dural tail as well as diffuse meningeal enhancement and thickening, both consistent with meningioma.

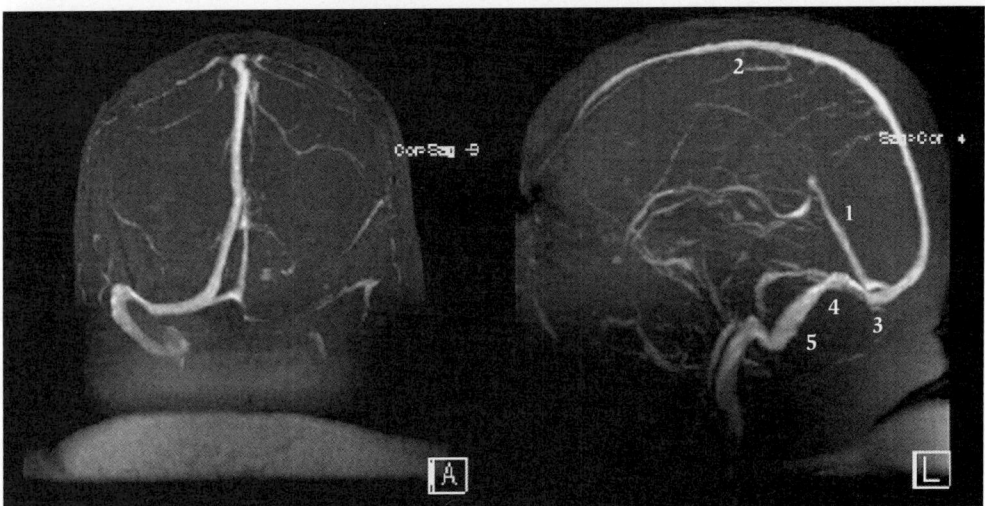

Figure 20-11 Axial and sagittal MRV showing the left venous sinus starting with the transverse sinus. **(1)** Straight sinus; **(2)** superior sagittal sinus; **(3)** confluence of sinuses; **(4)** transverse sinus; **(5)** sigmoid sinus.

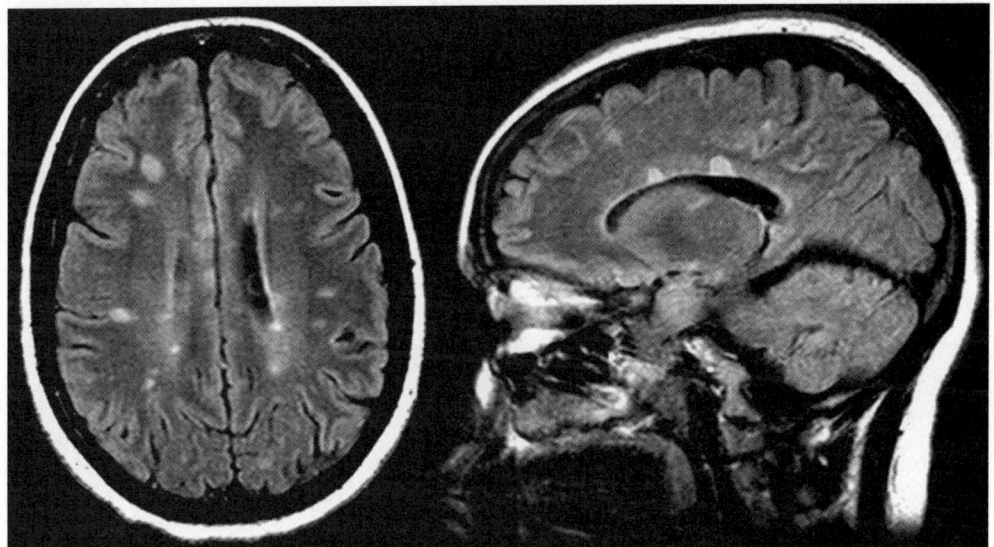

Figure 20-12 Axial **(left)** and sagittal **(right)** FLAIR MRI images showing multiple, discrete hyperintensities, including two linear hyperintensities extending from ventricle. These are Dawson fingers, indicating multiple sclerosis.

13. What is the most likely diagnosis of the lesions in Figure 20-12?

(A) Lymphoma
(B) Metastatic lesions
(C) Tuberculosis
(D) Sarcoidosis
(E) Multiple sclerosis

14. CT scans of a large hypertensive intracranial hemorrhage at days 1 and 3, Figure 20-13. Hypertensive hemorrhages occur most commonly in the following locations: caudate/putamen, pons, thalamus, cerebellum, and white matter (parietooccipital and temporal lobes). Match the location with the vessel that supplies it.

(A) Caudate/putamen
(B) Pons
(C) Thalamus
(D) Cerebellum
1. Branches of MCA
2. Branches of PCA
3. Branches of basilar artery
4. Branches of SCA

15. Which of the following is the *least* common endocrine dysfunction associated with the type of lesion seen in Figure 20-14?

(A) Prolactinoma
(B) Acromegaly
(C) Hyperthyroidism
(D) Cushing disease

16. Identify this lesion in a 58-year-old woman with HIV and hemoptysis seen in Figure 20-15.

(A) Pancoast tumor
(B) Metastatic prostate cancer
(C) Pott disease (tuberculosis)
(D) Neuroenteric cyst

17. Identify the etiology of this pontine lesion of acute onset, in Figure 20-16.

(A) Neoplastic
(B) Thrombotic
(C) Lead poisoning
(D) Inappropriate correction on metabolites

18. Identify the pathologic etiology of these three MRI FLAIR images seen in Figure 20-17 taken during the course of a month in this immunocompromised patient. Additional MRI images not shone revealed that the lesion did not enhance with gadolinium.

(A) Lymphoma
(B) Glioblastoma multiforme
(C) Progressive multifocal leukoencephalopathy
(D) Sarcoid

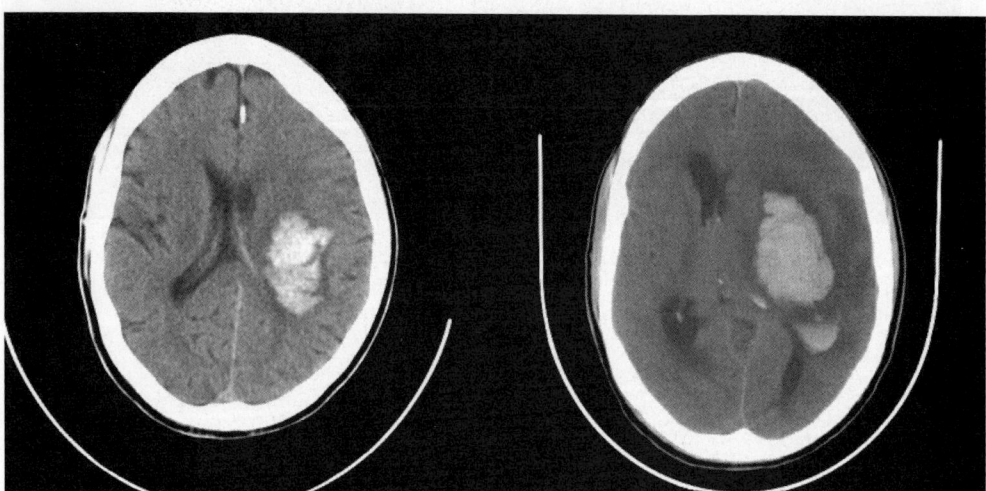

Figure 20-13 Axial CTs showing a putaminal bleed on days 1 and 3.

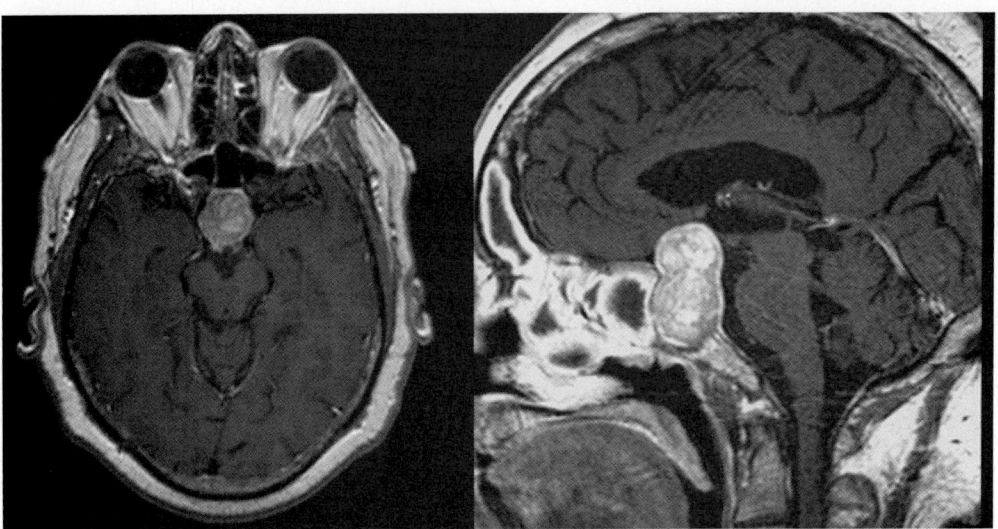

Figure 20-14 T1 axial **(left)** and postgadolinium sagittal **(right)** MRI showing a large pituitary adenoma.

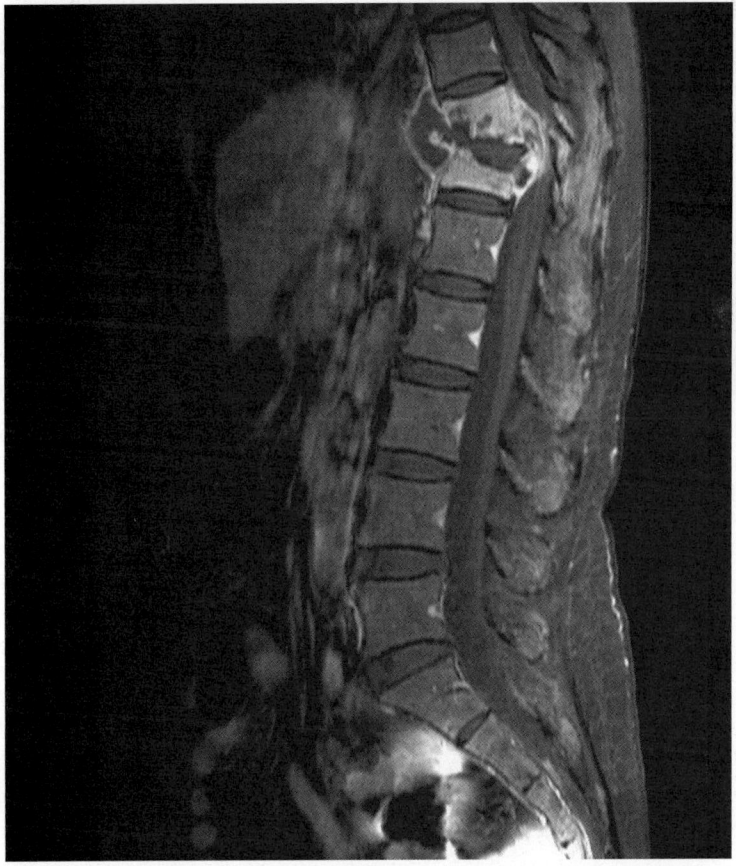

Figure 20-15 T1 sagittal MRI shows an encapsulated abscess and bone destruction consistent with Pott disease.

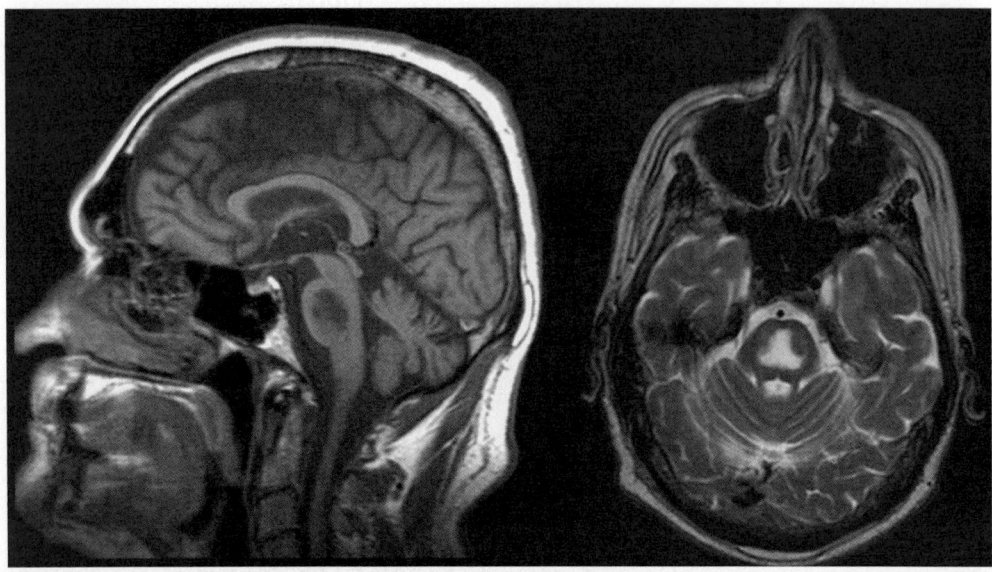

Figure 20-16 FLAIR sagittal **(left)** and T2 axial **(right)** MRI show a large lesion in the central pons, which is consistent with central pontine myelinolysis.

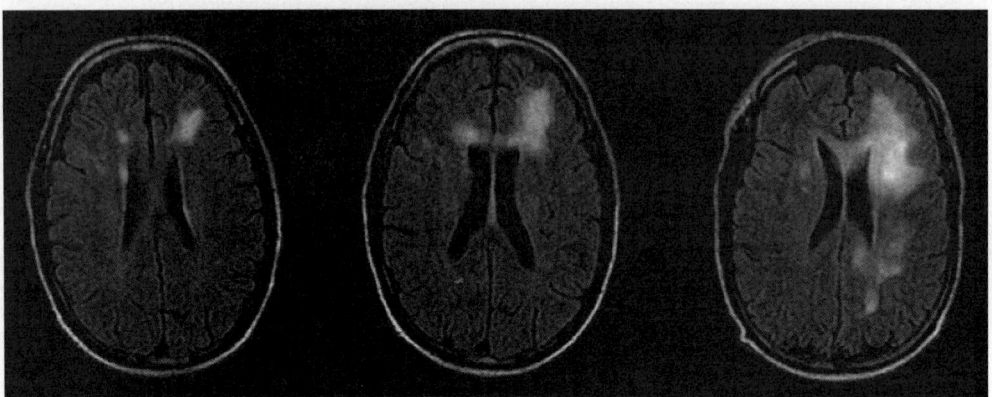

Figure 20-17 FLAIR MRI images show evolution over a month of a periventricular white matter lesion; lesion did not enhance. This is consistent with progressive multifocal leukoencephalopathy. In this case, the most prominent lesions are frontal; however in most PML cases, the lesions begin posteriorly.

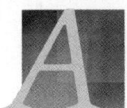# ANSWERS AND EXPLANATIONS

1. **The answers are:** 1 = B, 2 = A, 3 = C, 4 = D.

2. **D.** The most common locations for cerebral aneurysms to occur are: middle cerebral artery (29%), anterior communicating artery (15%), internal carotid artery (16%), and basilar artery (14%).

3. **B.** This infant has bilateral frontal hygromas and multiple posterior petechial hemorrhages due to excessive shaking. The skull is intact so there is no penetrating injury. Dandy-Walker malformation cannot be determined by the anatomic location of this image. This image does not portray schizencephaly, as there is no cleft extends across the entire cerebral hemisphere.

4. **C.** T1 MRI image of a calcified falx, which may contain a small incidental meningioma. This is a nonpathologic incidental finding.

5. **A**: MRI of a child with Arnold-Chiari type I malformation. Note the cerebellar herniation and syringomyelia. Arnold-Chiari type II malformation is associated with myelomeningocele and hydrocephalus. This is not Dandy-Walker or polymicrogyria, as the cerebellum and gyri are not small.

6. **D.** AV malformation. Comparison views of a T1 MRI and a cerebral angiogram. AV malformations often have a characteristic patchy appearance with poorly differentiated borders on MRI. The skull has no evidence of penetration. Intracerebral hemorrhage and ruptured aneurysms do not have this characteristic appearance.

7. **D.** MRI views of the same tumor. Clockwise from top left: T1 axial, T1 coronal, Contrast, FLAIR. It is not possible to determine if this ring-enhancing lesion is an infectious or neoplastic process on MRI imaging alone. Obtaining a tissue biopsy, SPECT, or PET scan could help determine if this lesion was infectious or neoplastic in nature. Due to the cerebral edema indicated by the sulcal effacement and slight midline shift, a lumbar puncture would not be recommended.

8. **A.** The image on the right is a diffusion-weighted image noting the recent stroke. The image on the left is an MRA noting absence of flow in the left ICA. The hypoperfused left MCA is receiving collateral flow originating from the right ICA. It is important to understand the difference between embolic and thrombotic strokes.
    - Embolic: 33% of ischemic strokes. Embolic events produce maximum neurologic deficit at onset and are most commonly due to an embolus from the heart, aortic arch, or large cerebral artery. The MCA is most commonly affected in the anterior circulation. The branch points of basilar artery or PCA are most commonly affected in the posterior circulation. When TIAs precede the event, the clinical symptoms vary as the embolus travels and lodges in different locations.
    - Thrombotic: 66% of ischemic strokes. Symptoms evolve over minutes to hours with the most common locations of occlusion including large cerebral arteries (ICA, MCA, basilar artery), small penetrating arteries (lacunar strokes), cerebral veins, and venous sinuses. Thrombotic events are commonly preceded by TIAs in recurrent territories causing similar deficits.

9. **C.** T1 sagittal (left) and T2 axial (right) of adult with Dandy-Walker malformation characterized by agenesis or hypoplasia of the cerebellar vermis, cystic dilation of the fourth ventricle, and enlargement of the posterior fossa.

10. D. This patient has orbitofrontal syndrome (disinhibited) associated with: disinhibited, impulsive behavior (pseudopsychopathic), inappropriate jocular affect, euphoria, emotional lability, poor judgment/insight, and distractibility. Confabulation is associated with chronic alcohol abuse and Wernicke-Korsakoff syndrome.

11. A. T1 axial and sagittal images with contrast of a meningioma. This lesion is consistent with meningioma due to the diffuse meningeal enhancement and dural tail (thin trailing segment at border of tumor and meninges on axial image). A dural tail occurs in 65% of meningiomas and only 15% of other peripheral tumors. Although it is not specific, it is highly predictive of the diagnosis.

12. The answers are: 1=B, 2=C, 3=A, 4=E, 5=C. This image is a MRV of left venous sinus thrombosis. Multiple pathophysiologic mechanisms and predisposing factors exist, although 25% present with no known predisposing risk factors. These factors include pregnancy, hypercoagulable state, dehydration, extrinsic compression or local invasion by tumor or infectious process, or low flow state. Venous sinus occlusion and subsequent congestion can lead to regional ischemia and infarction. These infarctions are often hemorrhagic and commonly occur at the gray–white matter junction.

13. E. MRI axial and sagittal FLAIR of a patient with multiple sclerosis. The multiple lesions appear to radiate from the lateral ventricles and corpus callosum (Dawson fingers).

14. The answers are: 1=A, 2=C, 3=B, 4=D.

15. C. Pituitary adenomas that are associated with thyroid-stimulating hormone (TSH) hypersecretion are uncommon. The following laboratory tests should be ordered if one of the subsequently noted endocrine dysfunctions in suspected:
- Prolactinoma: serum prolactin level.
- Acromegaly: serum growth hormone, serum insulinlike growth factor 1 (IGF-1), oral glucose tolerance test
- Cushing disease: 24-hour urine collection for free cortisol, dexamethasone suppression test, serum ACTH, metyrapone test

16. C. Pott disease: This patient is immunocompromised with active tuberculosis. The encapsulated abscess with destruction of bone can be noted on this sagittal MRI. This view reveals how only a single vertebra is affected with no involvement of the adjacent discs. Visible bone fragments within the swelling or abscess are strongly indicative of Pott disease as opposed to a cyst or malignancy.

17. D. Comparison views of sagittal FLAIR MRI and an axial T2 MRI in a patient with central pontine myelinolysis due to rapid correction of sodium.

18. C. These images are of a patient with progressive multifocal leukoencephalopathy (PML). Note how the lesion rapidly progresses over the course of a month and crosses the midline. JC virus is the etiologic infectious agent in this immunocompromised patient. Lymphoma, glioblastoma multiforme, and sarcoid are examples of other lesions that can cross the midline, although only PML would progress that rapidly and not enhance on a contrasted study.

CHAPTER 21

Sleep

I. Polysomnography

A. **Definition:** must include (usually in this order) an electroencephalography (EEG) channel that references the ear, an electroculogram (usually one channel, but can have a second channel), electromyogram (EMG) of the submentalis muscle, airflow, chest effort, pulse oximetry, electrocardiogram (ECG), EMG of anterior tibial muscles; unlike EEG, the windowing for the polysomnography is usually 30 seconds to one minute per page, so typical morphologic patterns of the EEG look very different
   1. Electrooculogram shows the eye movements. It mainly helps in distinguishing rapid eye movement (REM) sleep without atonia (usually horizontal) from blinks of wakefulness (vertical movements).
   2. EMG evaluates hypotonia; the tibialis anterior helps to show restless legs
   3. Airflow, chest effort, and pulse oximetry together allow one to characterize an apnea as central (>80% decrease of both airflow and respiratory movement), obstructive (decrease of airflow despite continued effort), or mixed (early central followed by obstructive component that reestablishes respiration). (Note: pulse oximetry desaturation or arousal is not needed to qualify.)
   4. ECG allows documentation of cardiac abnormalities with apneas.

B. **Indications:** excessive daytime sleepiness, unexplained nocturnal awakenings, unusual sleep behavior, and to initiate or titrate continuous positive airway pressure (CPAP).

C. **Interpretation**
   1. **Hypopnea** is a 30+% airflow decrease with a 4+% oxygen saturation decrease lasting at least 10 seconds.
   2. **Respiratory effect–related arousal** is an increase in negative esophageal pressure lasting at least 10 seconds followed by sudden increase in the pressure and an arousal. If >10 per hour with excessive daytime sleepiness, this is upper airway resistance syndrome.
   3. **Apnea–hypopnea index** (AHI) is the summated apneas (defined in the preceding text), hypopneas, (and respiratory effect related arousals by guideline that many do not follow) per hour. Any AHI >1 in children is abnormal, AHI >5 mild, >15 moderate, and >30 severe obstructive sleep apnea (OSA).
   4. **Periodic leg movement index with arousal** is the number of leg movements associated with arousal. >5 in adults is abnormal, >10 to 15 if >50 years old.

D. **Nap testing**
   1. **Polysomnography** is typically done the night before. The patient should discontinue any sleep altering medications 2 weeks prior to the test. The patient must be awake and not take any caffeine during segments of the test.

2. **Multiple sleep latency test:** four 20-minute nap trials 2 hours apart beginning 90+ minutes after awakening in the morning; a fifth nap trial is done if one sleep onset REM period is found. EEG and submentalis EMG are recorded. The patient is instructed to go to sleep and is fully dressed while in bed in quiet darkened room. The time to sleep is recorded. If patient sleeps during the 20 minutes, additional 15 minutes is allowed to see if patient achieves REM sleep. Mean sleep latency is average minutes to achieve sleep divided by the number of naps: <5 minutes is abnormal, 5 to 10 minutes is borderline, >10 minutes is normal. Two or more sleep-onset REM sleeps and mean sleep latency of <5 are the electrophysiologic criteria for narcolepsy.
3. **Maintenance of wakefulness test** is used to waiver noncommercial pilots so that they can continue to fly after a diagnosis of OSA. It is identical to mean sleep latency test except there is no fifth nap, and patient is instructed to stay awake. Mean sleep latency <11 is impairment, >18 is normal.

II. Night-Time Involuntary Limb Movements

A. **Restless legs syndrome** (RLS)
   1. **Diagnosis requires the following criteria:**
      a. Urge to move legs with uncomfortable sensation in the legs
      b. Unpleasant sensation/urge to move legs, worse during inactivity
      c. Relieved by movement
      d. Worse in evening or at night
      e. Although not part of diagnosis, should expect to have night to night variable severity
   2. **Pathophysiology:** likely due to dopamine as dopamine is naturally low at night, symptoms ameliorated by dopamine agonists and aggravated by dopamine antagonists
   3. **Secondary RLS** seen in iron deficiency anemia, dialysis patients, and pregnancy; normally resolves when underlying condition is relieved; all three may be due to the iron deficiency and may correct if iron deficiency is corrected
   4. **Drugs that can aggravate or even provoke RLS:** antihistamines, antipsychotics, selective serotonin reuptake inhibitors (SSRIs), tricyclics, dopamine antagonists, mirtazapine, venlafaxine
   5. **Treatment**
      a. Test iron, if deficient, give oral supplementation
      b. If symptoms intermittent: carbidopa/levodopa, clonazepam, or hypnotic for sleep
      c. If symptoms several times per week: dopamine agonist (Mirapex, Requip) and/or gabapentin

B. **Periodic limb movement disorder** (PLMD)
   1. **Diagnosis**
      a. Periodic limb movements are frequent occurrence with other sleep disorders and are merely a symptom of underlying disorder.
      b. If all other sleep disorders have been excluded and patient has movements at night that cause either frequent arousal or excessive daytime fatigue, send for sleep study. A sleep study is necessary because it is required criteria for diagnosis and the most frequent cause of PLMD is respiratory problems.
      c. The criteria for PLMD is four motor movements every 5 to 90 seconds.
   2. **Treatment:** utilize try dopamine agonists, gabapentin, and clonazepam

III. Excessive Daytime Sleepiness

A. **Narcolepsy** incidence 1:2,000
   1. **Symptoms:** excessive daytime sleepiness, partial to complete loss of muscle tone when faced with strong emotion positive emotions > negative emotions (cataplexy), hallucinations on

waking from sleep (hypnopompic) or falling to sleep (hypnagogic), feeling that cannot move while falling to sleep or waking up (sleep paralysis), nonsensical speech or behavior that the patient does not remember later (automatic behavior)
2. **Diagnosis:** most get a sleep study to assess if there are other aspects of the disorder aggravating it. Can also use a multiple sleep latency test, which tests for sleep-onset REM (also seen in sleep deprivation, obstructive sleep apnea, REM rebound) and sleep latency. Narcolepsy sleep latencies are often 2 to 3 minutes. Most patients have very low or no levels of hypocretin in their cerebrospinal fluid (CSF).

B. **Obstructive sleep apnea**
   1. **Symptoms/variable manifestations** including excessive daytime sleepiness, snoring, difficulty falling asleep, impaired memory, daytime headaches, BMI >28 kg/m^2.
   2. **Diagnosis** requires nocturnal polysomnography demonstrating AHI > 5 events per hour with respiratory effort during times of apnea/hypopnea with one additional feature including frequent sleep arousals, brady-tachycardia, or arterial oxygen desaturation.
   3. **Treatment**
      a. **Mild** OSA (AHI >5) treatment is first the following: weight loss if overweight; avoidance of things that may aggravate sleep including nicotine, sedatives, alcohol, and sleep deprivation; treatment of any comorbidities; and avoidance of supine posture while asleep. CPAP is used for any patients with excessive daytime sleepiness, hypertension, ischemic heart disease, coronary artery disease, or stroke. Second-line possibilities include stimulants and mouth appliances.
      b. **Moderate** (AHI >15) to severe (AHI >30) treated as mild, except that CPAP is given to everyone with severe disease, and surgery including tracheostomy and uvulopalatopharyngoplasty may be considered.
   4. **Childhood OSA** called obstructive sleep apnea hypoventilation syndrome—typically see continuous snoring, adenoidal-tonsillar hypertrophy, and behavioral problems rather than daytime sleepiness. Treatment is adenotonsillectomy in children with hypertrophy. In resistant cases, or without such hypertrophy, use CPAP, even though compliance is even less successful than in adults.
   5. AHI <5 without apneas is called **upper airway resistance syndrome**.
   6. **Central sleep apnea** defined as OSA without respiratory effort during times of apnea/hypopnea has a myriad of causes, both medical and neurologic. The question will give you hints as to the cause.
      a. Ondine curse = congenital central hypoventilation syndrome = failure of autonomic respiratory control. Half will have Hirschsprung disease. Of those who have both, one fifth will develop neuroblastoma or ganglioneuroma. Presentation is variable. All children should be referred for ophthalmologic evaluation. Sudden infant death syndrome (SIDS) is a risk for those with this condition.

C. **Menstrual related hypersomnia:** excessive sleepiness during the days before menstruation. If particularly burdensome, can try combined birth control pills.

D. **Idiopathic hypersomnia:** excessive daytime sleepiness, difficult to awake in the morning, can have sleep-related hallucinations, but no cataplexy. Sleep studies show shorted sleep latency, but no sleep-onset REM.

E. **Klein-Levin syndrome** is a disorder of adolescents with recurrent periods lasting days to weeks with excessive daytime sleepiness, daytime aggressiveness, hyperphagia, and hypersexuality. Treatment is usually not helpful, but typically the frequency diminishes with time.

F. **Treatment**
   1. The mainstays of treatment for all but OSA are four:
      a. **Modafinil** is a stimulant with unknown mechanism of action that seems to be well tolerated and effective but does not have some of the problems of the dopamine agonists.
      b. **Oxybate** (γ-hydroxybutyrate) very effective for both combating excessive daytime

sleepiness and cataplexy in narcolepsy, but the evidence is not nearly as good as for other agents. Also, it is only carried by one central pharmacy due to abuse potential.
- c. **Traditional dopamine agonists** do not appear to be as useful as either of the other agents due to risks of rebound hypersomnia, as the medication wears off and tolerance develops to the medication.
- d. **Antidepressants** ameliorate cataplexy, but tolerance can develop. In narcolepsy, use of antidepressants can start or exacerbate REM sleep behavior disorder.

IV. Parasomnias

A. Non-REM
1. Typically are more frequent during stage 3 or 4 of non-REM sleep; fairly common during childhood and decrease in frequency with age
2. **Night terrors:** can be familial, inconsolable waking from sleep with a scream, panic, and motor activity like running around the bedroom, complete or partial amnesia for the event may be present
3. **Sleep walking:** wildly varying prevalence make it impossible to know how common it is; also varies wildly in complexity, duration, and calmness
4. **Confusional arousal:** movements in bed while confused, sometimes with more aggressive motor activity
5. **Treatment:** generally all that is recommended is good sleep hygiene with avoidance of alcohol, drugs, or sleep deprivation; antidepressants or benzodiazepines can be tried if necessary; the best studied long-term treatment is hypnosis
6. **Nocturnal enuresis in children:** unable to establish consistent nocturnal continence by age 5; behavioral modification is successful in most cases, but can try imipramine or desmopressin for recalcitrant cases

B. REM
1. **REM sleep behavior disorder**
   - a. **Symptoms:** vivid dreams accompanied by vigorous and violent motor activity, >90% male, and usually after 60 years of age
   - b. **Acute form** usually caused by withdrawal, particularly from alcohol.
   - c. **Chronic form** is often a harbinger of neurodenerative disorders like Parkinson disease, Lewy body dementia, or multiple system atrophy, and may start more than 10 years before the symptoms of the neurodegenerative disease appears.
   - d. **Treatment standard** is clonazepam, which is effective in 90%, but consider trying melatonin first.
2. **Other disorders** include groaning during sleep (cataphrenia), stereotyped movements during sleep during childhood (rhythmic movement disorder), and propriospinal myoclonus (myoclonic jerks propagate in spine affecting different muscle groups). Only propriospinal myoclonus has a known treatment: clonazepam or anticonvulsants.

V. Nocturnal Seizures

A. **Benign Rolandic epilepsy** occurs in childhood with unilateral clonus and an EEG showing bilateral centrotemporal spikes that increase during non-REM sleep. These seizures remit in adolescence.

B. **Electrical status epilepticus** during sleep is a childhood disorder that shows normal EEG while awake and a virtually continuous epileptiform activity during sleep. It is asymptomatic and does not include any seizure manifestations.

C. Landau-Kleffner syndrome usually involves normal waking EEG and epileptiform activity in the temporal lobes while asleep. Affected children have acquired epileptic aphasia with variable deficits in expressive–receptive aphasia and seizures. They present from age 3 to 8 years and can have autistic-like attacks. Treatment needs to be aggressive because language can return with early intervention with steroids. If it does not return, children should be introduced to sign language. Antiepileptics can control the seizures.

VI. Circadian Rhythm Disorders

A. Delayed sleep pattern: Individuals fall asleep and wake up 3 to 6 hours after going to sleep at normal times, are often groggy in the morning, and their decreased mental alertness can have effects on work and school. Treat with 2 hours of 2,500 lux (a lux is the illumination of a single candle at a distance of one meter away from the candle) exposure in the morning and avoid light at night. Evening melatonin can also be tried.

B. Advanced sleep pattern: fall asleep and wake up several hours before conventional times. Associated with aging, can be autosomal dominant (AD) inherited. Bright light therapy in the evening, typically from 7 to 9 p.m. is the treatment.

C. Free running sleep pattern: sleep and waking up changes by 1 to 2 hours every day. Experienced by about 50% of blind people, very rare in sighted people. Can cause functional or social impairment. Treat with 0.5 to 1 mg of melatonin before bedtime and maintaining a regular sleep and work schedule.

D. Shift work sleep disorder: typical complaints are feeling unrefreshed upon awakening, sleepy at work, and symptoms persisting during days off. Usual etiology is working the night shift and inability to sleep the normal amount of time. First try: good sleep hygiene and wearing sun glasses/dark goggles on way home from work. If this doesn't work, can use melatonin or 3 to 6 hours of bright light exposure during the night shift. Last resort: sleeping medications (not that there is anything wrong with them, but this is a short-term solution to a chronic problem), caffeine, or modafinil

E. Jet lag: treat with bright light while awake, melatonin, and avoidance of bright light when trying to sleep.

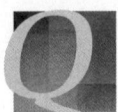 STUDY QUESTIONS FOR CHAPTER 21

Directions: Each of the numbered items or incomplete statements in this section is followed by answers or by completions of the statement. Select the ONE lettered answer or completion that is BEST in each case.

1. A 65-year-old man presents with several months of an uncomfortable sensation in his legs accompanied by an urge to move them. These symptoms are worse at night. Which of the following will improve his symptoms?

   (A) Paroxetine
   (B) Venlafaxine
   (C) Treatment of vitamin B_{12} deficiency
   (D) Treatment of iron-deficiency anemia
   (E) Rest

2. A 22-year-old woman comes to your clinic with one year of episodes of sleep attacks. She describes herself as excessively sleepy and notes that she frequently loses muscle tone when laughing. She also has hallucinations when awakening from sleep. Which of the following neurotransmitters is likely to be found at a low concentration in her cerebrospinal fluid?

   (A) Acetylcholine
   (B) Galanin
   (C) Glycine
   (D) Hypocretin
   (E) Taurine

3. A 12-year-old girl has been having difficulties in school as a result of excessive daytime sleepiness. A sleep study demonstrates obstructive sleep apnea. Which of the following features is similar in both adult and childhood obstructive sleep apnea?

   (A) Body habitus
   (B) Response to CPAP
   (C) Behavioral problems
   (D) Response to tonsillectomy
   (E) Response to SSRIs

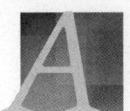# ANSWERS AND EXPLANATIONS

1. D. The patient has restless legs syndrome, which commonly improves upon treatment of iron-deficiency anemia. Paroxetine and venlafaxine may worsen symptoms of restless legs syndrome. Vitamin B_{12} deficiency is not associated with restless legs syndrome. Rest makes symptoms worse, and, in fact, leg movement improves the symptoms.

2. D. The patient described in the vignette has narcolepsy, which is characterized by excessive daytime sleepiness, partial to complete loss of muscle tone when faced with strong emotions, sleep paralysis, and hallucinations on falling asleep or awakening. It is associated with decreased cerebrospinal fluid levels of hypocretin. The other listed neurotransmitters are not affected by narcolepsy. Galanin is a neurotransmitter found in the part of the brain affected by Alzheimer's.

3. B. Both adult and childhood obstructive sleep apnea (OSA) respond to treatment with CPAP. Adults with OSA are typically overweight, whereas children are thin and have an "adenoidal" facies. Behavioral problems tend to predominate in children. Tonsillectomy is more useful in children. SSRIs are not used to treat OSA in either group.

CHAPTER 22

Neuroophthalmology

I. Eyelid Abnormalities

A. **Unilateral ptosis by paralysis of the levator muscle** (always check to see if old or new)
   1. **Aberrant regeneration:** upper lid retracts on lateral/downward gaze = pseudo von Graefe sign
   2. Sympathetic paralysis, that is, **Horner syndrome**
      a. Ptosis, miosis, and, sometimes, anhidrosis (if lesion above superior cervical ganglion)
      b. Verify miosis is worse in dark (miosis worse in light occurs in third cranial nerve palsy)
      c. Apply 1% hydroxyamphetamine to both eyes; normal side dilates; miotic side no effect if lesion is above superior cervical ganglion, dilates if below
      d. Top three causes if lesion is below superior cervical ganglion: (i) apical neoplasm (Pancoast tumor), (ii) transient Horner due to cluster or migraine headache, or (iii) carotid disease. If above superior cervical ganglion, likely congenital. No etiology found in 30%.
   3. **Myasthenia gravis**
      a. Overcompensation of the contralateral levator and frontalis muscle
      b. Transient retraction of upper lid with moving fixation from downward to straight ahead (sometimes called Cogan lid twitch)
   4. **Can be confused with trauma or lower lid sag** from seventh cranial nerve palsy
   5. **Can be due to infection or inflammation:** look at thickness of eyelid from below

B. **Inability to blink**, consider Bell palsy
   1. Trigeminal lesion no contralateral blink reflex, Bell palsy + contralateral blink reflex
   2. Aberrant regeneration of facial nerve; closure of eyelids with chewing or speaking
   3. Paralysis of both the levator oculi and the orbicularis oculi = myopathic disease

C. **Bilateral ptosis**
   1. **Causes:** muscular dystrophy; myasthenia gravis,; congenital ptosis, which can be redundant lid tissue; sagging of the upper lids of the elderly = normal; third nucleus or bilateral third nerve; external ophthalmoplegia
   2. **Localization of levator muscles:** midbrain central caudal nucleus

D. **Other signs**
   1. **Retraction of the upper lids** = proptosis with orbital tumors or thyroid disease
      a. Carotid sinus occlusion, carotid cavernous fistula, third cranial nerve palsy, or inflammation
      b. Unilateral proptosis: three most likely causes are thyroid disease, metastatic carcinoma, and hemangioma. In trauma, consider basilar skull fracture; in children, rhabdomyosarcoma.

c. With carotid cavernous sinus fistula, expect the proptotic eye to be pulsatile, with chemosis, visual impairment, and appreciation of buzzing noise (orbital bruit).
 2. **Retraction of both lids** = Collier sign, associated with dorsal midbrain lesions, hyperthyroidism, seen occasionally with chronic steroid use
    a. Dorsal midbrain with no lid lag on downward gaze (von Graefe sign) versus thyroid ophthalmopathy, which will have a positive von Graefe sign
 3. **Staring quality with Parkinson** and reduced blink rate, progressive supranuclear palsy, hydrocephalus

E. **Blinking:** normal is 12 to 20 times per minute
 1. **Increased** when patient does not feel comfortable, corneal irritation, blepharospasm
 2. **Decreased** when concentrating, supranuclear palsy, and Parkinson disease (PD)
    a. Myerson sign = inability to stop blinking with repeated forehead taps seen with PD
 3. **Two components of blink response**
    a. **Early** = slight move of upper lids, not in volitional control
    b. **Late** = eyelid closure, can be voluntarily inhibited

II. Pupils

A. **Noncircular shapes**
 1. **Oval:** neurosyphilis, glaucoma, congenital, Adie pupil
 2. **Pear-shaped:** surgical, congenital coloboma, anterior synechiae

B. **Marcus-Gunn pupil**: afferent pupillary defect; pupil dilates to consensual light reflex
 1. Nonspecific marker of any disease of retina or optic nerve

C. **Argyll-Robertson pupil:** can be irregularly shaped, usually bilateral
 1. Accommodates but does not react ("prostitute's" pupil); little effect with 4% cocaine
 2. Seen in many diseases, classically CNS syphilis, but also sarcoid, diabetes, alcoholism

D. **Adie tonic pupil:** can be oval, usually unilateral and mydriatic
 1. Absent/sluggish accommodation and poor reaction; dilation with 4% cocaine
 2. Benign finding, associated with decreased reflexes, visual blurring when reading

E. **Uncal herniation or third nerve dysfunction** in stages from initial to terminal
 1. **Early third nerve:** unilateral miosis, usually ipsilateral ⇒ test by contralateral Babinski
 2. **Late third nerve:** pupil fully dilates, once fully dilates, eye movements impaired = irreversible damage and stupor
 3. **Midbrain:** contralateral fixes; once both 5 to 6 mm and fixed, uniformly fatal if lasts longer than 30 minutes
 4. **Causes:** aneurysm, ischemia, trauma, herniation; order STAT CT
 5. **Compressive aneurysm to cranial nerve** (CN) III will cause abnormal reaction to light, whereas ischemic CN III lesion will have a normal pupillary reaction to light.

F. **Acute glaucoma** (this is a medical emergency)
 1. Pupil fixed 5 to 7 mm with red eyes and blurry vision
 2. Give intravenous (IV) mannitol or acetazolamide STAT, then call ophthalmology

G. **Bilateral pupillary problems**
 1. **Miosis + fixed:** medulla, severe hypoglycemia, post-anoxic, botulism, bilateral CN III nuclei
 2. **Miosis + reactive:** opiate withdrawal, albuterol nebulizers, if overdose use atropine, magnesium, tetracyclines, aminoglycosides, dopamine
 3. **Mydriasis:** diencephalic stage of tentorial herniation, pons, opiates

III. Vision

A. **Visual defects** are discussed in anatomy chapter

B. **Sudden visual change is a medical emergency, unilateral versus bilateral**

C. **Funduscopic examination essentials**
   1. Check for red reflex and then 2 to 3 feet from patient refocus to iris to verify that there are no opacities; if hazy call ophthalmologist to rule out interstitial keratitis; if round gray spots on posterior cornea, likely ocular sarcoid (but many other explanations)
   2. If unable to visualize fundus: opacities, severe astigmatism (ask patient to put on glasses)
   3. Locate the optic disc by going in direction of bifurcations of blood vessels.
      a. If venous pulsations present, CSF pressure likely normal; if not, normal in 20%
      b. Papilledema: initial changes are loss of disc margins and elevated disc often with splinter hemorrhages. Expect normal vision in acute papilledema. Need ophthalmologist with direct ophthalmoscope to verify.
         i. Many causes, including hemorrhage, increased intracranial pressure, retinal vascular disease, various poisons (carbon monoxide, lead, arsenic, vitamin A, ethylene glycol), and Guillain-Barré
         ii. Pseudo-papilledema: most commonly astigmatism or hypermetropia; tumor that obscures the disc; can be congenital defect of myelinated nerves; colloid bodies of the disc = drusen, hyaloid artery remnants
      c. Look for neovascularization.
      d. Look for glaucoma (any two): blood vessels disappear and reappear as they traverse the optic cup (do not be fooled by cilioretinal vessel, which does not reappear), optic cup >30% of total disc, most vessels appear on the nasal side, disc pallor, disc is vertically oval.
   4. Locate macula temporally. Best for microaneurysms. Uncomfortable, so do it last.
   5. Streaklike retina folded in on itself, retinal detachment, call ophthalmologist immediately

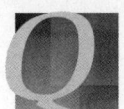# STUDY QUESTIONS FOR CHAPTER 22

Directions: *Each of the numbered items or incomplete statements in this section is followed by answers or by completions of the statement. Select the ONE lettered answer or completion that is BEST in each case.*

1. Your patient has anisocoria and ptosis on the left. You order hydroxyamphetamine (Paredrine) but the pharmacy calls to say only cocaine 4% is available. Knowing that cocaine blocks the reuptake of norepinephrine, what do you expect if you instill it in the patient's eyes?

   (A) It confirms the Horner syndrome, with no effect on affected pupil and other pupil dilating.
   (B) It confirms the syndrome, with both pupils dilating.
   (C) It confirms the syndrome, with dilation of affected pupil and no effect on other.
   (D) It would not be expected to confirm the syndrome.

2. You are examining a 79-year-old comatose patient in an intensive care unit. While testing the cranial nerves, you note that when the right eye is stroked gently with gauze, there is no corneal reflex in either eye, but when the left eye is stimulated, both eyes have a corneal reflex. A lesion at what site would produce this picture?

   (A) Right trigeminal nerve and its nuclei
   (B) Left trigeminal nerve and its nuclei
   (C) Right facial nerve and its nuclei
   (D) Left facial nerve and its nuclei
   (E) Right oculomotor nerve and its nuclei

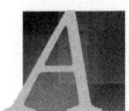 ANSWERS AND EXPLANATIONS

1. A. Only normal pupil is secreting norepinephrine, thus dilating a normal pupil. This will confirm Horner syndrome as it not be affected by cocaine. (B), (C) are opposites and are the expected results. (D) Distractor, as this test specifically confirms the condition.

2. A. A lesion of the trigeminal nerve and its nuclei can cause absence of the blink reflex on either side when the ipsilateral eye is stimulated. A lesion of the facial nerve and its nuclei causes absence of the blink reflex in the ipsilateral eye when either eye is stimulated. The oculomotor nerve is not involved in the blink reflex.

CHAPTER 23

Neurosurgery for the Neurologist

I. Trauma Basics

A. **300,000 Civilian head injuries per year** in the United States; 10% do not reach a hospital with early mortality

B. **Management**
  1. Of patients who do present to hospital, **Glasgow coma scale** (GCS) always measured on presentation to the emergency department
     a. 80% Mild head injury: GCS 13 to 15
     b. 10% Moderate head injury: GCS 8 to 12
     c. 10% Severe head injury: GCS <8, 50% will have one or more other major systemic injury; lowest score with no verbal or motor response or eye movements is 3.
     d. There are different, accepted classification schemes; we use the advanced trauma life support (ATLS) version; some neurologists may categorize GCS 13 as mild, ≤ 8 as severe.
  2. **Priorities**
     a. First establish an adequate airway, then appropriate fluid resuscitation and evaluation of circulatory status
     b. In trauma, cervical spine injury assumed until proved otherwise; 5% of head-injured patients have an associated spine injury, and 25% of spine-injured patients have at least a mild head injury; no head computed tomography (CT) until cervical injury excluded by plain radiogram
     c. Up to 20% of patients with a spine injury will have a second, possibly noncontiguous, spine injury; spine injuries are distributed as follows: 55% cervical spine and 15% each thoracic spine, thoracolumbar junction, and lumbar spine
  3. **Indications** for brain oxygen and intracranial pressure (ICP) monitoring
     a. GCS [9 after cardiopulmonary resuscitation plus either an abnormal head CT scan or two of the following: age >40 years, systolic blood pressure (BP) <90 mm Hg; decerebrate or decorticate motor posturing (unilateral or bilateral)
     b. Patients with altered level of consciousness (iatrogenic or otherwise) and multiple injuries whose treatments preclude effective neurologic examination that may adversely affect ICP [e.g., pharmacologic paralysis, large volumes of intravenous (IV) fluids, high levels of positive end-expiratory pressure (PEEP), etc.]. Invasive monitoring is generally deferred if the patient is able to localize or follow commands, as neurologic deterioration can be detected clinically.
  4. **Control of elevated ICP**
     a. General measures
        i. Very important: avoid hypotension and treat aggressively if present
        ii. Elevate head of bed 30 degrees
        iii. Keep head midline to avoid jugular vein kinking

iv. Light sedation with codeine or lorazepam
v. Avoid hyperglycemia, elevated temperature; hypoxia, hypercarbia
b. First-line therapy: ICP monitoring mandatory
  i. Heavier sedation with propofol, morphine, fentanyl, and/or lorazepam
  ii. Cerebrospinal fluid (CSF) drainage if external ventricular drain in place
  iii. Mannitol 0.25 to 1 g/kg IV bolus every 6 hours; measure serum osmolality with each dose and withhold next dose if osmolality exceeds 310
  iv. Brief hyperventilation to pCO_2 of 25 to 30 mm Hg
c. Second-line therapy: don't use corticosteroids as may worsen outcome
  i. High-dose barbiturates: titrate to burst suppression on EEG or bispectral index
  ii. Sustained hyperventilation to pCO_2 of 25 to 30 mm Hg (usually ineffective)
  iii. Hypothermia and/or decompressive craniectomy: controversial

II. Herniation Syndromes Due to Increased Intracranial Pressure

A. **Central (transtentorial) herniation:** diencephalon is forced downward through tentorial incisura, causing a rostrocaudal progression of brainstem ischemia from direct compression and shearing of perforators from the basilar artery.

B. **Uncal herniation:** as the medial uncus and hippocampal gyrus are pushed over the edge of the tentorium, oculomotor nerve becomes entrapped and midbrain is directly compressed. The posterior cerebral artery may also become injured. Expected findings are ipsilateral CN III deficit and contralateral hemiparesis. If midbrain is pushed to the opposite side, hemiparesis may be ipsilateral to pupillary dilatation (Kernohan notch).

C. **Subfalcine herniation:** usually identified radiographically, where one cingulate gyrus can be seen herniating across midline under the falx; usually clinically silent unless it causes kinking of the anterior cerebral arteries, which can produce bifrontal infarction

D. **Tonsillar herniation:** acute compression of cerebellar tonsils through foramen magnum compresses medulla, which precipitates respiratory arrest with increased BP, and bradycardia
  1. **Upward cerebellar herniation:** Cerebellar vermis ascends above tentorium, compresses the midbrain, and potentially compresses the bilateral superior cerebellar arteries.

III. Concussion

A. **Closed head injury** in a patient with a normal brain CT where there was transient disturbance in level of consciousness at the time of the injury
  1. The patient returns to full consciousness within 6 hours to satisfy the definition
  2. More severe if it is associated with retrograde and anterograde amnesia
  3. Postconcussion syndrome: headache, tinnitus, fatigue, blurred vision, double vision, nausea, dizziness, positonal vertigo, anosmia, memory difficulties, or other problems; usually self-limited; protracted course consider more serious etiology versus somatoform disorder

IV. Diffuse Axonal Injury

A. Prolonged posttraumatic coma not due to mass lesion or ischemic insults.

B. **CT** imaging may be normal but MRI may show widespread punctate hemorrhages, most prominently at the gray–white matter interface, corpus callosum, or hypothalamus.

C. **Mechanism** is thought to be disruption of axonal pathways from shearing forces.

D. **Patients** may be deeply comatose and often dysautonomia including hypertension, hyperhidrosis, hyperpyrexia. Motor posturing frequent; increased intracranial pressure possible. Clinical course long and complex, if patients survive, with recovery from comatose state very difficult to predict; most common cause of prolonged vegetative state

V. Cerebral Contusion and Traumatic Subarachnoid Hemorrhage

A. **Cerebral contusion:** usually associated with areas where sudden deceleration of the head causes the brain to impact on bony prominences, and both coup and contrecoup injuries may be seen from the same impact

B. **Delayed** traumatic intracerebral hemorrhage (ICH): incidence of 10% with GCS [8, usually manifests within 72 hours of injury, 12% of patients who experience acute neurologic deterioration in first 24 hours following injury; outcome generally poor

C. **Trauma** most common cause of subarachnoid hemorrhage; usually found focally on the cerebral convexities and rarely involving the basal cisterns

D. **Indications** for surgical intervention: controversial; same for hemorrhagic cerebrovascular accident (CVA); include surgically accessible location, large size, mass effect

VI. Epidural Hematoma (Figure 23-1)

A. **Classic clinical history** of acute epidural hematoma (EDH) is brief loss of consciousness immediately after traumatic injury, followed by lucid interval lasting several hours, then rapid deterioration to coma and herniation; actually seen in only 10% to 27% of patients with acute EDH.

B. **Men** are four times as likely as women to sustain this injury, and it is very rare in patients younger than the age of 2 years or older than the age of 60 years

C. **Most EDHs** result from bleeding from the middle meningeal or anterior meningeal artery, the majority of which are associated with an overlying linear skull fracture across middle meningeal artery groove

D. **Younger patients** are more vulnerable to EDHs in the absence of fracture, and are also more vulnerable to EDH from disruption of a venous sinus; venous EDHs are relatively rare, although they comprise the majority of the 5% of EDHs found in the posterior fossa

E. **Death usually from respiratory arrest, from uncal herniation causing midbrain injury**
   1. 60% with EDH have a unilaterally dilated pupil, of which 85% are ipsilateral due to transtentorial herniation
   2. Kernohan notch phenomenon: false localizing sign in 15% to 20%: brainstem shifts away from hematoma with compression of contralateral peduncle and ipsilateral hemiparesis

F. **Noncontrast CT scan:** in early stages, hyperdense biconvex mass adjacent to the skull with sharply defined edges, usually limited by cranial suture lines

G. **Emergent surgery** indicated for symptomatic or EDHs 1 cm in maximum thickness, as outcome best with early surgery

H. **Mortality** with EDH is highly dependent on prompt diagnosis and treatment, with rates of 5% to 10% reported in the CT era; poor prognostic factors include lack of a lucid interval, bilateral Babinski sign, preoperative decerebrate posturing, and concomitant presence of an underlying acute subdural hematoma

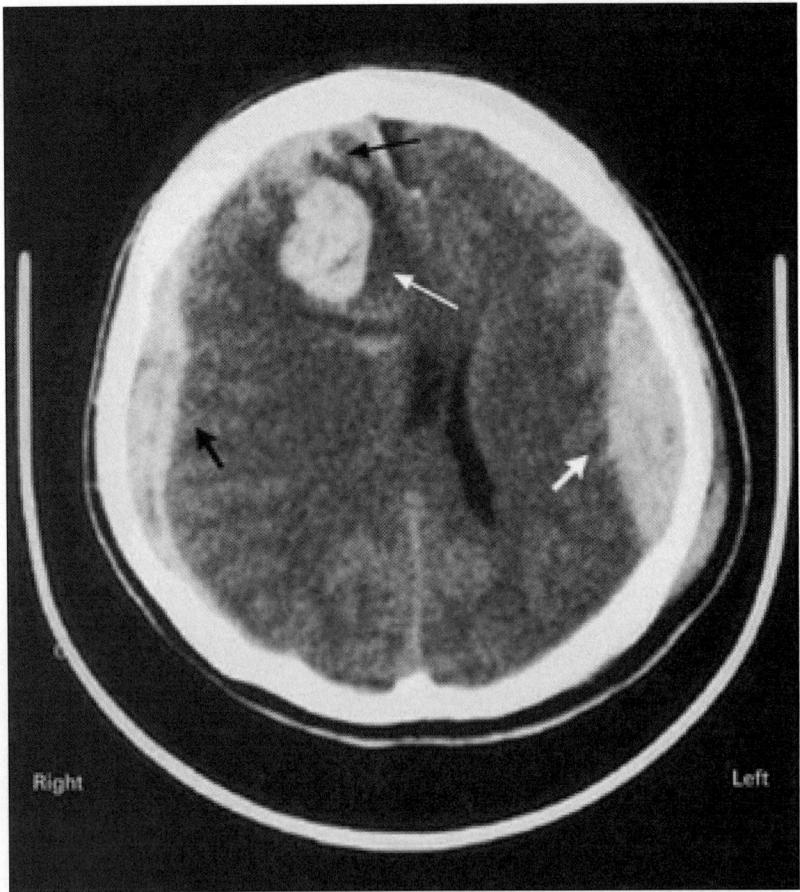

Figure 23-1 Four types of acute posttraumatic intracranial hemorrhage: an epidural hematoma *(thick white arrow)* and a squamous temporal fracture (which is not shown) on the left side, a laminated subdural hematoma *(thick black arrow)* on the right side, right-sided periventricular and frontal-lobe contusions containing an intraparenchymal hematoma *(thin white arrow)*, and a subarachnoid hemorrhage *(thin black arrow)* in the right frontal region. (Matiello JA, Munz M. Four types of acute post-traumatic intracranial hemorrhage. *New England Journal of Medicine* 2001; 344(8): 580. Copyright © 2001 Masssachustts Medical Society. All rights reserved.)

VII. Acute Subdural Hematoma (SDH)

A. Classically is disruption of bridging internal cerebral veins and superior sagittal sinus; anticoagulation increases risk of SDH sevenfold in males and 26-fold in females.

B. Appears as a hyperdense crescent-shaped mass adjacent to the inner table, and often generates midline shift greater than the thickness of the hematoma due to associated underlying brain edema.

C. Emergent surgical evacuation is indicated in symptomatic acute SDH where the midline shift or thickness of clot is 1 cm or greater (5 mm in pediatric patients).

D. Outcomes for SDH reflect the severity of associated brain injury. Mortality is generally reported at about 67%, with a range of 50% to 90% in the modern literature. Important factors that influence outcome include:

1. **Time to surgery:** patients who undergo operation within 4 hours of injury have better outcomes in terms of mortality and neurologic function.
2. **Age:** outcomes are significantly worse for age >65 years.
3. **Anticoagulation:** patients on therapeutic anticoagulation at the time of injury have a mortality of 90% or greater.
4. **GCS on admission:** GCS of 3, mortality >90% and functional survival <5%

VIII. Chronic Subdural Hematoma

A. **Precipitating head trauma**, sometimes trivial, is identified in 50% of cases; risk factors: elderly, alcohol abuse, seizure disorders, coagulopathies, or anticoagulation

B. **Patients generally present with minor symptoms** including headache, confusion, or TIA-like symptoms. Often, the diagnosis is unexpected prior to imaging.

C. **Appearance on CT scan:** crescent-shaped isodense or hypodense fluid collection between the brain and inside surface of skull, often with little or no mass effect evident

D. **Surgical evacuation if its thickness is greater than 1 cm or if the lesion is symptomatic**
   1. Iso- or hypodense appearance on CT scan indicates that subdural clot has liquefied and can be drained with simple burr holes, rather than an open craniotomy
   2. Overall mortality is reported at 4% or less.

IX. Cranial Nerve Palsies Dysfunction with Skull Base Fractures

A. **CN VII or VIII:** associated with temporal bone fracture; delayed presentation of CN VII palsy associated with better outcome; treatment with steroids, serial facial EMGs; surgical nerve decompression considered if EMG studies show continued deterioration

B. **CN I:** usually associated with cribriform plate fracture; anterior fossa fractures affecting olfaction may extend to the optic canal and potentially injure CN II

C. **CN VI:** associated with clivus fractures

D. **Look for battle sign** (discoloration behind ear over mastoid process) and raccoon eyes (blood leaking into periorbital tissue)

E. **Risk of meningitis** due to dural tear; if rhinorrhea, most resolve spontaneously

X. Penetrating Head Injury

A. **Gunshot wound** most common mechanism, incidence: men 5 times > females.

B. **Suicide attempts** are associated with the highest mortality.

C. **Initial GCS strong predictor of mortality:** 3 to 5, 94%, survivors neurologically devastated; 6 to 8, 59% overall, 9 or greater, 3% to 15%, and surgery is generally undertaken

D. **Emergent noncontrast** CT mandatory prior to surgical exploration; ominous findings on imaging include midline shift, significant missile fragmentation, compressed basal cisterns, and transventricular injury

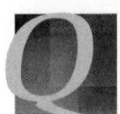# STUDY QUESTIONS FOR CHAPTER 23

Directions: *Each of the numbered items or incomplete statements in this section is followed by answers or by completions of the statement. Select the ONE lettered answer or completion that is BEST in each case.*

1. A 45-year-old man is brought to the emergency department after falling and landing on back of his head. The patient demonstrates bilateral flexor posturing of his upper extremities and does not open his eyes or make any attempt at speech. What is the most appropriate first step in management?
   (A) Endotracheal intubation
   (B) Start two large-bore IV lines and infuse warmed crystalloid
   (C) Noncontrast CT scan of the brain
   (D) Placement of a hard cervical collar

2. Which of the following is not appropriate as an initial management step in the patient with suspected elevated intracranial pressure?
   (A) Cooling blanket to treat temperature of 38.6°C
   (B) Intravenous codeine for light sedation
   (C) Intravenous mannitol bolus
   (D) Elevate head of bed 30 degrees
   (E) Dopamine to treat systolic blood pressure of 70 mm Hg refractory to fluid resuscitation

3. Which of the following injuries has the highest mortality?

   (A) Epidural hematoma from an unhelmeted motorcycle accident
   (B) Acute subdural hematoma from a high-speed motor vehicle collision
   (C) Chronic subdural hematoma of unknown etiology
   (D) Gunshot wound to the head in a patient with a GCS of 11 on initial presentation

4. Fracture of what structure has the highest risk of potentially impairing vision?
   (A) Clivus
   (B) Cribriform plate
   (C) Temporal bone
   (D) Parietal bone

5. Which of the following scenarios illustrate the Kernohan notch phenomenon?
   (A) Right-sided EDH, pupils midposition and sluggish, left hemiparesis
   (B) Left-sided SDH, left-sided extensor posturing, right-sided flexor posturing
   (C) Right-sided coup and contrecoup cerebral contusions, bilateral flexor posturing
   (D) Left-sided SDH, left blown pupil, left hemiparesis

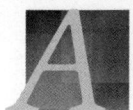 ANSWERS AND EXPLANATIONS

1. A. Glasgow coma scale score of 5 (3 motor, 1 verbal, 1 eye opening); therefore, severe head injury category. (B,D) While initiation of IV fluids and placement of a hard cervical collar are appropriate steps in acute management, first priority is establishment of definitive airway. (C) CT scanning deferred until patient is hemodynamically stabilized.

2. C. Intermittent mannitol is very effective as acute therapy but should be deferred until general management implemented. Exceptions: if ICP monitor is in place showing elevated pressure or if patient is clinically demonstrating signs of herniation. (E) Rapid correction of hypotension is mandatory. (A,B,D) Are all general management steps.

3. B. Mortality from acute subdural hematoma overall is between 50% and 90%, which represents highest mortality among injuries listed. For others described, associated mortalities are 4% for chronic SDH (C), 5% to 10% for EDH (A), and 3% to 15% for gunshot wound to the head in which the patient's presenting GCS is 9 or greater (D).

4. B. Fractures of the cribriform plate can potentially extend into the optic canal and injure the optic nerve. (A,C,D) can also impair vision by damaging the optic pathways, but have a much, much smaller chance of affecting vision.

5. D. Kernohan notch phenomenon is mass lesion on one side causing shift of brainstem, which compresses contralateral cerebral peduncle, leading to hemiparesis ipsilateral to lesion. Most commonly with EDH but possible with any expanding intracranial mass. (A,B) show contralateral hemiparesis; (C) shows bilateral abnormalities.

Internal Medicine for the Neurologist

I. Medical Issues Complicating Neurology Patients

A. Stroke
1. **Atrial fibrillation** complicates about 15% of stroke. This means that in searching for a source, the finding of atrial fibrillation is not enough, as a further 15% will have a second cardiac risk for stroke. All patients with chronic or recurrent paroxysmal atrial fibrillation should be placed on warfarin with an internal normalized ratio (INR) goal of 2 to 3, unless there is a compelling reason otherwise, unless there is lone atrial fibrillation [defined as: <65 years of age, no coronary artery disease (CAD), normal electrocardiogram (ECG), normal echocardiogram (ECHO), no hypertension/diabetes mellitus (DM)], in which case anticoagulation is not indicated because the risk of stroke is not increased.
    a. There are three cardiology atrial fibrillation trials that neurologists should know:
        i. **AFFIRM** showed that among patients with atrial fibrillation, anticoagulation should be continued even in those patients in whom the rhythm had been suppressed.
        ii. **RACE** showed that there was a nonsignificant trend toward worse outcome with rhythm control. Post hoc analysis showed a significant worsened effect with women and hypertensive patients experiencing rhythm control.
        iii. **SPAF** identified stroke/transient ischemic attack (TIA) as a risk factor for recurrence and is the main reason almost everyone with an ischemic stroke/TIA is put on warfarin.
    b. There is no convincing evidence of increased thrombotic events after initiation of warfarin without heparin (warfarin induced protein C and S deficiency) unless using high doses of warfarin
    c. Immediate anticoagulation with heparin/heparinoids is not necessary, as the daily risk of stroke is 0.02% in high-risk patients.
    d. Unless symptomatic, the cornerstone of treatment should be rate control (<100) with β-blockers. Some caveats exist: asthmatics should get calcium channel blockers; for patients with congestive heart failure (CHF), try esmolol to see if patient can tolerate a β-blocker and consider digitalizing; second-line agent calcium channel blocker
2. **Cardiac abnormalities** include S-T changes, Q-T prolongation, and left-axis deviation. These changes are present in 15% to 20% of ischemic stroke and 60% of subarachnoid hemorrhage and suggest that cardiac monitoring might be considered for all stroke patients.
3. **Hypercoagulability work-up** is expensive, costing about $3,000, so it should be done only when indicated such as when stroke is of venous origin (venous sinus thrombosis). Different authors have different ideas, but an age <55 years without a clear cause is generally accepted as young for stroke. Some series suggest that up to 5% to 8% of ischemic strokes are complicated by a hematologic abnormality. The two most important causes of hypercoagulability in arterial stroke are malignancy and antiphospholipid antibody.

a. Test for protein C, protein S, antithrombin III, lupus anticoagulant, factor V Leiden, and anticardiolipin in venous origin stroke.
   b. Activated protein C inactivates factors Va and VIIIa. In acute stroke, low concentrations are fairly normal. Repeat testing in 3 months. If still low, consider testing family members.
      i. Factor V Leiden is a point mutation of factor V, where activated protein C inactivates Va. It is the most common inherited hypercoagulable state. There is some controversy among epidemiologists over whether this is truly a risk factor; in the medical community it is treated as established fact.
   c. Antithrombin III inhibits IXa, Xa, XIa, XIIa, and thrombin. Dysfunction and deficiency are both inherited (autosomal dominant, occurs in 0.05%) and acquired [nephritic syndrome, disseminated intravascular coagulation (DIC), heparin, leukemia, diabetes] forms.
   d. Antiphospholipid antibody (anticardiolipin and lupus anticoagulant) INR should be >3.0 (by retrospective analysis).

II. Medical Consults

A. Delirium
   1. **Probably the most common consult.** Key facts to know: can be caused by a combination of minor medical abnormalities, 15% of unexplained altered mental status is subclinical seizures (often misquoted by emergency department staff, because unexplained means the work-up has been done)
   2. **Differential diagnosis:** M-I-N-D-E-T-H H-I-S P-I-P-E-S (Table 24-1).
   3. **When should a neurologist be involved?** When there are focal neurologic findings or when the work-up has failed to produce an etiology.

B. Renal
   1. **Von Hippel-Lindau:** autosomal dominant where 80% of the mutations can be localized in genetic testing, central nervous system (CNS) hemangioblastomas, renal cell carcinomas
      a. Retinal hemangioblastoma often the first disease manifestation
      b. Cerebellar hemangioblastomas occur in one half of cases, can cause erythrocytosis; screening: brain MRI every 3 years until age 50 then every 5 years (at risk relative 15 to 40 years every 3 years then every 5 years until age 60); ophthalmologic and medical screening appointments yearly

Table 24-1 *Differential Diagnosis of Delirium*

M—metabolic: renal/hepatic	Drugs known to induce delirium:
I—infectious: UTI, pneumonia, etc.	antiarrhythmics, anticholinergics
N—neoplastic: edema or lesion	barbiturates, β-blockers,
D—drugs and intoxicants (see below)	calcium channel blockers,
E—electrolytes: calcium and sodium	digoxin, dopamine agonist,
T—trauma: head	ethanol, hallucinogens,
H—hypoxia	isoniazid, MAO inhibitors,
H—hemodynamic cardiac output or volume	lithium, muscle relaxants,
I—inflammatory: autoimmune	narcotics
S—seizure/postictal	phenothiazines
P—psychiatric	salicylates
I—intracranial hemorrhage	stimulants
P—porphyria	theophylline
E—endocrine: hypoglycemia, thyroid, adrenal, B12, folate	
S—stroke	

MAO, monoamine oxidase; UTI, urinary tract infection.

2. **Polycystic kidney disease:** intracranial aneurysm in 5% to 15%; no guidelines but MRA every 3 years is reasonable; hypertension: treat aggressively.
3. **Uremic encephalopathy:** symptoms variable changing rapidly, progresses in stages: early—fatigue, impaired concentration; middle—labile, forgetful, sleep inversion, frontal lobe dysfunction; late—delirium, coma, convulsions; can see hypertonia, increased reflexes, meningismus, clonus, Babinski, asterixis, coarse tremor; these findings can be asymmetric, with hemiparesis common, even alternating sides
   a. Electroencephalogram (EEG): acute stage generalized slowing often greatest frontally; chronic = bilateral spike and wave without seizure activity in about 10%
   b. Poor correlation of level of azotemia with course of disease
4. **Uremic neuropathy**
   a. Rare in children, but complicates many chronic renal insufficiency patients; does not seem to develop if glomerular filtration rate (GFR) >12 mL/minute and can be reversed with transplantation
   b. Usually axonal sensory and motor distal > proximal with burning; can be pure sensory or pure motor; foot dorsiflexion often first motor symptom; patients are at an increased risk of compressive neuropathies; patients may also experience hearing loss that may reverse with initiation of dialysis
5. **Dialysis**
   a. **Dialysis dysequilibrium syndrome:** now typically occurs only during initiation of dialysis/emergent dialysis when an osmotic gradient develops between the plasma and the brain; patients have restlessness, cramps, and headaches; if it worsens, dysequilibrium, myoclonus, delirium, or other seizures can develop
   b. **Dialysis dementia:** occurs in about 1% of dialysis patients; starts with dysarthria, dysphasia, and dysgraphia, often with stuttering speech after dialysis; myoclonus develops in most, later hallucinations, seizures, and finally become immobile and mute; caused by aluminum; newer systems do not have this risk, although some sporadic cases occur; treat with desferrioxamine

C. **Hepatology**
   1. **Hepatic encephalopathy.** (Please see Table 24-2 for stages and symptoms.) Consult may take place because of the deliriumlike qualities. One quick way of assessing whether it is hepatic encephalopathy is to give flumenazil intravenous (IV) 0.3 to 0.5 mg; in about 60% of cases, there will be a great improvement of mental status in 5 minutes or less; to follow subclinical mental status changes, can either use the number connection test or use the poor man's version of it: ask the patient to draw a five pointed star. NH_3 is elevated—must be arterial or free-flowing venous (no tourniquet) blood. EEG shows triphasic waves.
   2. **Wilson disease.** Disorder of copper metabolism where copper accumulates; neurologic findings include an initial deterioration of functioning then incoordination, tremor, dysarthria, ataxia evolving into dystonia, spasticity, and seizures; the symptoms are generally reversible with treatment; in untreated patients with neurologic manifestations, Kayser-Fleischer rings occur if CNS signs present
      a. If appears to have the disease, order a ceruloplasmin concentration

Table 24-2 *Hepatic Encephalopathy*

Stage I: mild confusion, well preserved verbal ability, decreased attention
Stage II: lethargy, personality change, unable to cooperate, somewhat disoriented
Stage III: somnolent, unable to perform tasks, amnesia, worsened disorientation
Stage IVA: coma responsive to painful stimuli
Stage IVB: coma unresponsive to painful stimuli

b. Treatment is with D-penicillamine 250 to 500 mg q.i.d. before meals. Warn patients that symptoms may worsen during the first month of treatment. In addition, new manifestations of the disease may appear. In such cases, decrease the dose and slowly taper upward. Trientine or oral zinc are alternatives.

D. Pregnancy
1. **Common problems**
   a. Restless legs syndrome may complicate up to 20%. Test for iron and folate deficiency.
   b. **Carpal tunnel syndrome:** rates of symptoms are increased. Usually resolves after pregnancy, so conservative treatment is the rule. Other focal compressive neuropathy is facial nerve dysfunction.
2. **Headaches:** commonly are reduced but can worsen or even occur for the first time. Acetaminophen is safe but may cause delayed onset of labor as well as premature closure of the ductus arteriosus. No increases in birth defects have been seen. Sumatriptan is not recommended, as there have been >1% of birth defects in pregnancies that used triptans. For frequent or disabling migraines, use propanolol. Headache worsening in later stage.
   a. eclampsia
   b. venous sinus thrombosis
   c. idiopathic intracranial hypertension
3. **Epilepsy:** increases the risk of fetal malformations. If taking an enzyme-inducing drug, give 10 mg IV vitamin K at the onset of labor. Treat status normally. Breast feeding is probably safe, because although many anticonvulsants are excreted in breast milk, the amount excreted is small.
4. **Uncommon problems**
   a. **Bell palsy:** treat with short course of steroids
   b. **Chorea gravidarum:** multiple possible causes, do not treat unless disabling; can try low dose haloperidol if patient is aware of teratogenic potential.
5. **Seizures:** most commonly eclampsia, but also consider intracerebral hemorrhage, cerebral venous thrombosis, tumor, intracerebral infection, metabolic disturbances, and autoimmune sources; treat with magnesium 5 g over 20 minutes, followed by 2 g per hour, and checking the patient frequently (hourly) for side effects; recurrent seizure merits 2 g bolus over 2 minutes; another recurrence should get benzodiazepines and intensive care unit (ICU) admission should be considered

E. Critical illness consults
1. **Difficulty weaning from the ventilator:** neurologic cause can be found in about 40%; this will generally either be critical illness polyneuropathy or myopathy or central drive defect, often in combination with one or more other neurologic problems; patient should get a good physical examination to exclude localizing lesion suggesting brain or spinal cord pathology; due to the high rates of neurologic basis for difficulty weaning, consider getting electrophysiologic work-up for all such patients; if electrophysiologic testing is negative, consider magnetic resonance imaging (MRI) and EEG
2. **Weakness before ICU admission:** generally includes one of Guillain-Barré, myasthenia-gravis, or Lambert-Eaton syndrome; conditions not to miss include a high cervical spinal cord compression or transverse myelitis; any suggestion of these mandates emergency MRI; also do not be fooled by chronic polyneuropathies, which can occasionally include rapid respiratory failure, such as diabetic neuropathy or chronic inflammatory demyelinating polyradiculoneuropathy (CIDP); it may be one of the rare instances that needle electromyogram (EMG) of the diaphragm is useful
3. **Weakness after ICU admission:** all patients should get a creatine kinase (CK) and nerve conduction study (NCV)/EMG
   a. Critical illness polyneuropathy: normal CK, depression of sensory nerve action potential (SNAP) amplitude and CMAP; if only decrease in compound muscle action potential (CMAP), then a motor neuropathy; patients should have single fiber repetitive stimulation to exclude neuromuscular transmission block
   b. Disuse myopathy if NCV/EMG normal

c. If needle EMG shows a primary myopathy (i.e., short duration motor unit potentials with polyphasic waves), likely to be thick-filament myopathy. Expect markedly diminished CMAP amplitudes. Look for ophthalmoplegia, steroids treating asthma, especially in a history of receiving neuromuscular blocking agents. Recovery is usually rapid. Recommend discontinuing steroids and neuromuscular blocking agents, and start physical therapy for both prevention of contractures and strengthening. Always consider checking for myoglobin in the urine, and if positive, likely to be critical illness necrotizing myopathy, which is rare; check phosphate levels.

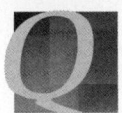

STUDY QUESTIONS FOR CHAPTER 24

Directions: *Each of the numbered items or incomplete statements in this section is followed by answers or by completions of the statement. Select the ONE lettered answer or completion that is BEST in each case.*

1. A 43-year-old male alcoholic with hepatitis C presents to your office with his wife, somewhat out of sorts and somewhat inattentive, 2 weeks after discharge from the hospital. Your nurse checks his vital signs, which are normal. You saw him just after his discharge and he was asymptomatic. What can you do to prevent the patient from being sent to the emergency room and then likely admitted?

(A) Mini-mental status examination
(B) Check a uremia level
(C) Administer flumazenil
(D) Tell the patient to come back tomorrow

2. Same patient as in number 1. What do you expect the patient's forward digit span to be?

(A) 7
(B) 5
(C) 2
(D) 1
(E) 0

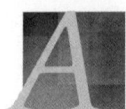# ANSWERS AND EXPLANATIONS

1. C. Flumazenil may reverse his symptoms if they are due to stage I hepatic encephalopathy, and one could follow the patient closely with an increased amount of lactulose. Close follow-up is probably not sufficient for a patient who likely has hepatic encephalopathy.

2. B. Forward digit span in normal adults is 7±2. It is a test used both in intelligence testing and as a surrogate for attention; 2 or lower would likely indicate someone severely inattentive; 5 would be low normal and might be expected for someone described as somewhat inattentive.

CHAPTER 25

Neuropsychiatry

I. Neuropsychiatric Evaluation

A. **Mental status examination:** Observe patient behavior throughout examination.
 1. **Consciousness and attention:** test by observation and formal tests, for example, digit span, serial seven subtractions
 2. **Memory**
    a. Immediate memory is attention.
    b. Short-term memory (verbal and visual): have patient learn three to five objects or a short story and test recall after 2 to 5 minute distraction; hide objects, ask patient to find; tests of orientation; ask about recent personal history or current events
    c. Long-term memory: more remote personal history or facts of common knowledge
 3. **Language and related functions**
    a. Spontaneous speech: listen; note fluency, word choice, meaning
    b. Verbal comprehension: note response to yes–no questions and commands
    c. Repetition: test phrase, for example, "no ifs, ands, or buts"
    d. Naming: ask patient to name objects such as "watch" and parts of object
    e. Reading: test comprehension
    f. Writing: a complete sentence, not signature; if aphasic, writing dysfunction is small as verbal
 4. **"Constructional ability":** test by copying figures, for example, superimposed pentagons or draw a clock
 5. **Other higher cortical functions:** includes neglect; right–left orientation; praxis; agnosia
 6. **Frontal lobe** (executive) functions and abstract thinking; word fluency tests (letter or category); proverb interpretation; finding similarities between related words; alternating sequences tests, "go–no go"

B. **Neuropsychological testing:** useful in diagnostically difficult cases and to chart progression of symptoms over time; also important in research. Hundreds of tests to choose from, some as standard batteries (e.g., Wechsler Intelligence Scale, California Verbal Learning Test), others used only by individual examiners. Let neuropsychologist know what the question is; results must be interpreted in context of each individual patient.

C. **Neuroimaging and other laboratory tests**
 1. Help diagnose specific illness, not neuropsychiatric syndromes
 2. Computed tomography (CT) and magnetic resonance imaging (MRI) play essential role in localizing lesions in circumscribed syndromes
 3. No consistent CT or MRI abnormalities reported yet in traditional psychiatric disorders but scan needed to exclude potential structural brain disease; dynamic imaging still largely experimental; electroencephalography helpful in seizure-related syndromes

II. Common Neuropsychiatric Syndromes

A. **Circumscribed neuropsychiatric syndromes:** deficits predominantly in one domain of function; often localizable
  1. **Disorders of arousal:** see section on coma
  2. **Disorders of perception:** ("organic") hallucinatory syndromes; often associated with sensory deficits or delirium
  3. **Disorders of attention**
     a. Global inattention: delirium
        i. May also have somatic symptoms, for example, tremor, and hallucinations
        ii. Usually caused by medical conditions, drugs, withdrawal states
        iii. Rarely from focal central nervous system (CNS) disease, for example, brainstem, right parietal cortex
     b. Restricted inattention: neglect
        i. Overwhelmingly, left side of space; with right hemisphere lesion; may be in visual, auditory, or somatic modality; sometimes associated with anosognosia ("denial of illness")
  4. **Disorders of language and related functions**
     a. **Aphasia:** left hemisphere disease in most cases (right and left handers)
        i. **Nonfluent aphasias:** halting speech with reduced phrase length and grammatical complexity; lesions anterior to central sulcus
           (a) **Broca aphasia:** nonfluent speech, poor repetition; relatively better comprehension; usually have right hemiparesis and hemisensory defect and apraxia; typically from lesions; in dorsolateral frontal, opercular, and anteroparietal cortex, with subcortical extension
           (b) **Transcortical motor aphasia:** repetition better; lesion farther from Sylvian fissure, sparing opercular cortex; can also be subcortical
        ii. **Fluent aphasias:** normal phrase length but paraphasic, with phonemic or semantic word substitutions and neologisms; lesions posterior to central sulcus
           (a) **Wernicke aphasia:** poor comprehension, repetition, many paraphasias; lesion in posterior superior temporal gyrus (Wernicke area) usually accompanying right visual field defect
           (b) **Transcortical sensory aphasia:** repetition is relatively intact; lesions surround Wernicke area, that is, middle and inferior temporal gyri
           (c) **Conduction aphasia:** disproportionately poor repetition; lesion in arcuate fasciculus
           (d) **Anomic aphasia:** word finding problems, impaired naming, relatively intact comprehension and repetition; various localizations, including posterior association cortex; common residual aphasia
        iii. **Global aphasia:** combination of Broca and Wernicke with limited word output; from large perisylvian lesion
     b. **Acquired dyslexia:** two common subtypes are
        i. Pure alexia (without agraphia); lesion in visual association cortex and adjacent corpus callosum
        ii. Alexia with agraphia; usually occurs in context of an aphasia
     c. **Agraphia:** two common subtypes are
        i. Agraphia as part of an aphasic syndrome
        ii. Pure agraphia; various locations of lesions
  5. **Amnestic syndrome**
     a. Anterograde (short term) and, nearly always, some retrograde (long term) memory impairment; retrograde amnesia may show temporal gradient
     b. Lesion is in medial temporal lobe (hippocampal region, perirhinal, parahippocampal gyrus), amygdala, or diencephalon (mammillary bodies, medial dorsal nucleus of the thalamus); bilateral, if persistent
     c. Etiologies include: posterior circulation strokes, head injury, Wernicke-Korsakoff disease,

herpes simplex encephalitis, cerebral anoxia; transient global amnesia, sudden onset with preserved awareness, improves spontaneously, seldom recurs
6. **Apraxias:** inability to perform a learned movement despite normal comprehension and adequate motor function
   a. **Ideomotor apraxia:** worse pantomiming than imitating act; lesion in corpus callosum, left inferior parietal lobule or supplementary motor cortex, depending upon the pattern of deficit
   b. **"Ideational" apraxia:** trouble with complex sequence of actions; often not easily localized; usually associated with dementia
7. **Agnosia:** impaired ability to recognize objects despite intact elementary sensory perception; usually visual, with lesion in occipitotemporal visual association cortex
   a. **"Apperceptive":** visual discrimination and perception problem; cannot copy or match visual object
   b. **"Associative":** perception is normal but object is not recognized; can copy or match, but not name visual object
8. **Other high order visual deficits**
   a. **Balint syndrome:** several components, most salient is simultanagnosia, inability to attend to more than one part of the visual field at a time; right or bilateral occipitotemporal lesions
   b. **Prosopagnosia:** impaired recognition of faces; lesions in medial temporal or occipital cortexes; right hemisphere more than left, or bilateral
   c. **Visuospatial and constructional disorders:** usually demonstrated by difficulty copying drawings; likely the result of disruption in multiple visual, motor, attentional networks; either hemisphere, frontal or parietal lobes
9. **Frontal lobe and frontal lobe network syndromes:** pathology in frontal lobes and interconnected subcortical structures
   a. **Compartmental syndromes** (can be mixed; more obvious with bilateral disease)
      i. **Frontal disinhibition:** impulsive, poor judgment; orbito- and medial frontal cortex
      ii. **Frontal "abulia":** apathy, emotional blunting; dorsolateral frontal lesions
   b. **Cognitive slowing** ("subcortical dementia"); frontosubcortical connections
   c. **Disorders of "executive function":** inability to plan and successfully carry out complex activities

B. **Major neuropsychiatric syndromes** (excluding dementia)
   1. **Delirium:** see preceding text
   2. **Attention deficit/hyperactivity disorder:** maladaptive combination of inattention, hyperactivity, and impulsivity; usually appearing in childhood, boys more than girls; comorbid conditions include conduct and oppositional defiant disorders, learning disorders, pervasive developmental disorders, tics, and mood disorders
   3. **Reading and other learning disorders:** specific deficits in various academic cognitive skills (e.g., reading, mathematics, written expression) without general intellectual or neurologic impairment
   4. **Autism and pervasive developmental disorder**
      a. **Autism:** impaired social interaction and communication abilities, with restricted, repetitive, and stereotyped behaviors and interest
      b. **Rett disorder:** progressive development of autism in girls
      c. **Asperger syndrome:** milder form of autism
   5. **Substance abuse:** significant impairment and distress resulting from maladaptive pattern of substance use; manifested by preoccupation with and excessive use of agent, evidence of tolerance or withdrawal symptoms, inability to cut down use
   6. **Disorders of mood**
      a. **Clinical syndromes:** all must be sufficiently severe to impair function
         i. **Major depressive episode:** sadness and loss of pleasure, weight loss, sleep disturbance, loss of energy and interest, sense of worthlessness, difficulty concentrating, feelings of guilt, morbid thoughts, psychomotor retardation, suicidal ideation

ii. **Manic episode:** elevated, expansive, or irritable mood; sometimes, decreased sleep, over talkative, flight of ideas; grandiosity
iii. **Hypomanic episode:** less severe than manic episode
  b. **Specific mood disorders**
     i. **Unipolar** mood disorders
        (a) Major depressive disorder: depression symptoms in absence of mania; with or without delusions or hallucinations
        (b) Dysthymic disorder: less severe than major depression
     ii. **Bipolar** mood disorders
        (a) Depression alternating or mixed with mania or hypomania
        (b) Recurrent mania only
        (c) Cyclothymic disorder: less severe
  c. **Mood disorders associated with medical illness or medication**
7. **Anxiety disorders:** common syndromes include
  a. **Panic disorder with agoraphobia:** recurring panic attacks and fear of being in situation where attack may occur and escape is impossible
  b. **Panic disorder without agoraphobia**
  c. **Generalized anxiety disorder:** persistent anxiety and worry, often with somatic symptoms, for example, muscle tension, fatigue, sleep disturbance
  d. **Social phobia:** excessive fear of social or performance situations, often associated with avoidance and anxious anticipation
  e. **Specific phobia:** excessive fear of a specific object or situation
8. **Schizophrenia and related disorders:** hallucinations and delusions not easily attributed to medical condition or brain disease
  a. **Schizophrenia:** delusions (often bizarre) or hallucinations (usually well-formed) or both; thought disorder manifested by disorganized behavior and speech ("positive symptoms"); flattened affect and lack of social engagement ("negative symptoms")
  b. **Schizophreniform disorder:** 1 to 6 months of schizophrenic symptoms; some people question whether this is a distinct entity
  c. **Delusional disorder:** nonbizarre, encapsulated delusion (often persecutory) without other symptoms of schizophrenia
9. **Personality disorders:** patterns of inflexible and maladaptive personality traits that cause subjective distress and significant functional impairment; three clusters include
  a. **"Odd, eccentric":** paranoid (everyone is out to get them, often start law suits), schizoid (loners with no interest in having friends), schizotypal (bizarre beliefs and speech but not psychotic), avoidant (no friends but want them, inferiority complex)
  b. **"Dramatic, emotional, erratic":** borderline (unstable moods, behavior, relationships, people are all good or all bad), histrionic (overly dramatic, seductive, need to be the center of attention), narcissistic (egocentric, lack empathy, sense of entitlement), antisocial (long criminal records, tortured animals/set fires as children; pediatric conduct disorder required), lying (without remorse or conscience)
  c. **"Anxious, fearful: avoidant":** dependent (cannot be/do anything alone), obsessive-compulsive (cheap, stubborn, restricted affect, anal-retentive, not obsessive compulsive disorder)

C. **Neurologic conditions** (excluding dementias) with prominent behavioral and emotional symptoms
  1. **Stroke**
     a. Poststroke depression: common, severity varies, more likely after left sided and anterior lesions
     b. Pathologic laughing and crying; not always mood congruent; usually from bilateral disease, usually part of pseudobulbar palsy
  2. **Epilepsy**; behavioral problems mainly found in temporal lobe forms
     a. **Ictal** manifestations can include feelings of familiarity (déjà vu) or strangeness, fear, joy, obsessive thoughts, and symptoms of psychosis
     b. **Interictal** manifestations can include schizophreniform disorder, depression, and a particular type of personality disorder (Geschwind syndrome)

3. **Multiple sclerosis:** high incidence of depression, disproportionate to disability
4. **Traumatic brain injury:** behavioral and cognitive problems; severity varies
   a. Cognitive symptoms, for example, amnesia, aphasia
   b. Mood and behavior symptoms, for example, depression, agitation with aggression; personality changes
5. **Klüver-Bucy syndrome:** combination of placidity, hyperorality, hypersexuality, and hyperphagia can occur from bilateral temporal lesions that affect bilateral hippocampi, medial temporal lobe but spare the amygdaloid nuclei; can also rarely occur from a variety of diseases or dementias
6. **Movement disorders**
   a. **Parkinson disease** and related disorders
      i. Dementia in 40% (mainly elderly); depression in 40% to 50%
      ii. Hallucinations, from, for example, Lewy body disease, or from medications
   b. **Huntington disease:** depression, suicidal thoughts, personality disorder; may precede chorea and formal diagnosis; cognitive impairment
   c. **Tic disorder:** often comorbid obsessive-compulsive or attention deficit

III. Treatment of Neuropsychiatric Disorders (except Cognitive Impairment)

A. **Nonpharmacologic treatments**
   1. **Psychotherapies:** helpful in all patients with reasonably intact cognitive function
   2. **Behavioral and cognitive therapy:** especially for panic disorder and phobias; also helps in other anxiety disorders and depression
   3. **Speech and occupational therapies:** speech therapy for aphasias and other language-related symptoms; occupational therapy can be helpful for higher order visual and motor abnormalities
   4. **Electroconvulsive therapy:** reserved for severe, medication resistant depression, imminent danger of suicide

B. **Pharmacologic treatments**
   1. **Antidepressants:** used for depressed mood, anxiety, panic disorder, obsessive-compulsive disorder, social and other phobias; start with monotherapy; if this is unsuccessful, consider combining two antidepressants with different mechanisms of action, for example, a selective serotonin reuptake inhibitor and a serotonin 2A antagonist antidepressant; may also supplement with anxiolytic or hypnotic; a patient with bipolar disease, misdiagnosed as unipolar depression, may be worsened by antidepressants
      a. Monoamine oxidase (MAO) inhibitors: for example, phenelzine, tranylcypromine, isocarboxazid—block enzyme that destroys monoamine neurotransmitters; significant side effects, used only as second-line agents
      b. Tricyclic antidepressants, for example, imipramine, amitriptyline, nortriptyline, block reuptake pump of serotonin, norepinephrine, and dopamine; block muscarinic cholinergic receptors, H1 histamine receptors, and alpha-1 adrenergic receptors; also used for nonpsychiatric conditions, for example, chronic pain, bladder disturbances
      c. Selective serotonin reuptake inhibitors, for example, fluoxetine, sertraline, paroxetine, fluvoxamine, citalopram, escitalopram; start at maintenance dose, onset of response generally delayed
      d. Norepinephrine and dopamine reuptake inhibitors, for example, bupropion
      e. Dual serotonin and noradrenergic reuptake inhibitors, for example, venlafaxine, duloxetine
      f. Drugs with dual serotonin and norepinephrine actions via alpha 2 antagonism, for example, mirtazapine
      g. Dual serotonin 2A antagonists/serotonin reuptake inhibitors, for example, nefazodone, trazodone

2. **Anxiolytics and sedative-hypnotics:** for generalized anxiety and anxiety subtypes and insomnia; may also be helpful for depression
   a. Serotonergic anxiolytic, for example, buspirone
   b. Noradrenergic anxiolytics, for example, clonidine
   c. Benzodiazepines, for example, alprazolam, clonazepam, diazepam, chlordiazepoxide, lorazepam, oxazepam, temazepam, flurazepam; effect is on γ-aminobutyric acid (GABA) receptors; also helpful for sleep
   d. Barbiturates
3. **Antipsychotics:** used for schizophrenias, delusional disorder, unipolar and bipolar mood disease, behavioral disturbances associated with dementia; may be combined with mood-stabilizing drugs
   a. Conventional antipsychotics, for example, chlorpromazine, clozapine, fluphenazine, haloperidol, loxapine, perphenazine, thioridazine, thiothixene, trifluoperazine; block dopamine 2 receptors and other actions; numerous side effects including extrapyramidal symptoms such as akathisia, parkinsonism, tardive dyskinesia, and neuroleptic malignant syndrome due to effect on nigrostriatal pathway
   b. Atypical, for example, risperidone, olanzapine, quetiapine, ziprasidone, aripiprazole; serotonin-dopamine antagonists that work differently in nigrostriatal, mesocortical, and tuberoinfundibular pathways; fewer side effects
4. **Mood stabilizing drugs:** used in major mood disorders, acutely and for maintenance; frequently combined with antipsychotics
   a. Lithium: action probably occurs beyond the receptor; can cause tremor
   b. Anticonvulsants, for example, valproic acid, lamotrigine, carbamazepine; effect on ion channels may influence GABA activity

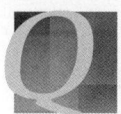 STUDY QUESTIONS FOR CHAPTER 25

Directions: *Each of the numbered items or incomplete statements in this section is followed by answers or by completions of the statement. Select the ONE lettered answer or completion that is BEST in each case.*

1. A patient presents with halting speech, consisting of only short and grammatically simple phrases. Comprehension is relatively intact but there is some problem naming objects. The patient can, however, repeat a few test phrases and when the examiner begins reciting the Pledge of Allegiance, the patient completes the recitation flawlessly. Minimal, if any, right-sided weakness is present. Which of the following aphasia type/localization combinations is the most likely diagnosis and anatomic correlation?

   (A) Anomic aphasia; lesion in posterior association cortex
   (B) Broca aphasia, lesion dorsolateral frontal lobe and frontal operculum
   (C) Transcortical sensory aphasia, lesion middle and inferior temporal gyri
   (D) Transcortical motor aphasia, lesion caudate nucleus and surrounding white matter of internal capsule
   (E) Transcortical motor aphasia, lesion dorsolateral frontal lobe sparing frontal operculum

2. A patient presents with severe depression. There is no history of manic episodes. The patient is resistant to initial treatment with an SSRI antidepressant, even becoming somewhat worse. What is the next best pharmacotherapeutic maneuver?

   (A) Switch to using another SSRI
   (B) Add another SSRI
   (C) Add a benzodiazepine
   (D) Add an atypical antipsychotic
   (E) Switch to a dual serotonin and noradrenergic reuptake inhibitor

3. A 72-year-old man is brought to the emergency room by his family because of "confusion" and visual hallucinations. Earlier in life he had had several admissions to a psychiatric hospital for schizophrenia but he has been living at home for at least 15 years. He takes care of all of his own basic activities of daily living but does not drive, do his finances, or perform any household chores. He is treated currently with a low dose of an atypical antipsychotic; he may have been on a conventional antipsychotic in the past. He is also being treated for diabetes, hypertension, and gout. On examination he is alert but disoriented with impaired attention and short-term memory. The patient may be hallucinating. He has a mild tremor and some increased tone at both wrists. CT scan shows cortical atrophy with white matter changes. He has a few minor metabolic abnormalities revealed by biochemistry. What is the most likely diagnosis?

   (A) Dementia of the Alzheimer type with behavioral and psychiatric symptoms
   (B) Delirium
   (C) Exacerbation of schizophrenia
   (D) Lewy body disease
   (E) Neuroleptic malignant syndrome

4. After a motorcycle-related head injury, a 23-year-old man becomes disinhibited, impulsive, and aggressive, requiring 24-hour care and physical restraint. What is the most likely localization of the lesion that is producing this behavior?

   (A) Dorsolateral frontal lobes
   (B) Orbitofrontal cortex
   (C) Dorsomedial frontal lobes
   (D) Parietal lobes
   (E) Medial temporal lobes

5. A 32-year-old woman is being treated for depression. Which of the following antidepressants works by noradrenergic reuptake inhibition in addition to serotonin reuptake inhibition?

   (A) Bupropion
   (B) Nefazodone
   (C) Nortriptyline
   (D) Sertraline
   (E) Venlafaxine

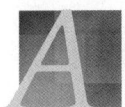# ANSWERS AND EXPLANATIONS

1. E. Transcortical motor aphasia because, despite basically nonfluent speech, repetition is relatively preserved, suggesting sparing of the frontal operculum; intact repetition excludes answer (B) (Broca aphasia), where the lesion involves the frontal operculum and repetition is impaired. Although patients with transcortical sensory aphasia (C) also have intact repetition, they have impaired comprehension, which was not the case with this patient. Patients with anomic aphasia (A), a residual category, would be expected to have fluent, not nonfluent, speech. The form of transcortical motor aphasia caused by a caudate nucleus/internal capsule lesion (D) is excluded by the absence of motor signs. The border zone of internal carotid perfuses the region causing transcortical sensory and motor aphasia. These deficits indicate need for carotid angiogram.

2. D. Although many possible drug-treatment scenarios are possible, worsening after using an antidepressant, with an agitated response, often suggests that the underlying diagnosis might actually be bipolar disease even without a history of manic episodes. Trying another SSRI (A) might not be effective; adding another SSRI (B) or an antidepressant drug with dual serotonin and noradrenergic properties (E) might further worsen the situation. The addition of a benzodiazepine (C) might improve anxiety or sleep problems but have no effect on depression. The best solution (D) would be to add an atypical antipsychotic or mood stabilizing drug.

3. B. Patient has inattention and visual hallucinations, more consistent with delirium than exacerbation of psychosis (C). In the absence of clear-cut history of dementia (patient's life style could be consequence of schizophrenia or medical conditions rather than evidence of dementia), presence of inattention precludes concomitant diagnosis of dementia, including Alzheimer disease (A). Motor findings are compatible with delirium or nonspecific and not enough to diagnose Lewy body disease (D) or neuroleptic malignant syndrome (E) (and patient is currently on an atypical antipsychotic, which is much less likely to cause the syndrome).

4. B. The lesion that produces disinhibited, impulsive, and aggressive behavior is located in the orbitofrontal cortex. Dorsolateral frontal lobes produce problems with working memory, whereas dorsomedial lesions produce abulia. Parietal lobes would not be expected to produce the problems that this patient has; rather, they could produce sensory deficits, apraxia, or neglect. Medial temporal lobe lesions are associated with amnesia but not disinhibited or aggressive behavior.

5. E. Venlafaxine is a serotonin and noradrenergic reuptake inhibitor. Bupropion is a norepinephrine and dopamine reuptake inhibitor. Nefazodone is a dual serotonin 2A antagonist and serotonin reuptake inhibitor. Nortriptyline works as a reuptake inhibitor for serotonin, norepinephrine, and dopamine. Sertraline is a selective serotonin reuptake inhibitor.

Vertigo and Dizziness

I. Anatomy and Physiology of Vertigo

A. Definitions
1. The visual, vestibular, cerebellar, and somatosensory systems contribute to feeling of balance. Mismatched information from these systems leads to sensation of **vertigo**—defined as delusion of a motion. The patient reports a sensation of motion—for example, the environment is spinning or patient is spinning around.
2. **Dizziness** is a general term. Patients can use it to mean the following:
   a. Vertigo—spinning; need to distinguish between vestibular peripheral, peripheral nerve, and central dysfunction
   b. Dysequilibrium—cerebellar
   c. Lightheadedness—presyncopal
   d. Vague symptoms—"big head" or psychiatric (part of panic/anxiety)

B. The sensation of vertigo may be caused by activation of the vestibular system from the periphery (vestibular apparatus) to the central connection (temporal cortex). This triggers the vestibuloocular (causes nystagmus), vestibulospinal (causes ataxia), and vestibuloautonomic (causes vomiting via the medullary vomiting center) reflexes.

C. Useful tests for diagnosing cause
1. Spin patient around with eyes closed, and then stop; this simulates sensation of vertigo.
2. Cold and warm caloric testing (COWS—cold opposite, warm same—the fast phase of nystagmus beats toward normally warm stimulus—absent/defective ipsilaterally in vestibular disease
3. Have patient focus on examiner's nose and rapidly move the head. The development of saccades and indicates peripheral vestibular dysfunction (head thrust test).
4. Hallpike and Barany maneuver: Move the patient from sitting to lying with the head back 30 degrees off table and turned to the side 30 to 45 degrees. When the pathologic ear is turned toward the floor, nystagmus is induced.
5. Have patient squat for several minutes, then stand: simulates the sensation of presyncope
6. Hyperventilation for several minutes: simulates the sensation of "lightheadedness"

D. Look for systemic causes including hypertension (HTN), chronic obstructive pulmonary disease (COPD), endocrine disorders (hypoglycemia, hyperglycemia, thyroid disease), upper respiratory infection (URI), sinusitis, drugs, medications, alcohol, psychiatric disorder.

II. Vertigo

A. The false sensation of one's person or the environment moving (often rotating). There is concurrent nystagmus. Generally there is nausea, vomiting, and difficulty walking, possibly with feeling of being pulled or thrown to the ground. If horizontal semicircular canals are affected, the patient experiences spinning around the environment; if vertical canals are affected, the patient experiences rocking up and down as on rough seas.

B. Peripheral vestibular disease: nausea, vomiting common, but no other brainstem findings; nystagmus is unidirectional horizontal or rotatory with the slow phase toward the side of the lesion; there is past pointing and the gait falls toward the lesion; symptoms and nystagmus may improve or resolve with being stationary, visual fixation, looking toward the lesion, and with time (as central compensation occurs); caloric testing shows vestibular paresis (impaired caloric testing without associated vertigo); positive head thrust test

1. **Benign paroxysmal positional vertigo**
   a. Common cause of episodic vertigo that lasts for seconds and recurs over months
   b. Turning the head quickly, for example, rolling over in bed, may precipitate symptoms.
   c. Nystagmus is inducible with Hallpike maneuver, has a latency of a few seconds, fatigues with repetition, and worsens with looking contralateral to the lesion.
   d. Generally idiopathic, injury to temporal bone or viral labyrinthitis possible; origin otolith debris in endolymph, usually in posterior semicircular canal; differentiate from lightheadedness due to postural hypotension, which also occurs with change in position
   e. Treatment: most spontaneously resolve; however, the canalith repositioning [Epley] procedure reduces symptoms in most; the Hallpike maneuver is performed, inducing symptoms; then, the head is turned to opposite side at 45 degrees; the body is then rotated to same side and head turned another 45 degrees; head is rotated final time so patient is looking toward the floor; the patient then sits up and must stay vertical for 24 hours

2. **Acute peripheral vestibulopathy/acute labyrinthitis/vestibular neuritis**
   a. Single bout of (often rotatory) vertigo that gradually subsides over days to weeks
   b. Often with preceding URI; may be caused by a virus such as herpes simplex type 1
   c. Treatment: symptomatically in the acute period with antihistamines or scopolamine; some evidence exists for use of steroids and/or acyclovir

3. **Ménière disease**
   a. Acute, limited (minutes to hours) episodes of severe vertigo, low-frequency hearing loss (speech discrimination intact), tinnitus, and a feeling of fullness in the ear; some patients have falling attacks; with increased attacks comes increased sensorineural deafness; episodes stop when the patient is completely deaf in the pathologic ear
   b. Horizontal nystagmus (slow phase toward affected ear) ± rotatory component
   c. May be due to an increase in endolymph and stretching of this system
   d. Tullio's phenomenon: increased vertigo with loud noises
   e. Treatment: bed rest, antihistamines, scopolamine, and antiemetics; for refractory cases, endolymphatic–subarachnoid shunt, surgical sectioning of vestibular portion of cranial nerve (CN) VIII, transtympanic gentamicin, or ablation of labyrinth (when completely deaf); some utilize diuretics

4. **Acoustic neuroma:** tumor of the vestibular portion of CN VIII
   a. Loss of high-pitched hearing (sensorineural deafness with diminished speech discrimination patient complaints often difficulty understanding speech in a loud room or talking on telephone) followed by vertigo
   b. Palsies of CN V or CN VII, ipsilateral ataxia, headache, or signs of increased intracranial pressure (ICP) may also be present, with tumor expansion into the cerebellopontine angle
   c. Other pathology of the petrous bone or cerebellopontine angle may mimic this
   d. Diagnosis: magnetic resonance imaging (MRI) with gadolinium, brainstem auditory evoked response (BAER), lengthening or loss of expected peaks
   e. Totally intracanalicular tumor may have only acoustic and vestibular signs. Imaging shows enlarged internal acoustic meatus.

5. **Bilateral vestibular failure**
   a. Causes include ototoxic drugs such as aminoglycosides, meningitis, autoimmune disorders, neuropathy, and cerebellar degeneration
   b. Oscillopsia with head movement and gait instability (especially without visual cues); no symptoms if stationary; caloric and vestibuloocular reflexes are absent

6. **Other peripheral causes:** purulent labyrinthitis as a complication of otitis media or meningitis; drug (alcohol, aspirin) intoxication; motion sickness (physiologic vertigo); head trauma, concussion, or whiplash (without hearing loss, improves over days to weeks); temporal bone fractures (may have hearing loss); and chronic vestibular imbalance (destruction of labyrinthine branch of internal auditory artery). If vertigo does not have identified etiology and does not respond to therapy, refer to ENT as endolymph fistula; may require surgery.

C. **Central vestibular disorders:** 2% of vertigo complaints; involves vestibular nuclei or connecting tracts; nystagmus may be any direction including vertical, and it is exacerbated by visual fixation and looking to ipsilateral side; on Hallpike maneuver, nystagmus has no latency period, occurs for more than a few seconds, does not fatigue with repetition; dysequilibrium may be seen, with gait falling to ipsilateral side; other brainstem, cranial nerve signs common; hearing usually normal; diagnosis of etiology necessitates computed tomography (CT), MRI, and/or BAER; for symptomatic relief, benzodiazepines
   1. **Localization of lesions** by the direction of nystagmus
      a. **Horizontal:** unilateral vestibular nuclei (pontomedullary area)
      b. **Vertical:** bilateral involvement; if upbeat, then medulla or pontomesencephalon [as in medial longitudinal fasciculus (MLF)]; if downbeat, then flocculus or commissural fibers (that connect the vestibular nuclei); also seen with metabolic etiologies or ingestions
      c. **Rotatory:** contralateral pontomesencephalon or ipsilateral pontomedullary region
   2. **Posterior circulation vascular:** Wallenberg syndrome is due to ischemia of the medial branch of the posterior inferior cerebellar artery (PICA), which supplies the lateral medulla and cerebellum; vertigo occurring as isolated symptom does *not* represent verebro-basilar
      a. Bi-directional horizontal nystagmus and dysequilibrium
      b. Common focal neurologic findings include vertigo, limb ataxia, past pointing, deficits of pain and temperature sensation on the ipsilateral face and contralateral body, Horner syndrome, dysphagia, and dysarthria.
      c. Sudden dizziness with or without hearing loss is internal auditory artery occlusion
   3. **Multiple sclerosis:** never seen with dizziness alone
   4. **Basilar artery migraine:** vertigo often occurs before the onset of headache.
   5. **Cerebellar pathology:** with acute problems such as hemorrhage or viral infection
   6. **Seizures:** activation of the posterior superior temporal lobe may cause vertigo or dysequilibrium. Vertigo may be seen in pure vertiginous epilepsy (rare), as an aura, or in temporal lobe epilepsy (along with hallucinations, aphasia, and visual changes).
   7. **Familial vestibulocerebellar syndrome:** attacks of vertigo and truncal dysequilibrium, often induced by exertion or strong emotion; treat with acetazolamide

III. Presyncope or Syncope

A. **The (usually sudden) sensation of being about to faint,** with or without actual loss of consciousness; the patient may also have dimmed vision, scotomas, and weakness

B. **Etiology** is decreased cerebral blood flow due to decreased blood pressure and/or bradycardia; causes include orthostatic hypotension [remember gastrointestinal (GI) bleeding, anemia, infection], arrhythmias, increased vagal tone (micturition syncope, carotid sinus hypersensitivity), aortic stenosis, or myocardial infarction

C. **Diagnosis:** electrocardiogram (ECG), arrhythmia (Holter) monitoring, transthoracic echocardiogram (TTE), orthostatics, and cardiology consult

D. **Convulsive syncope:** asymmetric myoclonic jerks and incontinence may be present, but there is no postictal-like state. Antiepileptic drugs are not indicated—they can worsen symptoms. Remember that 5–10% of normal and syncope population have nonspecific EEG abnormalities; therefore, syncope + EEG does not equate to epilepsy.

E. **Neurocardiogenic syncope:** decreased preload leads to an abnormally high increase in sympathetic C fiber activation, which inappropriately increases vagal tone. Diagnose with a tilt-table test. Treat with β-blockers, midodrine, or selective serotonin reuptake inhibitors (SSRIs).

IV. Dysequilibrium

A. **The sensation of being unbalanced,** often felt in the trunk and limbs and not in the head; may be worse with standing or ambulation and better with sitting or lying down; tends to be constant rather than episodic; often seen in the elderly

B. **Multiple sensory deficits** may lead to disorientation. The sensation of imbalance is worse when walking and turning, although the patient is not ataxic.
  1. Deficits include those that are visual, neuropathic, or vestibular, or cervical spondylosis.
  2. Treatment: increase sensory cues: lighting, walkers, glasses, cataract removal, hearing aids
  3. Rapid vision correction (cataract removal or new glasses) may also cause dizziness

C. **Motor deficits also contribute**; examples include orthopedic disorders, gait impairment, cerebellar dysfunction, and neuromuscular diseases

V. Other

Other, including lightheadedness and giddiness: any other sensation like floating, swimming, dissociation, patient may say it is hard to describe; symptoms often continuous or chronic; if symptoms occur in the same situation or location, consider anxiety, panic attacks

A. **Lightheadedness:** often consistent with the feeling one has after hyperventilation
  1. Associated with paresthesias, classically circumoral or digital, and pain
  2. Often with comorbid anxiety or depression; consider panic attack if there is also shortness of breath, palpitations, fear of another attack, and no focal neurologic signs
  3. Treatment: anxiolytics, antidepressants

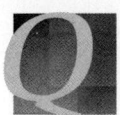 STUDY QUESTIONS FOR CHAPTER 26

Directions: Each of the numbered items or incomplete statements in this section is followed by answers or by completions of the statement. Select the ONE lettered answer or completion that is BEST in each case.

1. Which finding is not consistent with Wallenberg syndrome?
 (A) Dysarthria
 (B) Nystagmus
 (C) Loss of 2-point discrimination, vibration sense, proprioception on contralateral body
 (D) Loss of pain and temperature on ipsilateral face
 (E) Horner syndrome

2. A 20-year-old college student presents with 2 days of dizziness, nausea, and vomiting. He describes his dizziness as "spinning," continuous, worse on moving but not with any particular movement. He has not been able to go to class due to the severity of his symptoms. He has not fainted and does not have a headache, difficulty hearing, or vision changes. He had "a cold" about one week ago. On examination, he appears diaphoretic but has normal vital signs. His mucous membranes are moist. He has unidirectional horizontal nystagmus with the slow phase to the left, and ataxia with gait pulling to the left. The remainder of his neurologic examination, including ophthalmologic examination, is normal. What is the most appropriate next step at this time?
 (A) Obtain a CT of the head
 (B) Fluid resuscitation with normal saline
 (C) Obtain an ECG and transthoracic echocardiogram
 (D) Perform canalith repositioning maneuver
 (E) Prescribe a short course of scopolamine

3. During the course of evaluating a 79-year-old man with vertigo, you perform a Dix-Hallpike maneuver. Which of the following responses during the performance of this maneuver is suggestive of central rather than peripheral origin of his symptoms?
 (A) Latency of nystagmus of greater than a few seconds
 (B) Lack of fatigue with repetition
 (C) Production of nausea and vomiting
 (D) Nystagmus that predominates in one direction and disappears in the opposite direction
 (E) An upbeat torsional waveform

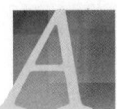# ANSWERS AND EXPLANATIONS

1. C. Wallenberg syndrome results from ischemia of dorsolateral branch of the posterior inferior cerebellar artery, causing damage to the lateral medulla and cerebellum. Answer C is not part of this syndrome because loss of 2-point discrimination, vibration, and proprioception is due to involvement of the dorsal-column-medial lemniscus system. At the level of the medulla, the medial lemniscus is *medial*, and therefore not affected occlusion of the arteries supplying the lateral medulla. However, there may be loss of pain and temperature sensation on the contralateral body from involvement of the spinothalamic tract.

2. E. His age (young adult) and history of a preceding upper respiratory infection (URI) are classic for acute labyrinthitis. He should be treated symptomatically with antihistamines or scopolamine, as the symptoms tend to be disabling. His symptoms should resolve over the next several days. Imaging of the brain is not indicated at this time. Fluid resuscitation would be appropriate if the patient were hypotensive or orthostatic. An EKG and TTE are part of the workup for syncope, which this patient does not describe. The canalith repositioning maneuver is indicated for benign paroxysmal positional vertigo. This patient describes continuous vertigo that is not related to position, making benign paroxysmal positional vertigo less likely.

3. B. The characteristics of nystagmus on Dix-Hallpike maneuver produced by a central nervous system lesion include short latency, lack of fatigue with repetition, change in direction of the nystagmus, and nystagmus that lasts longer than a minute. Nausea and vomiting do not distinguish central from peripheral nystagmus. Upbeat torsional nystagmus is the classic waveform seen in patients with benign paroxysmal positional vertigo.

Autonomic Nervous System and Hypothalamus

I. Autonomic Nervous System

A. Autonomic neuropathies: complete autonomic paralysis (dysautonomic polyneuropathy, pure pandysautonomia); *presentation/diagnosis:* onset one to several weeks, develop combination of anhidrosis, orthostatic hypotension, loss of pupillary reflex, loss of lacrimation/salivation, impotence, impaired bowel/bladder, flushing/heat intolerance; usually severe fatigue; due to lymphocytic infiltrate in autonomic nerves; cerebrospinal fluid (CSF) normal or mildly increased; *treatment:* none; usually recover within several months to baseline; amyloid and diabetic neuropathy most likely etiologies
  1. **Paraneoplastic form**, and rarely after Epstein-Barr virus (EBV), HIV, rubella, herpes zoster, or vaccinations

B. Riley-Day syndrome (autonomic neuropathy in infants and children): familial autosomal-recessive (AR) disease; presents with postural hypotension, poor temperature regulation, decreased hearing, hyperhydrosis, blotchy skin, pain insensitivity, emotional lability, vomiting

II. Orthostatic Hypotension due to Autonomic Causes

A. Orthostatic hypotension: rapid decrease in blood pressure upon standing without compensatory tachycardia; may be cardiovascular or due to impaired autonomic reflex; *causes:*
  1. **Idiopathic orthostatic hypotension**: can be peripheral (degenerative; dysfunction of postganglionic sympathetic neurons) or central (damage to cerebellum/basal ganglia; associated with Parkinson disease)
  2. **Secondary to peripheral neuropathy:** impaired autonomics due to damaged to baroreceptors and sympathetic fibers in spinal nerves; occurs commonly with neuropathy of Guillain Barré syndrome (GBS), alcoholic/nutritional, porphyric, diabetic, amyloid
  3. **Secondary to aging:** due to loss of sensory ganglion cells; treatment: physical maneuvers (standing slowly, sleep with head elevated, tensing and crossing legs while standing), support stockings, increase sodium and water intake; fludrocortisone, sympathomimetic agents

III. Horner Syndrome

Presentation/diagnosis: miosis, drooping eyelid, enophthalmos, unilateral sweating of face; caused by interruption of sympathetics; *common causes:* cervical lymph node mass, surgical trauma, carotid artery dissection, brachial plexus neoplasm/trauma, lateral medullary infarct (Wallenberg), idiopathic hereditary variant

A. **Heterochromia:** iris on lesion side does not pigment if Horner occurs early in development; looks blue/gray

B. **Lesion of stellate ganglion:** presents as Horner with loss of sympathetic innervation to arm

IV. Autonomic Dysfunction with Spinal Cord Lesions

Note: Lesions above T6—patients lose sympathetic and sacral parasympathetics; lesions below T6—sympathetic remains intact, lose descending sacral parasympathetic; spinal shock and mass reflex, see Chapter 9

A. **Sympathetic storm** (acute autonomic crisis): *presentation/diagnosis:* acute overexcitation of ANS can cause severe hypertension, mydriasis, seizure, ST-T wave abnormalities; *causes:* cocaine/PCP, tricyclic antidepressant (TCA) overdose (with ventricular arrhythmia) tetanus, severe head trauma, cerebral hemorrhage; *treatment:* β-blockers
   1. **Cushing response:** triad of hypertension, bradycardia, and change in breathing pattern after brainstem distortion

B. **Raynaud syndrome:** *presentation/diagnosis:* digital artery spasm causing episodic painful blanching of fingers; usually in cold temperatures or during emotional stress; hands turn red with rewarming; *cause:* patients may have systemic disease (i.e., connective tissue disorder) or local trauma (usually vibratory injury); also arterial disease, ergots, β-blockers, cold agglutinins; treatment: prevention of exposure to stimuli

V. Bladder Dysfunction

A. **Interruption of sensory afferents from bladder** (tabes dorsalis), and cord destruction below T12: paralyzed bladder (no sensation or control); bladder distends, overflow incontinence occurs; patients "control" urination by Credé maneuver of abdominal compression/straining; disease of sacral motor neurons same but sensation is retained

B. **Interruption of afferent and efferent innervation** (diabetes mellitus, cauda equina compression): flaccid bladder

C. **Upper spinal cord lesions:** reflex neurogenic (spastic) bladder (micturition and incontinence with decreased bladder capacity)

D. **Mixed type neurogenic bladder** (due to lesions at multiple levels; found in multiple sclerosis, subacute combined degeneration, syphilitic meningomyelitis): combined sensory/motor/spastic types; *treatment:* flaccid—bethanechol; spastic-propantheline, oxybutynin; self-catheterization

VI. Bowel Problems

A. **Bowel ileus:** common in spinal shock, reflex neurogenic colon, Guillain Barré (GBS); treatment; cisapride

B. **Congenital megacolon (Hirschsprung disease):** *presentation/diagnosis:* male infants/children; absence of ganglion cells in myenteric plexus; no relaxation of bowel; no peristaltic waves; high mortality from endocarditis; *treatment:* surgical excision

VII. Sexual Function Disorders

A. Impotence: *presentation/diagnosis:* inability to attain/sustain erection; causes: depressive state most common (patients still have nocturnal erections); prostatectomy, sacral cord disease (tumors, tabes, diabetes mellitus); treatment: phosphodiesterase inhibition

VIII. Respiration

A. Ondine curse: *presentation/diagnosis:* loss of automatic respiration during sleep with preserved voluntary breathing; *causes:* brainstem infarcts, hemorrhage, encephalitis, Leigh syndrome; treatment: mechanical ventilation at night
  1. **Idiopathic form** (congenital central hypoventilation syndrome) begins in infancy with apnea/sleep disturbances

B. Hyperventilation: anxiety states or with many diverse widespread lesions

C. Hiccup: poorly understood mechanism; occurs often in patients with brain lesions; treatment: none; sometimes phenothiazines

IX. Swallowing

A. **Both voluntary and reflexive**; defects occur in the following:
  1. **Initiation of swallowing:** weakness of tongue (myasthenia, motor neuron disease), CN XII palsy (metastasis to base of skull)
  2. **Nasal regurgitation of liquids due to failure of velopalatine closure:** with myasthenia, CN X palsy, bulbar/pseudobulbar palsy; usually nasal speech with air escaping from nose
  3. **Aspiration due to muscle weakness:** with vagus lesion, myopathy, motor neuron disease [amyotrophic lateral sclerosis (ALS), myasthenia gravis], medullary lesion; also occurs with diseases of corticospinal (hemispherical stroke) or basal ganglia (Parkinson disease); can alter timing of swallowing/breathing and lead to decreased swallowing causing pooling of saliva; high aspiration risk; most severe in initial poststroke phase; diagnosis: bedside observation; video fluoroscopy; treatment: speech therapy for recommendations about diet, postural adjustments, possible need for tracheostomy or feeding tube

X. Global Hypothalamic Syndromes

Signs of reduced pituitary function plus diabetes insipidus: caused by many lesions including sarcoid granulomatous disease, idiopathic inflammatory disease, germ cell tumors; sarcoid—sometimes primary manifestation occurs in hypothalamus; also causes facial palsy, hilar lymphadenopathy; diagnosis: increased angiotensin-converting factor, especially in cerebrospinal fluid (CSF); magnetic resonance imaging (MRI)

XI. Partial Hypothalamic Syndromes

A. Diabetes insipidus: *presentation:* polyuria, decreased blood volume, and polydipsia; *causes:* central—lack of antidiuretic hormone (ADH) due to lesion on neurohypophysis, or acquired diabetes insipidus through brain masses, head injury, intracranial surgical trauma, granulomatous; or nephrogenic—resistant renal tubular epithelium; congenital or associated with lithium toxicity; *diagnosis:* low urine osmolality and specific gravity with high serum sodium and osmolality; vasopressin injection can distinguish between neurogenic and nephrogenic diabetes insipidus; *must* *rule out osmotic dehydration secondary to diabetes mellitus or glucosuria; treatment:* central—desmopressin; nephrogenic—thiazide diuretics, nonsteroidal anti-inflammatory drugs (NSAIDs), low salt/low protein diet; patients with partial ADH function can take chlorpropamide, clofibrate, or carbamazepine to stimulate ADH release

B. **Syndrome of inappropriate ADH secretion (SIADH):** *presentation/diagnosis:* increased urine osmolality, low serum sodium and osmolality; resultant hyponatremia causes confusion, cramping, weakness, and seizures; *cause:* usually transient feature of underlying illness; also: cerebral lesions and local hypothalamic disease, subarachnoid hemorrhage; GBS, ventilatory patients; medications: chlorpropamide, clofibrate, carbamazepine, NSAIDs, vincristine; *treatment:* correct sodium by restricting water intake to 400 to 800 mL/day; if sodium is <115 mEq/L or drowsiness/confusion/seizure occur, then infuse isotonic or 3% NaCl over 3 to 4 hours with furosemide (Lasix); raise <12 mEq/L in first 24 hours and no more than 20 mEq/L in 48 hours or risk cerebral pontine myelinosis
  1. **Neurogenic (cerebral) salt wasting:** often combined with SIADH; common in patients with acute intracranial disease including SAH, and status post neurosurgery; must determine intravascular volume and urine sodium before treating

C. **Precocious puberty:** *presentation/diagnosis*: early-onset secretion of sex hormones; premature development of secondary sexual characteristics as well as spermatogenesis or cyclic ovarian secretion; can be central (pituitary) or due to exogenous steroid production; *causes*: von Recklinghausen disease, teratoma of pineal gland, hormone secreting tumor; *diagnosis:* serum luteinizing hormone (LH) [basal and post gonadotropin-releasing hormone (GnRH) challenge] increase in gonad-dependent precocious puberty; need CT/MRI of hypothalamus, ovaries, adrenals; *treatment*: central-GnRH analogs to suppress pituitary-gonadal feedback; some give with growth hormone (GH); exogenous—specific to cause

D. **Hypothalamic disease associated with weight alterations:** satiety center in ventromedial nuclei and appetite center in ventrolateral nuclei of hypothalamus; lesions in either can affect eating/growth; causes tumors, trauma, inflammatory disease, hydrocephalus
  1. **Rare:** diencephalic syndrome in infants: failure to thrive despite normal food intake in alert/cheerful infant; caused by astrocytoma of anterior hypothalamus or optic nerve

E. **Abnormalities of growth:** retardation can be deficiency of GnRH or GH if severe, but healthy unusually short children are likely familial with no hormone defect; controversial use of GH shows spurt during first year, but long-term effects not studied

F. **Gigantism:** increased GH before epiphysial closure; usually secondary secreting pituitary adenoma (increased GH after closure causes acromegaly)

G. **Disorders of temperature regulation**
  1. **Hyperthermia:** *presentation/diagnosis:* anterior hypothalamic lesions impair heat dissipating mechanisms (vasodilation, sweating); temperature rises to ≥41°C until death or recovery; *causes*: rupture of anterior communicating artery, any trauma/surgery to third ventricle; *diagnosis:* sedation, cooling by evaporation; medications ineffective
  2. **Malignant hyperthermia:** *presentation/diagnosis:* autosomal dominant, inherited susceptibility to develop hyperthermia (1 to 2°C per 5 minutes) and muscle rigidity in response to inhaled anesthetics and succinylcholine; *treatment:* dantrolene; premonitory symptom: trismus/masseter spasm, next symptom hypercapnia
     a. **Neuroleptic malignant syndrome:** similar to malignant hyperthermia; occurs with neuroleptics; treat with dantrolene and/or bromocriptine
  3. **Hypothermia:** *presentation/diagnosis:* posterior hypothalamic lesion leads to hypothermia (<35°C) or poikilothermia (equilibrium of body temperature to environmental temperature); associated confusion, somnolence, hypotension; *treatment:* rewarming
  4. **Spontaneous periodic hypothermia:** associated with third ventricle or corpus callosum disturbances; random attacks lasting minutes to hours; temperature as low as 30°C with

autonomic disturbances (nausea/vomiting/sweating/salivation)

5. **Chronic hypothermia:** occurs with hypothyroidism, hypoglycemia, uremia; intoxication with barbiturates/phenothiazines/alcohol; also in elderly

H. Cushing syndrome: *presentation* includes truncal obesity, hypertension, baldness, extremity skin mottling, osteoporosis, and purplish cutaneous striae; happens with adrenal hyperplasia secondary to pituitary adenoma (increased ACTH), primary adrenal tumor (increased cortisol), ACTH-producing tumor, prolonged glucocorticoid administration

I. Cushing disease: *presentation*: basophil adenoma produces ACTH or corticotropin, stimulates adrenals; *diagnosis*: 24-hour urine cortisol secretion; low or high dose dexamethasone suppression testing; MRI or high resolution CT can be used to visualize tumor; usually microadenoma and sella is not enlarged; *treatment:* transsphenoidal microsurgery if microadenoma can be visualized; or pituitary irradiation if tumor not found or fertility a concern; last option: adrenalectomy—medical or surgical, which requires extensive hormone replacement to compensate

J. Addison disease (adrenocortical insufficiency): *presentation*: pigmented skin/mucous membranes, nausea/vomiting/weight loss, muscle weakness, hypotension; *causes:* most primary are idiopathic, likely autoimmune, often associated with diabetes mellitus and Hashimoto thyroiditis; secondary: pituitary or hypothalamic lesion; *diagnosis*: hyperkalemia, decreased sodium, low serum cortisol; *treatment:* lifelong replacement of glucocorticoid and mineralocorticoid; important to follow patients closely during stress periods (i.e., postoperative, infections)

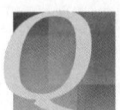 STUDY QUESTIONS FOR CHAPTER 27

Directions: Each of the numbered items or incomplete statements in this section is followed by answers or by completions of the statement. Select the ONE lettered answer or completion that is BEST in each case.

1. The parents of an infant with Riley-Day syndrome are interested in conceiving and wish to know the chance that a second baby will have the same condition. You inform them that the probability is:

(A) <1%
(B) 25%
(C) 50%
(D) 75%
(E) 100%

2. You are asked to evaluate a 38-year-old woman with anisocoria after placement of a central line, and note a Horner syndrome. Which of the following findings is most consistent with a congenital origin of Horner syndrome?

(A) Decreased perspiration of the face only
(B) Decreased perspiration of the face and ipsilateral trunk and arm
(C) Enophthalmos
(D) Loss of pigment in the affected eye
(E) Blindness in the affected eye

3. A 4-year-old girl is brought to a pediatric endocrinologist because she has developed secondary sexual characteristics. Which of the following neurocutaneous syndromes is associated with precocious puberty?

(A) Neurofibromatosis type 1
(B) Tuberous sclerosis
(C) Incontinentia pigmenti
(D) Sturge-Weber syndrome
(E) Von Hippel-Lindau disease

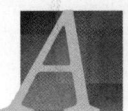

ANSWERS AND EXPLANATIONS

1. B. Riley-Day syndrome is inherited as an autosomal-recessive condition. Both parents are carriers of the gene, so the probability that a second child will have the condition is 25%.

2. D. Horner syndrome is characterized by miosis, ptosis, anhidrosis, and apparent enophthalmos. It is due to interruption of the oculosympathetic pathways. Common causes include cervical lymph node masses, surgical trauma, carotid artery dissections, brachial plexus trauma, and lateral brainstem infarction. Heterochromia iridis, a gray or blue discoloration of the affected iris, points to a congenital origin of Horner syndrome. The pattern of perspiration may help to localize the lesion, but does not help to define its onset. Similarly, enophthalmos does not help to date the onset of the lesion. Blindness is not a component of Horner syndrome.

3. A. Neurofibromatosis type 1 can be associated with precocious puberty. The other choices listed are not known to produce this syndrome.

CHAPTER 28

Special Senses

I. Smell

A. **Hyposmia:** decreased sense of smell, most commonly smoking, allergic rhinitis, dementia, but could be any cause of anosmia (see subsequent text)

B. **Anosmia:** loss of smell
   1. **Unilateral** usually not noticed by patient: consider cribriform meningioma
   2. **Bilateral:** patient will usually complain of loss of sense of taste; verify sense of taste is preserved by testing tongue with salty/sweet tastes
   3. **Testing:** use nonirritating odors (coffee, peanut butter both can sit in bag a long time) without degrading
   4. **Five Groups**
      a. **Nasal:** odors do not reach epithelium: chronic atrophic rhinitis, rhinitis, nasal polyps
      b. **Neuroepithelial:** receptors damaged: atrophic rhinitis, influenza, herpes, hepatitis, radiation
      c. **Central:** pathway lesion: 6% closed head injury, stroke, tumor, immune-mediated disorders (Wegener)
      d. **Hormonal/nutritional/systemic**
         i. **Hormonal:** many women have differences in smell during threshold period
         ii. **Nutritional/systemic:** vitamin A or thiamine deficiency, chronic renal failure or cirrhosis
      e. **Malingering:** often do not complain of loss of taste

C. **Hyperosmia:** rule out migraine or aseptic meningitis

D. **Dysosmia or parosmia:** usually unpleasant odor distortion: rule out severe sinusitis and depression

E. **Phantosmia:** odors no one else can detect—usually amygdala nuclei even if psychological
   1. If brief, likely to be temporal lobe seizure; often described as burning plastic
   2. Patient who thinks he smells bad and washes excessively likely has psychiatric disorder
   3. Patient who thinks that those around him smell likely has schizophrenia
   4. If with senile dementia, consider depression evaluation

II. Taste

A. **Ageusia:** loss of taste

B. **Hypogeusia:** most likely post influenza, also consider tumor, vitamin A/B deficiency, hepatitis, myxedema, scleroderma, adrenal insufficiency
   1. **Taste alteration** accompanies many medications.

C. **Bilateral ageusia:** most commonly normal aging, heavy smoking, especially pipe smoking
   1. **Need saliva for taste to function:** xerostomia, Sjögren, cystic fibrosis, radiation
   2. **Dysautonomia:** either global or familial (Riley-Day syndrome)

D. **Unilateral ageusia:** Bell palsy

E. **Hallucinations:** consider thalamic, parietal stroke or frontoparietal or uncal seizure

F. **Burning mouth syndrome:** mainly postmenopausal female who complains of burning mouth but has completely normal examination—consider diabetes, vitamin B_{12} deficiency, depression

III. Vision

Any vision complaint must include a retinal examination.

A. **Papilledema**
   1. **Stages**
      a. **Early** with disc elevation, blurring of disc margin, especially superior/inferior aspects
         i. The blurring of disc margins can be seen with hypermetropia
         ii. Venous pulsations = intracranial pressure (ICP) 19 cm H_2O, absent in 10% to 15% of normals
      b. **Moderate** with edema, vessel obscuration at disc margins, hemorrhages
      c. **Advanced** is almost always bilateral
      d. **Chronic** with increased pallor, disc pallor, and decrease in size of disc
   2. **Differential diagnosis**
      a. **Increased ICP:** headache, blurred binocular vision and/or increased blind spot, usually normal pupil examination; visual loss may occur
         i. Differential diagnosis: lymphoma, intracranial structural lesion, hydrocephalus, central nervous system (CNS) neoplasm, migraine, transient ischemic attack (TIA), CNS infection, chronic lung disease with hypercarbia, leukemia, arteriovenous malformation (AVM), polycythemia
      b. **Pseudopapilledema:** hyaline bodies, can have progressive blind spot enlargement or even inferior arcuate nasal defect, afferent pupillary defect possible
      c. **Optic neuritis:** pain on ocular movement, usually monocular rapid visual loss, afferent pupillary defect
      d. **Anterior ischemic optic neuropathy:** headache (if temporal arteritis), usually monocular visual loss, altitudinal defect possible, afferent pupillary defect
      e. **Foster-Kennedy syndrome:** papilledema on one side and optic atrophy on the other; can include anosmia; frontal tumor, olfactory meningioma on side of atrophy

IV. Pupillary Defects

Pupillary defects covered in neuroophthalmology section

V. Eye Movements

Patient complains of **diplopia** (Table 28-1). For diplopia or abnormal eye movement unexplained by localizing neurological lesion, consider myasthenia, thyroid disease, and Wernicke syndrome.

A. **Simple ophthalmoplegias**
  1. **Find the direction where there is greatest diplopia**; the red glass test is handy, because the direction of separation localizes the paresis. Remember the "p" rule: the peripheral image belongs to the paretic muscle.
  2. **Need to understand the description of movements for the boards**
     a. Medial rectus adducts, lateral rectus abducts
     b. Both superior and inferior recti move temporally, superior moves superiorly and inferiorly
     c. Superior oblique moves inferior and medial, whereas the inferior oblique moves superior and medial
  3. **Superior oblique palsy:** often has a head tilt to the opposite shoulder; patient may complain about difficulty walking down steps; differential diagnosis is trochlear lesion, torticollis, and nystagmus
  4. **Cranial nerve deficits** can be central or peripheral; if central, you should be able to find other focal deficits; if peripheral, the causes are numerous; the most likely causes are tumors, diabetes, head trauma, and aneurysms
     a. **Abducens nerve (CN) VI:** most common adult tumor nasopharyngeal cancer metastasis—that is, you must check nasopharynx carefully and possibly biopsy; most common child tumor—pontine glioma; can be diabetic ischemic infarction or associated with any number of causes of increased ICP, as well as pregnancy
     b. **CN IV:** most likely head trauma or congenital other causes, herpes zoster ophthalmicus, diabetes, increased ICP; rare causes include lupus, Sjögren, and superior oblique myokymia (recurrent diplopia with monocular visual blurring; treatment: carbamazepine); often remains idiopathic after investigation
     c. **CN III:** most likely neoplasm then aneurysm; diabetic infarction does not involve the pupil
  5. **Pseudo-inferior oblique palsy:** Brown syndrome of rheumatoid arthritis = superior oblique tendon tenosynovitis; eye gets stuck, when released hear a clicking
  6. **Weakness of near accommodation** is Mobius sign of hyperthyroidism
  7. **Isolated medial or inferior rectus restriction:** likely Graves disease

B. **Other ophthalmoplegias**
  1. **Painful usually unilateral:** aneurysm, tumor, or inflammation
     a. **Tolosa-Hunt syndrome** = inflammation of the superior orbital fissure/anterior cavernous sinus; pain both in and behind the eyes; treatment: steroids
     b. **Orbital pseudotumor** = inflammation of extraocular muscles; conjunctival and lid injection, slight proptosis, visual loss possible; treatment: steroids
     c. **Cavernous sinus syndrome** = periorbital pain and chemosis with CN III and CN VI deficits, can include CN IV and can occur both bilaterally and include sensory loss in CN V_1; obtain MRI/magnetic resonance angiography (MRA); most common causes: trauma, tumor, and re-emergence of previous condition
     d. **Rare causes:** temporal arteritis, thyroid ophthalmopathy, and Brown syndrome (mechanical restriction due to pulley of the superior oblique tendon; often includes clicking with sudden release)

Table 28-1	Diplopia
CN III	Expect ptosis unless diabetic infarction
CN IV	Head tilted to opposite direction; complains of difficulty walking down steps
CN VI	Unable to look past midline on affected eye
Pseudo-IO palsy	Brown syndrome of rheumatoid arthritis Eye gets stuck
Accommodation	Mobius sign of hyperthyroidism

2. **Bilateral ophthalmoplegias**
   a. **Chronic**
      i. Progressive external ophthalmoplegia; can begin at any age; ptosis initially followed by unremitting progressive ophthalmoplegia; if includes atypical pigmentary degeneration, heart block, short stature = a mitochondrial disorder called Kearns—Sayre syndrome
      ii. Thyroid ophthalmoplegia; often includes pain, proptosis, and lid retraction but is variable, can involve one eye or even a single muscle; always test for antibodies even if thyroid stimulating hormone (TSH)/thyroxin (T4) levels are normal, as infrequently can be normal
      iii. Restricted muscular dystrophy to extraocular muscles
   b. **Acute:** most likely causes include brainstem infarction, Wernicke, Guillain-Barré, tuberculous meningitis, myasthenia gravis, botulism, cavernous sinus tumor
3. **Internuclear ophthalmoplegia** (INO)
   a. **Symptoms:** ipsilateral rectus paralysis and contralateral conjugate gaze palsy; if the left eye does not adduct when the patient looks to the right, this is called left INO, because it is localized to left CN VI nucleus and median longitudinal fasciculus; also, dissociated nystagmus that affects the abducting eye
   b. If includes loss of convergence, lesion in high midbrain and called anterior INO
   c. If includes skew deviation, lesion in lateral medulla
   d. Most common cause of unilateral INO is paramedian pontine infarction.
   e. Most common cause of bilateral INO is multiple sclerosis.
   f. One and a half syndrome (Fisher syndrome): one eye fixed midline for all horizontal movements and the other can only adduct; pontine localization

VI. Hearing

A. **Tinnitus** affects 37 million Americans
   1. **Classification**
      a. **Tonal**, which can be heard only by patient
         i. Most normals have physiologic tinnitus heard when ambient noise is <20 dB (normal ambient noise is about 35 dB)
         ii. Low frequency often described as blowing, likely conductive hearing loss
         iii. High frequency often described as chirping, likely sensineuronal hearing loss
         iv. Fluctuating tinnitus with episodic deafness in one ear without vertigo is Ménière
         v. Rhythmic clicking: palatal myoclonus or contraction of stapedius/tensor tympani
         vi. Medications like gentamicin or vancomycin
      b. **Non-tonal** are real and pulsatile
         i. Most normals can hear pulse while lying with one ear compressed by hand or bed
         ii. Many causes: most common are intracranial hypertension, glomus tumors, and carotid disease and should be ruled out before looking for other conditions

B. **Hearing loss** affects 28 million Americans with 2 million deaf. Your job is to classify and send to appropriate specialist.
   1. **Classification**
      a. **Conduction defects:** otosclerosis (most common cause in young adult), cerumen, chronic otitis media, tympanic membrane thickening, external auditory canal atresia; often described as partial inability to hear low pitched sounds
      b. **Sensineuronal deafness:** due to cochlear or cranial nerve deficit; often described as partial inability to hear high pitched sounds; if you raise your voice and the patient thinks that you're shouting, lesion is localized to cochlea (this is called recruitment)
      c. **Central deafness:** bilateral cochlear nuclei or temporal lobe; most likely form is tone deafness, an autosomal dominant condition

C. **Hallucinations**
   1. Older patients with long duration neurosensory deafness can hear song-like sounds
   2. Pontine lesions can produce musical or loud ZZZ-like sounds, likely focal neurologic examination

D. **Psychogenic deafness**
   1. Diagnosis of exclusion, after temporal lobe seizure has been ruled out
   2. Corroborate by checking reflex blinking (can be suppressed) and sweating in response to loud sounds; can check brainstem auditory evoked response (BAER) to be sure

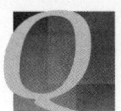 STUDY QUESTIONS FOR CHAPTER 28

Directions: Each of the numbered items or incomplete statements in this section is followed by answers or by completions of the statement. Select the ONE lettered answer or completion that is BEST in each case.

1. A 28-year-old complains of 2-week loss of taste sensation and no other complaints or medical history, no history of recent illness, and otherwise nonfocal neurologic examination. You verify his loss of taste. Which of the following lab tests do you not order?

(A) TSH
(B) Acute hepatitis panel
(C) Morning cortisol
(D) MRI brain

2. An 83-year-old complains of occasional double vision. On examination, you notice that the right eye only has nystagmus on looking to the right. You would most likely also observe which of the following:

(A) Right eye can not abduct on looking to right
(B) Left eye can not adduct on looking to right
(C) Right eye can not adduct on looking to left
(D) Left eye can not abduct on looking to left

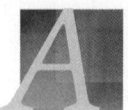 # ANSWERS AND EXPLANATIONS

1. C. Without any suggestive cause of decrease in taste, one would want to rule out reversible causes: A, B, D. An MRI of the brain might be ordered if no reversible causes could be found.

2. B. This is left INO, in which the left eye cannot abduct on looking to right is expected finding. The question states that the right eye can look to the right (abduct), so eliminate A. There should be no problem looking to the left: C, D.

CHAPTER 29

Final Exam

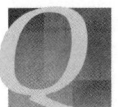

Directions: Each of the numbered items or incomplete statements in this section is followed by answers or by completions of the statement. Select the ONE lettered answer or completion that is BEST in each case.

1. Which of the following is most consistent with Lennox-Gastaut syndrome?
   (A) Male gender
   (B) Mental retardation
   (C) Prior febrile seizure
   (D) Family history of complex partial seizures
   (E) EEG frequency during absence seizures of 3 Hz

2. You are asked to provide a second opinion on a 48-year-old man with frequent seizures, cognitive decline, and ataxia. On examination, you additionally note decreased reflexes and tendinous xanthomas. Which intervention will most probably improve his seizure frequency?
   (A) Chenodeoxycholic acid
   (B) Vitamin E supplementation
   (C) Dietary phytanic acid restriction
   (D) Biotin
   (E) Niacin

3. A 44-year-old man is noted by his primary care physician to have anisocoria. He is referred to you for further evaluation and you note that his right pupil is 3 mm and reacts to 2 mm, whereas his left pupil is 7 mm and reacts to 2 mm. His anisocoria is greater in the light than the dark. You apply a 1% hydroxyamphetamine solution to both eyes. The right eye remains at 3 mm while the left eye dilates to 10 mm. The right eyelid is 1 mm lower than the left. All eye movements are normal. What is the diagnosis?
   (A) Right Horner syndrome below the superior cervical ganglion
   (B) Right Horner syndrome above the superior cervical ganglion
   (C) Left third nerve palsy
   (D) Right third nerve palsy
   (E) Physiologic anisocoria

4. A 19-year-old woman develops painful visual loss in her right eye, weakness in the left hand, and an unsteady gait. Her weakness progresses over several days and she is admitted to the hospital. While in the hospital, she is confused and has three seizures. A diagnosis of acute disseminated encephalomyelitis is made. Which clinical feature is most suggestive of acute disseminated encephalomyelitis rather than multiple sclerosis?
   (A) Her young age
   (B) Presence of pain with her visual loss
   (C) Onset of symptoms referable to multiple neurologic locations
   (D) Progression of symptoms over several days
   (E) Seizures

5. An 85-year-old woman is brought to the emergency room by her daughter with the sudden onset of confusion. When she is examined, it is noted that she is capable of writing sentences, but cannot read any of the sentences that she has just written. What other neurologic deficit might be expected in this patient?
   (A) Right homonymous hemianopia
   (B) Left homonymous hemianopia
   (C) Right hemiparesis
   (D) Left hemiparesis
   (E) Transcortical motor aphasia

6. A 41-year-old man with lower back pain develops worsening low back and leg pain and mild weakness in his lower extremities after a

CT myelogram. Which of the following conditions is most likely to account for the worsening of his pain and weakness?

(A) Fibrocartilaginous embolus
(B) Lumbar disk herniation
(C) Vacuolar myelopathy
(D) Adhesive arachnoiditis
(E) Transverse myelitis

7. A 48-year-old woman is referred to you for evaluation of headache of 6 months' duration. Her physical examination is normal with the exception of papilledema in the left eye and optic atrophy in the right eye. What is the most likely diagnosis?

(A) Left frontal meningioma
(B) Right frontal meningioma
(C) Left optic neuritis
(D) Right optic neuritis
(E) Hydrocephalus

8. A 48-year-old alcoholic is found unconscious in a poorly ventilated garage. Despite their best efforts, the emergency medical service is not able to revive him. He is brought to autopsy and is found to have massive cerebral edema and putaminal necrosis. What is the most likely cause of death?

(A) Carbon monoxide
(B) Thiamine deficiency
(C) Methanol
(D) Ethylene glycol
(E) Central pontine myelinolysis

9. A 67-year-old right-handed man presents to the emergency room with the sudden onset of flinging of his right arm. The most likely location for a stroke producing this problem is:

(A) The left subthalamic nucleus
(B) The left globus pallidus internus
(C) The left globus pallidus externus
(D) The left caudate nucleus
(E) The left substantia nigra

10. A 36-year-old man comes to your clinic with reports of 6 months of acting out his dreams. His wife reports that 3 to 4 hours after sleep onset, he screams out, punches at the air, and appears to be having violent conversations with people who are not present.

(A) Most patients who develop this condition are in their 30s and 40s
(B) This condition predisposes to Alzheimer disease
(C) Clonazepam is usually successful in treating the symptoms
(D) Alcohol intoxication increases the frequency of episodes
(E) Treatment of an underlying mood disorder is effective

11. A 52-year-old man is brought to the emergency room with fever to 103.4°F, neck stiffness, and lethargy. He has a witnessed seizure in the emergency room. A noncontrast head CT is normal and a lumbar puncture contains 512 WBCs, 99% polymorphonuclear cells, 113 protein mg/dL, and 54 glucose mg/dL. Gram-positive cocci are found in the CSF. Which of the following features makes encephalitis rather than meningitis the likely diagnosis?

(A) Fever greater than 102°F
(B) Positive Gram stain
(C) CSF WBC >500
(D) CSF glucose 60

12. A 69-year-old man is brought to the emergency room after sustaining a head injury in a motor vehicle accident. On presentation, his GCS is 8. Which of the following would prompt insertion of an ICP monitor?

(A) His age
(B) Hypotension
(C) Decerebrate posturing
(D) Decorticate posturing
(E) Evidence of intracranial hemorrhage

13. A 30-year-old surgery resident has difficulty awakening in time for morning rounds. He falls asleep at approximately 2 a.m. every morning and wakes up at 9 a.m. Although he has tried to go to sleep earlier in the evening, he is unable to do so. Which medication is most likely to help him?

(A) Clomipramine
(B) Clonazepam
(C) Melatonin
(D) Modafinil
(E) Trazodone

14. A 67-year-old woman comes to your office with a complaint of multiple episodes of dizziness, by which she means that the room is spinning around her. These are provoked by turning over in bed or reaching up for an object on a high shelf. Some of the episodes are severe enough to produce vomiting. The Dix-Hallpike maneuver produces upbeat torsional nystagmus. What is the most likely site of pathology?

(A) Utricle
(B) Saccule
(C) Anterior semicircular canal
(D) Posterior semicircular canal
(E) Horizontal semicircular canal

15. A 52-year-old alcoholic man is brought to the emergency department with symptoms of alcohol intoxication. You are called to examine him because his gait is unsteady. What part of the cerebellum is most affected by chronic alcohol abuse?

(A) Deep nuclei of the hemispheres
(B) Flocculonodulus
(C) Hemispheres
(D) Middle cerebellar peduncle
(E) Vermis

16. You are called to the emergency room to evaluate an 83-year-old woman for the possibility of stroke. She says that she woke up in the morning with dizziness, which has persisted for about 6 hours. Which of the following is most likely to suggest a peripheral cause of vertigo as an alternative explanation?

(A) Double vision
(B) Facial numbness
(C) Facial weakness
(D) Hearing loss
(E) Vomiting

17. You are called to see a patient with visual loss in the right eye. In addition to acuity of 20/200 in the right eye, you note right proptosis with pulsatility and injection of the right eye. The patient has no other medical history. What is the likely diagnosis?

(A) Optic neuritis
(B) Angle closure glaucoma
(C) Carotid-cavernous sinus fistula
(D) Orbital trauma
(E) Hyperthyroidism

18. While on call in the pediatric emergency room, you admit a 3-month-old infant with tonic spasms. An EEG obtained the next day demonstrates predominantly delta frequency background. What can you conclude from this EEG?

(A) The parents overreacted: these events were not seizures.
(B) Delta frequency indicates status epilepticus.
(C) This likely represents an artifact.
(D) Delta frequency indicates that this infant is encephalopathic.

(E) Delta frequency is the predominant background frequency in infants.

19. A 78-year-old nursing home resident is brought to the emergency room because of fever, headache, neck stiffness, and lethargy. His examination additionally discloses mild left hemiparesis. You suspect bacterial meningitis. What is the appropriate sequence of actions at this time?

(A) No head CT, immediate lumbar puncture, start antibiotics if Gram staining is positive
(B) Head CT, lumbar puncture if head CT is normal, start antibiotics if Gram staining is positive
(C) Head CT, start antibiotics, lumbar puncture if head CT is normal
(D) Start antibiotics, head CT, lumbar puncture if head CT is normal
(E) Start antibiotics, head CT, no lumbar puncture needed because antibiotics will reduce its sensitivity

20. A 9-month-old is brought to your office for the assessment of developmental delay. You perform a complete neurologic examination including reflex testing. The presence of which of the following reflexes would be most worrisome?

(A) Moro reflex
(B) Asymmetric tonic neck reflex
(C) Symmetric tonic neck reflex
(D) Babinski reflex
(E) Foot grasp reflex

21. A 44-year-old woman is referred to you by a pulmonologist for further evaluation of dyspnea. The tests that have been ordered thus far are consistent with a restrictive deficit, but no source has been found. You perform an EMG, and while the limb muscles appear normal, there are multiple myopathic-appearing units in the diaphragm. What is the most likely diagnosis?

(A) Acid maltase deficiency
(B) Becker muscular dystrophy
(C) Central core disease
(D) Emery-Dreifuss dystrophy
(E) Limb-girdle dystrophy

22. After a motor vehicle accident, a 32-year-old man complains of double vision. The double vision is mostly vertical. On examination he is noted to have vertical diplopia greatest when he looks downward. His diplopia is also greatest in leftward gaze and his head tilts to the left shoulder. Which muscle is most likely dysfunctional?

(A) Right inferior oblique
(B) Right inferior rectus
(C) Right superior oblique
(D) Right superior rectus
(E) Right medial rectus

23. An 84-year-old diabetic man presents with sudden onset of hearing loss in the left ear. Occlusion of which of the following vessels is most likely to produce this deficit?

(A) Right middle cerebral artery
(B) Left middle cerebral artery
(C) Left superior cerebellar artery
(D) Left anterior inferior cerebellar artery
(E) Left posterior inferior cerebellar artery

24. A 45-year-old woman undergoes an MRI/MRA of her head for evaluation of headaches for 3 years. A 4-mm aneurysm of the posterior communicating artery is noted. How should you counsel her?

(A) The risk of bleeding of this aneurysm is less than 1% per year.
(B) This is likely an inherited condition.
(C) She should be investigated for connective tissue disorder.
(D) The aneurysm is the cause of her headache.
(E) This is an emergency and should be treated immediately.

25. While on call, a medical intern asks you to urgently see an 84-year-old comatose patient with an unreactive left pupil. You arrive and find that the left pupil is 2 mm and pear shaped. The right pupil is 3 mm and reacts to 2 mm. Cold caloric stimulation produces tonic deviation of the eyes to either side. Because the patient is comatose, you cannot establish the presence or absence of ptosis. What additional history would most likely help establish the diagnosis?

(A) Cataract surgery
(B) Syphilis
(C) Sudden-onset severe headache
(D) Apical lung cancer
(E) Atropine administration during resuscitation

26. A 54-year-old woman has had multiple episodes of vertigo lasting hours at a time, low-frequency hearing loss, tinnitus, and a feeling of fullness in the ear. Which of the following is most likely to produce vertigo in this patient?

(A) Bright lights
(B) Loud noises
(C) Laughter
(D) Fright
(E) Change in altitude

27. A 42-year-old man with AIDS (CD4 count 63) develops headaches, blurry vision, and ataxia over a period of several months. You obtain an MRI of his head. Which of the following locations is most likely to be abnormal?

(A) Optic nerves
(B) Frontal lobes
(C) Occipital lobes
(D) Pons
(E) Cerebellum

28. A 23-year-old woman comes to your office with a complaint of facial heaviness and slurred speech. On examination, she has weakness of the left side of her face in a lower-motor neuron distribution. You make a diagnosis of Bell palsy. Which of the following sensory modalities would be most commonly affected?

(A) Perception of high-frequency hearing in the left ear
(B) Taste on the anterior two thirds of the tongue
(C) Gross touch on the left side of the face
(D) Pinprick sensation on the left side of the face
(E) Pinprick sensation on the right side of the body

29. A 19-year-old man has sustained a head injury in a motorcycle accident. His initial GCS score was 3 and he is intubated and sedated. An intracranial pressure monitor is placed and the initial reading is elevated. Which of the following interventions is most likely to be beneficial?

(A) Hyperventilation to a pCO_2 25 mm Hg
(B) Flattening the head of his bed
(C) Increasing his sedation
(D) Corticosteroids
(E) Intravenous fluids

30. At the onset of his typical seizure, a 16-year-old boy turns his head and eyes forcefully to the left side and contracts his right hand.

What is the most likely location of this seizure focus?

(A) Left frontal lobe
(B) Right frontal lobe
(C) Left temporal lobe
(D) Right temporal lobe
(E) Generalized onset

31. A 53-year-old heroin-abuser is brought to the emergency room for evaluation of pain in the middle of his back and progressive lower extremity weakness. He has a fever to 101°F, mid-back tenderness, and 4+/5 weakness in his lower extremities in his lower extremities in a pyramidal pattern. Which of the following tests is most helpful to evaluate the possibility of an epidural abscess?

(A) MRI with contrast
(B) ESR
(C) WBC
(D) Lumbar puncture
(E) Blood cultures

32. An 82-year-old man is admitted to the cardiac care unit after a myocardial infarction. Per the ambulance report, he had no pulse for 15 minutes prior to defibrillation. You are asked to provide prognostic information and order an EEG. Which of the following patterns would suggest the worst prognosis?

(A) Alpha coma
(B) Beta coma
(C) Spindle coma
(D) Periodic lateralized epileptiform discharges
(E) Triphasic waves

33. A 29-year-old man relates that he has a long history of being a loner with no desire to make friends or form relationships. He is not bothered by these symptoms. What is the most appropriate personality disorder?

(A) Avoidant personality disorder
(B) Schizoid personality disorder
(C) Schizotypal personality disorder
(D) Borderline personality disorder
(E) Obsessive compulsive personality disorder

34. A 3-year-old boy is brought to your office because of loss of language development milestones. Six months ago he was able to string together three- and four-word sentences and had an appropriate vocabulary for age, but now he communicates mostly with sounds and gestures rather than words. Which of the following is true concerning his condition?

(A) His EEG is likely to show spike-wave discharges during the daytime
(B) His EEG is likely to show frontal spikes during sleep
(C) He may respond to treatment with corticosteroids
(D) His behavior is otherwise likely to be normal
(E) His primary deficit is likely to be audiologic rather than neurologic

35. A 3-year-old boy is brought to your office for evaluation of headache, vomiting, and falls for 3 weeks. Examination discloses papilledema and left limb ataxia. An MRI is performed and a left cerebellar hemispheric mass is seen. What is the most likely diagnosis?

(A) Medulloblastoma
(B) Choroid plexus papilloma
(C) Ependymoma
(D) Pilocytic astrocytoma
(E) Subependymoma

36. A 76-year-old woman with small cell lung cancer presents with dry mouth and fatigable proximal muscle weakness. What is the most likely pathophysiology of her condition?

(A) Antibodies to the acetylcholine receptor
(B) Inability to package and release presynaptic acetylcholine
(C) Antibodies to voltage-gated calcium channels
(D) Antibodies to muscle-specific tyrosine kinase
(E) Myositis secondary to neoplastic infiltration

37. A 78-year-old man visits his primary care physician complaining of bifrontal squeezing headaches. He is given a diagnosis of tension headaches and is sent home. The next day, he is found dead in his kitchen. At autopsy, he is found to have a Rathke cleft cyst. Which of the following is true?

(A) The Rathke's cleft cyst was likely responsible for his headaches.
(B) Rathke cleft cysts are derived from remnants of the neurohypophyseal bud.
(C) The Rathke cleft cysts do not enhance on MRI.
(D) Rathke cleft cysts are frequently large and space-occupying.

(E) Rathke cleft cysts are less common than craniopharyngiomas.

38. A 9-year-old boy is brought to your office with a history of one year of weakness and falls. On examination you note that he has absent reflexes and a cerebellar ataxia. Of the following choices, which is the most likely diagnosis?

(A) Abetalipoproteinemia
(B) Episodic ataxia 1
(C) Infectious cerebellitis
(D) Medulloblastoma
(E) Spinocerebellar ataxia 1

39. You are asked to evaluate a 31-year-old woman with a headache who is 8 weeks pregnant. The woman tells you that she has had a diagnosis of pseudotumor cerebri in the past, but has not had symptoms for 8 years. You perform a funduscopic examination, looking for evidence of papilledema. What is the first change that you would expect to see in a patient with papilledema?

(A) Absence of venous pulsations
(B) Elevated disc margins
(C) Splinter hemorrhages
(D) Increased cup-to-disc ratio
(E) Drusen

40. A 38-year-old woman is referred to you for evaluation of diplopia. When she moves her eye, she occasionally hears a click. After evaluation, it appears that she has isolated inferior oblique palsy. Her neurologic and ophthalmologic examinations are otherwise normal. What is the most likely cause of this palsy?

(A) Grave disease
(B) Brown syndrome
(C) Aneurysmal rupture
(D) Diabetes
(E) Intraocular tumor

41. A 76-year-old woman comes to the emergency room for evaluation of weakness. She is noted to have difficulty abducting the left eye and a right hemiparesis. Which of the following localizations is most likely?

(A) Left paramedian midbrain
(B) Left medial superior pons
(C) Left medial mid pons
(D) Left medial inferior pons
(E) Left medial medulla

42. A comatose 89-year-old woman is admitted to the hospital confused with a fever of 103°F. As part of her fever evaluation, a lumbar puncture is performed. She is placed in an upright position and the opening pressure is measured at 290 mm CSF. Which of the following is true concerning her opening pressure?

(A) The pressure is suggestive of bacterial meningitis.
(B) The pressure was increased by placement in the upright position.
(C) This value is normal for a woman of her age.
(D) She should receive acetazolamide to reduce the pressure.
(E) The elevated pressure places her at risk for herniation.

43. The concerned parents of a 2-month-old infant bring him to your office for evaluation of constant head nodding and jerky eye movements. On examination, you find that the infant is floppy and has head titubation and spontaneous nystagmus. What is the likely pattern of inheritance of this condition?

(A) Autosomal dominant
(B) Autosomal recessive
(C) X-linked recessive
(D) Sporadic
(E) Mitochondrial

44. A 35-year-old man with epilepsy who has recently moved to your town is referred to you by his psychiatrist. He has a history of temporal lobe epilepsy, which has been well-controlled by carbamazepine. What is the most likely psychiatric disorder for which this patient is treated?

(A) Depression
(B) Mania
(C) Temporal lobe epilepsy personality
(D) Schizophrenia
(E) Psychosis

45. A 70-year-old man with diabetes complains of double vision. He says that the images are purely side-by-side rather than up-and-down. The diplopia is greater when he looks to the right side. Which of the following cranial nerves is most likely involved?

(A) The right oculomotor nerve
(B) The right trochlear nerve
(C) The right abducens nerve
(D) The left oculomotor nerve
(E) The left abducens nerve

46. Which of the following pairs of cranial nerves might be expected to be abnormal in a patient with acoustic neuroma?
(A) CN III and V
(B) CN V and VII
(C) CN VI and VII
(D) CN VII and IX
(E) CN IX and X

47. A 41-year-old woman with glioblastoma multiforme is brought to the emergency room with a worsening in her mental status. A head CT is urgently obtained and demonstrates uncal herniation. Which structure is likely to be compressed by uncal herniation?
(A) Cerebellar tonsils
(B) Sixth cranial nerve
(C) Posterior cerebral artery
(D) Anterior cerebral artery
(E) Basilar artery perforators

48. A 46-year-old woman has been treated for ocular myasthenia for 2 years. She has responded to pyridostigmine but occasionally has diplopia at the end of a long day. She has not developed proximal muscle weakness, dysarthria, or dysphagia. What is the most likely clinical course for this patient?
(A) Limitation of disease to her eyes
(B) Resolution of disease upon discontinuation of pyridostigmine
(C) Progression to include bulbar weakness
(D) Progression to include proximal limb weakness
(E) Progression to include bulbar and proximal limb weakness

49. Nerve conduction studies are performed to evaluate numbness and tingling in the toes of a 48-year-old woman. Which of the following patterns of sensory nerve action potentials (SNAPs) is most consistent with demyelination without conduction block?
(A) Decreased amplitude, decreased conduction velocity
(B) Decreased amplitude, normal conduction velocity
(C) Normal amplitude, decreased conduction velocity
(D) Normal amplitude, normal conduction velocity
(E) Increased amplitude, decreased conduction velocity

50. A 57-year-old man is brought to your office for difficulties with sleep. His wife reports that he acts out his dreams, talking and fighting in his sleep, and injuring her on one occasion. This man is at risk for development of which form of dementia?
(A) Alzheimer disease
(B) Frontotemporal dementia
(C) Lewy-body disease
(D) Primary progressive aphasia
(E) Vascular dementia

51. A 54-year-old man is brought to the emergency room in a state of confusion. In addition to his confusion, he cannot abduct either eye and has bilateral limb ataxia. What is the most appropriate initial step in his management?
(A) Non-contrast CT of the head
(B) Lumbar puncture
(C) Intravenous thiamine administration
(D) Intravenous diphenhydramine (Benadryl) administration
(E) Neurosurgical consultation

52. A 12-year-old girl is brought to your office by her mother because she has had two episodes of awakening from sleep accompanied by left facial twitching in the last 3 months. She has never had a frank convulsion or an event during the daytime. Her neurologic examination is normal. What is the most appropriate next step?
(A) MRI of her head
(B) EEG
(C) Initiate treatment with carbamazepine
(D) Initiate treatment with lamotrigine
(E) Hyperventilation to attempt to reproduce the episode

53. A 52-year-old man with a temporal lobe astrocytoma is brought into the emergency department in a coma. He is noted to have a fixed and dilated left pupil and withdraws his left side less briskly than his right side. What is most likely responsible for this presentation?
(A) Left-to-right uncal herniation with compression of the left oculomotor nerve and left cerebral peduncle
(B) Left-to-right uncal herniation with compression of the left oculomotor nerve and right cerebral peduncle
(C) Right-to-left uncal herniation with compression of the left oculomotor nerve and left cerebral peduncle

(D) Right-to-left uncal herniation with compression of the left oculomotor nerve and right cerebral peduncle
(E) Right-to-left uncal herniation with compression of the left oculomotor nerve and right basis pontis

54. A 38-year-old man with chronic diarrhea and abdominal pain comes to your office with ataxia, which has developed over the last 6 months. He reports a 45-pound weight loss in the 3 years of his diarrhea. In addition to his ataxia, you note that he has rhythmic movements of his face and jaw and a supranuclear gaze palsy. What is the best method to establish a diagnosis in this patient?

(A) Blood cultures
(B) Stool cultures
(C) Jejunal biopsy
(D) Genetic testing
(E) Brain MRI

55. A 38-year-old man is admitted to the hospital with flaccid paralysis that developed over a period of 10 days. He is intubated, has 0/5 strength in all appendicular muscles, and has no reflexes. In the course of evaluation of this condition, you obtain laboratory studies including CSF analysis. Which of the following laboratory findings is most likely?

(A) Elevated white blood cell count
(B) Hyponatremia
(C) Hyperglycemia
(D) Elevated transaminases
(E) Increased opening pressure during lumbar puncture

56. A 32-year-old woman is brought to the emergency room by her husband for 2 days of fever, headache, and malaise. She has meningismus on examination. Lumbar puncture is performed: the opening pressure is 250 mm H$_2$O, WBC 633/mL, RBC 5/mL, protein 96 mg/dL, and glucose 52 mg/dL. Her serum glucose is 119. What is the most likely organism responsible for her presentation?

(A) *Escherichia coli*
(B) *Haemophilus influenzae*
(C) *Neisseria meningitides*
(D) *Staphylococcus aureus*
(E) *Streptococcus pneumoniae*

57. A 4-month-old girl is brought to your office for evaluation of frequent infantile spasms. On funduscopic examination, you note retinal lacunae. To further evaluate this patient, you order an MRI with request for specific attention to which structure?

(A) Pineal body
(B) Posterior commissure
(C) Thalamus
(D) Corpus callosum
(E) Hippocampus

58. While examining a 4-year-old girl with headache, you note that her left pupil is 8 mm and does not react to light, whereas the right pupil is 8 mm and reacts briskly to 4 mm. The pupil dilates when you apply a dilute solution of pilocarpine. Her eyes move normally. The remainder of her examination is normal with the exception of decreased deep tendon reflexes. What is the correct diagnosis?

(A) Aneurysm of the posterior communicating artery compressing the left third nerve
(B) Left Horner syndrome
(C) Left Adie tonic pupil
(D) Miller-Fisher variant of Guillain-Barré syndrome
(E) Left Argyl-Robertson pupil

59. A 28-year-old woman is referred to your neurogenetics clinic for evaluation of ataxia. She has had slurred speech, difficulty walking, and clumsiness for 3 years. Her 31-year-old brother has the same condition. On examination, you find scanning speech, areflexia, dorsal column sensory loss, areflexia, and upgoing toes. Which element of her presentation suggests a diagnosis other than Friedreich ataxia?

(A) Age of onset
(B) Her affected brother
(C) Dorsal column sensory loss
(D) Areflexia
(E) Upgoing toes

60. A 92-year-old woman has developed a gradually worsening left hemiparesis after a fall at her nursing home. On examination, she is also found to be mildly confused. Head CT demonstrates a 1.3-cm hypodense crescent-shaped clot in the right hemisphere. What is the appropriate management?

(A) Repeat the head CT in one week to look for expansion
(B) Repeat the head CT in one day to look for expansion

(C) MRI to confirm the location of the clot and exclude other sources of her presentation
(D) Drainage of the clot through burr holes
(E) Open craniectomy

61. During a stress test, a 73-year-old man feels lightheaded. His blood pressure drops from 160/110 to 90/50 mm Hg and his heart rate falls from 110 to 60 bpm. He is observed to fall to the ground, shake his arms, and lose continence of urine. He recovers very quickly, and his blood pressure recovers to 140/90 mm Hg and his pulse to 90 bpm. Which of the following interventions is most likely to prevent recurrence of such an event?

(A) Anticonvulsants
(B) β-blockers
(C) Correction of underlying cardiac defect
(D) Epilepsy surgery
(E) Salt tablets

62. Six months after a right anterior temporal lobectomy for epilepsy, a 39-year-old woman returns to her neurologist for examination. Which of the following pieces of her visual field is most likely to be missing?

(A) The entire left hemifield
(B) The superior part of the left hemifield
(C) Left inferior part of the left hemifield
(D) The entire left hemifield sparing the macula
(E) The entire right hemifield sparing the macula

63. Each time an 18-month-old boy is frightened, he passes out and appears to shake. His mother has obtained a video of one of these episodes, and the child appears to hold his breath, turns blue, lose consciousness, and then have tonic extension of his arms with rolling of his eyes upward. The entire event lasted less than 10 seconds. What is the most likely EEG finding during one of these episodes?

(A) 2-Hz Spikes and waves
(B) 3-Hz Spikes and waves
(C) Hypsarrhythmia
(D) Flattening of the EEG
(E) Background delta rhythm

64. A 42-year-old woman is brought to the emergency room for evaluation of double vision. She cannot adduct the left eye and has no horizontal movements of the right eye. Vertical eye movements are normal. What is the most likely location of her lesion?

(A) Left midbrain
(B) Right midbrain
(C) Left pons
(D) Right pons
(E) Left medulla

65. You are performing a neurologic examination on a healthy 3-month-old infant and are about to test the Moro reflex. Which of the following movements do you expect to see?

(A) Flexion of the arms
(B) Abduction of the arms
(C) Pronation of the hands
(D) Flexion of the knees
(E) Extension of the feet

66. A 3-year-old boy is admitted to the pediatrics service with bacterial meningitis. Which cranial nerve dysfunction is most likely as a consequence of this meningitis?

(A) CN III
(B) CN IV
(C) CN VI
(D) CN VII
(E) CN VIII

67. An 81-year-old right-handed man experiences the sudden onset of right hemiparesis and aphasia. A head CT shows a large infarct involving the entire territory of the left middle cerebral artery. Two days later, his hemiparesis worsens to a hemiplegia and a CT scan demonstrates a large amount of edema surrounding the infarct. Which of the following is true about the edema and its appropriate treatment?

(A) It is cytotoxic edema and should decrease with steroid administration
(B) It is cytotoxic edema and should not decrease with steroid administration
(C) It is vasogenic edema and should decrease with steroid administration
(D) It is vasogenic edema and should not decrease with steroid administration
(E) It is interstitial edema and should decrease with steroid administration

68. A 62-year-old man is brought by his wife to your office with the complaint of depression after a stroke. He has no interest in his old hobbies, is frequently found crying by his wife, and wakes up early in the morning. He has few other sequelae from his stroke. What is the most likely localization of his stroke?

(A) Right frontal
(B) Left frontal
(C) Right parietal
(D) Left parietal
(E) Right temporal

69. A 43-year-old man with excessive daytime sleepiness is suspected of having obstructive sleep apnea and is referred for a sleep study. The diagnostic impression in the sleep study report is that he actually has central sleep apnea. What finding on the sleep study distinguishes central from obstructive sleep apnea?

(A) Airflow decreases greater than 10 seconds
(B) Respiratory effort absence during an apneic episode
(C) Oxygen saturation decrease during an apneic episode
(D) Apnea-hypopnea index >15
(E) Airflow decreases by 50% during an apneic episode

70. A 68-year-old hypertensive man sustains a left thalamic hemorrhage. Which of the following sensory modalities would be preserved?

(A) Olfaction
(B) Vision
(C) Hearing
(D) Touch
(E) Taste

71. After an upper respiratory tract infection, a 35-year-old man develops the abrupt onset of exquisite pain in the right shoulder followed by weakness in the right arm. On examination, you find 3/5 weakness in the deltoid, biceps, triceps, and finger extensors. What will be the most likely course of this patient's illness?

(A) Permanent deficit
(B) Improvement with corticosteroids
(C) Improvement with intravenous immunoglobulin
(D) Spontaneous improvement in several months
(E) Progression to the contralateral arm

72. After an assault with a crowbar, a 76-year-old woman has developed vertigo. She has the sensation that the room spins around her every time she changes position. The vertigo has a latency of about one minute and then lasts about 30 seconds before returning to normal. Which bone was most likely fractured during the assault?

(A) Cribriform plate of the ethmoid bone
(B) Occipital bone
(C) Temporal bone
(D) Parietal bone
(E) Clivus

73. In the evaluation of multiple sclerosis, a 19-year-old woman undergoes brainstem auditory evoked potentials. She is noted to have prolonged latency between waves I and V. Which structure is responsible for wave V?

(A) Cochlear nucleus
(B) Principal sensory nucleus of the trigeminal nerve
(C) Lateral lemniscus
(D) Superior olivary nucleus
(E) Inferior colliculus

74. You are asked to see a 54-year-old man who was recently fired from his job for poor performance. He was behaving inappropriately at meetings, showing up late, and insulting clients. The event that ultimately led to his dismissal was public urination. His wife relates that he was normally a quiet man until the last 3 years. He gradually became more outgoing, swearing more, and misbehaving at social events. What is the most likely diagnosis?

(A) Alzheimer disease
(B) Frontotemporal dementia
(C) Lewy-body disease
(D) Bipolar disorder
(E) Schizophrenia

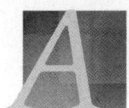 # ANSWERS AND EXPLANATIONS

1. B. Lennox-Gastaut syndrome is characterized by a variety of seizure types including atonic seizures and atypical absence seizures. Mental retardation is seen in 90% of children with Lennox-Gastaut syndrome. Male gender, prior febrile seizures, and family history of complex partial seizures do not predispose to Lennox-Gastaut syndrome. The characteristic EEG finding during an atypical absence seizure of Lennox-Gastaut syndrome is 2 to 2.5 Hz spike and wave.

2. A. The patient described in the vignette most likely has cerebrotendinous xanthomatosis. The most effective treatment for this disorder is chenodeoxycholic acid. Vitamin E supplementation can improve the symptoms of abetalipoproteinemia. Phytanic acid restriction is effective for Refsum disease. Biotin may help improve biotinidase deficiency. Niacin is used in the treatment of Hartnup disease.

3. B. This man has a larger left pupil with the anisocoria greater in the darkness. This is consistent with right-sided sympathetic dysfunction, that is, a right Horner syndrome. Failure of the affected eye to dilate after application of a 1% hydroxyamphetamine solution is diagnostic of a right Horner syndrome above the superior cervical ganglion. Third nerve palsies may produce anisocoria, but anisocorias are worse in light and are often (though not always) associated with other eye movement abnormalities. Anisocoria of 5 mm is unlikely to be physiologic.

4. E. Seizures, encephalopathy, stupor, coma, and meningismus are more suggestive of acute disseminated encephalomyelitis than multiple sclerosis. Onset in young adulthood, painful visual loss, multiple foci of involvement, and relatively rapid progression of symptoms are all features shared by multiple sclerosis and acute disseminated encephalomyelitis.

5. A. This patient has alexia without agraphia. This is caused by infarction in the territory of the left posterior cerebral artery, affecting occipital cortex and adjacent splenium of corpus callosum. It is usually accompanied by right homonymous hemianopia. The pyramidal fibers are not affected and no hemiparesis will be seen. Transcortical motor aphasia is produced by left frontal lobe lesions, rather than by occipital lesions.

6. D. The risk for developing adhesive arachnoiditis is increased after CT myelography, or any procedure in which medication is injected into the subarachnoid space. Fibrocartilaginous embolism typically occurs in healthy young adults, and is not associated with CT myelography. Although lumbar disk herniations are quite common, CT myelography does not cause them. Vacuolar myelopathy is secondary to HIV infection. Transverse myelitis is an autoimmune process, not one produced by CT myelography.

7. B. This woman has Foster-Kennedy syndrome, which is classically caused by a frontal meningioma. Foster-Kennedy syndrome produces optic atrophy ipsilateral to the tumor and papilledema contralateral to the tumor. Optic neuritis typically produces normal funduscopic findings in the acute setting and optic atrophy in the chronic setting. It is also unlikely to be a chronic condition. Hydrocephalus may produce bilateral papilledema.

8. C. Methanol intoxication produces massive brain swelling, edema, and necrosis of the optic nerves, claustrum, and putamen. Carbon monoxide characteristically affects the globus pallidus. The classic site of pathology thiamine is the mamillary bodies. Ethylene glycol intoxication does not usually affect the putamen. As its name suggests, central pontine myelinolysis affects the central portion of the pons.

9. A. The patient presented with hemiballismus. The most likely localization for this problem is the contralateral subthalamic nucleus. The other locations listed are not likely to produce hemiballismus.

10. C. The patient in the vignette is suffering from REM sleep behavioral disorder; this usually responds to treatment with clonazepam. Most patients who develop REM sleep behavioral disorder are older than 60 years of age. REM sleep behavioral disorders predisposes to synucleinopathies such as Parkinson disease, Lewy body dementia, or multiple system atrophy, but not to Alzheimer disease. Alcohol withdrawal rather than intoxication is likely to make REM sleep behavioral disorder worse. Treatment of an underlying mood disorder is not likely to affect the outcome of REM sleep behavioral disorder.

11. C. Encephalitis is characterized by parenchymal infiltration. Mental status changes and seizures are clinical signs that suggest encephalitis rather than meningitis. The other features listed may be seen in either meningitis or encephalitis.

12. E. The combination of GCS [9 plus an abnormal head CT would prompt insertion of an ICP monitor. Although all the other choices would favor placement of an ICP monitor in combination, the abnormal head CT is the only finding in isolation that would mandate placement of an ICP monitor.

13. C. This man has delayed sleep pattern, a circadian rhythm disorder characterized by falling asleep and waking up 3 to 6 hours after conventional times. Patients with this condition are often groggy in the morning and have decreased mental alertness. The most effective treatments are light exposure in the morning and evening melatonin. The other listed medications are not likely to help improve the symptoms of delayed sleep pattern disorder.

14. D. This patient's symptoms and signs are most consistent with benign paroxysmal positional vertigo. The upbeat torsional nystagmus is characteristic for nystagmus produced by the posterior semicircular canal.

15. E. The principal site of pathology in alcoholic cerebellar degeneration is the anterior superior vermis.

16. D. Central causes of vertigo are frequently associated with other cranial nerve deficits, and may produce double vision, facial numbness, and facial weakness. Hearing loss is more commonly seen with peripheral causes of vertigo. Vomiting does not distinguish between a central and peripheral cause of vertigo.

17. C. The classical presentation of carotid-cavernous sinus fistula is visual loss with proptosis, pulsatility, and chemosis. Optic neuritis may cause mildly painful visual loss but proptosis, orbital pulsatility, and chemosis are not seen. Angle closure glaucoma is also not associated with these findings. Orbital trauma should be accompanied by an appropriate history and examination findings of trauma. Hyperthyroidism may produce proptosis, but the other features listed are typically absent.

18. E. Delta frequency is the predominant background frequency in infants. Although the EEG is normal at this time, it may be abnormal at a later date or during a seizure. Delta frequency does not indicate status epilepticus or an artifact. Although delta frequency may indicate an encephalopathy in an adult, it does not mean the same thing in an infant.

19. D. This patient's clinical history is consistent with meningitis, but he is lethargic and has a focal neurologic examination. He should be given antibiotics as a first measure, a head CT because of his lethargy and focal neurologic examination, and then a lumbar puncture. The administration of antibiotics will not change the sensitivity of the lumbar puncture if it is performed quickly.

20. A. The Moro reflex should disappear by 3 to 6 months. The asymmetric tonic neck reflex disappears between 4 and 10 months, the symmetric tonic neck reflex disappears between 8 and 9 months, the Babinski reflex disappears at about 10 months, and foot grasp reflex disappears at about 10 months.

21. A. Isolated respiratory failure caused by myopathic disease in an adult is most consistent with acid maltase deficiency. In infants, this disorder causes a floppy baby with cardiomegaly and hepatosplenomegaly, whereas in children, acid maltase deficiency presents as prominent muscle weakness. Becker muscular dystrophy affects proximal muscles, and usually has onset by age 11. Central core disease is a hereditary myopathy that may appear in adulthood, but not with isolated diaphragmatic weakness. Emery-Dreifuss dystrophy is characterized by early onset of elbow and ankle contractures. Limb-girdle dystrophy predominantly affects the limb-girdle muscles, as its name suggests, not respiratory muscles.

22. C. Right superior oblique dysfunction produces vertical diplopia greatest on downgaze with the eye in adduction. A patient with superior oblique dysfunction will also tilt his head to the opposite side of dysfunction. Right inferior oblique and superior rectus dysfunction produce vertical diplopia greatest on upgaze. Right inferior rectus dysfunction should result in diplopia greatest in rightward gaze. Right medial rectus dysfunction does not produce vertical diplopia.

23. D. The anterior inferior cerebellar artery supplies the dorsal cochlear nucleus, which can result in ipsilateral deficits. Although the middle cerebral arteries supply auditory cortex, infarction does not cause hearing loss. Superior cerebellar artery and posterior inferior cerebellar artery infarctions do not cause hearing loss.

24. A. Aneurysms greater than 7 mm in diameter have about a 1% annual risk of bleeding, but aneurysms of this size bleed less commonly. Most intracranial aneurysms are sporadic rather than inherited or associated with connective tissue disorders. This aneurysm is unlikely to cause her headache. Management of aneurysms of this size is by no means emergent.

25. A. This patient likely has a surgical pupil, commonly seen after cataract surgery. Syphilis should produce an irregularly shaped pupil but is usually bilateral. Sudden-onset severe headache would suggest subarachnoid hemorrhage, possibly secondary to a ruptured aneurysm. In this case, the unreactive pupil should be the larger one. Atropine should also produce large rather than small pupils. Apical lung cancer can produce a Horner syndrome, but the pupil is typically round.

26. B. The patient described in the vignette has symptoms most consistent with Ménière disease. The Tullio phenomenon refers to increased vertigo precipitated by loud noises. The other choices listed do not typically produce vertigo in a patient with Ménière disease.

27. C. This patient's history is most consistent with progressive multifocal leukoencephalopathy (PML), a demyelinating disease of the CNS occurring in people with AIDS. PML lesions occur most commonly in the parieto-occipital lesions, although all the other listed locations may also be affected by PML.

28. B. Bell palsy is caused by a lesion of the ipsilateral seventh cranial nerve. Taste on the anterior two thirds of the tongue is mediated by the seventh nerve. Hearing would be impaired in a lesion of the eighth cranial nerve. Although a seventh nerve palsy could cause increased sensitivity to high-frequency tones, the perception of these tones is not diminished. Both gross touch and pinprick sensation on the face are functions of the fifth cranial nerve. Pinprick sensation on the body is not mediated by the cranial nerves.

29. C. Sedation is the most likely intervention to decrease intracranial pressure. Hyperventilation to a pCO_2 <25 mm Hg may cause vasoconstriction and ischemic strokes. Brief hyperventilation to a pCO_2 of 25 to 30 mm Hg may be beneficial. Flattening the head of the bed is likely to increase intracranial pressure. The ideal position of the head of the bed is about 30 degrees. Corticosteroids and intravenous fluids may worsen the patient's outcome.

30. B. Frontal lobe seizures can produce tonic deviation of the head and eyes to contralateral side with forced contraction of ipsilateral hand. In this case, right frontal lobe seizure is most likely. Temporal lobe seizures and seizures with generalized onset do not typically produce tonic head and eye deviation at seizure onset.

31. A. Although elevated ESR, increased WBC, CSF leukocytosis, or positive blood cultures are useful to establish diagnosis of epidural abscess, MRI with contrast is most sensitive and specific test, particularly in early, mild cases.

32. A. Alpha coma is associated with the worst prognosis. Beta coma can be seen after drug toxicity or anesthesia, spindle coma is associated with a somewhat hopeful prognosis, periodic lateralized epileptiform discharges are characteristic of stroke or herpes encephalitis, and triphasic waves are seen in encephalopathies.

33. E. This man has schizoid personality disorder, characterized by emotional detachment and preference for solitude. Avoidant personality disorder shares several features with schizoid personality disorder, with principal difference being the desire for intimate personal contact expressed by people with avoidant personality disorder. Patients with schizotypal personality disorder are described as odd and eccentric. Borderline personality disorder is characterized by overly dramatic behavior, with patients having the need to be the center of attention. Obsessive-compulsive personality disorder is characterized by perfectionism and an excessive requirement for order.

34. C. This boy's history is most consistent with Landau-Kleffner syndrome, or acquired epileptic aphasia. This condition may respond to corticosteroids if anticonvulsants are ineffective. His daytime EEG is likely to be normal, but he will have temporal spikes during sleep. Children with Landau-Kleffner syndrome often have autistic-type behaviors. As noted, he has acquired epileptic aphasia, and his problem is likely to be neurologic rather than audiologic. Audiometry, however, should still be performed as part of his evaluation.

35. D. The pilocytic astrocytoma is the most frequent posterior fossa tumor in children. All of the other tumors are found in posterior fossa but are less likely than pilocytic astrocytoma.

36. C. The most likely diagnosis is Lambert-Eaton myasthenic syndrome. This disorder is caused by antibodies to voltage-gated calcium channels, which prevent release of acetylcholine. Myasthenia gravis is caused by antibodies to the acetylcholine receptor. The inability to package and release presynaptic acetylcholine is characteristic of botulism. Antibodies to muscle-specific tyrosine kinase (MuSK) are seen in minority of patients with myasthenia gravis. Widespread myositis secondary to neoplastic infiltration would be unlikely.

37. C. Rathke cleft cysts are derived from the hypophyseal pouch rather than neurohypophyseal bud. They are common findings at autopsy and are usually small, asymptomatic, and do not enhance on MRI. It is unlikely that this man's headaches were secondary to the Rathke cleft cyst.

38. A. Abetalipoproteinemia (Bassen-Kornzweig disease) is the most likely diagnosis. Friedreich ataxia can also produce similar symptoms, but is not among the choices. Episodic ataxia is characterized by ataxia, and possibly myokymia and epilepsy. Infectious cerebellitis does not usually last for one year and is not associated with absent reflexes. Medulloblastoma should not produce absent reflexes. In addition to ataxia, spinocerebellar ataxia is associated with ophthalmoparesis, pyramidal, and extrapyramidal signs, but not absent reflexes.

39. A. Loss of venous pulsations is the first sign of papilledema. Elevated disc margins and splinter hemorrhages are later findings. An increased cup-to-disc ratio is suggestive of glaucoma. Drusen are colloid bodies seen in the optic disc and may be confused with papilledema but does not represent intracranial hypertension.

40. B. Brown syndrome is superior oblique tendon tenosynovitis, which, due to restriction of superior oblique muscle mimics inferior oblique palsy. Graves disease may cause a restrictive ophthalmoplegia, but usually affects the medial or inferior rectus. Aneurysmal rupture is unlikely to produce isolated inferior oblique palsy; other structures supplied by third cranial nerve are likely to be affected. Diabetes can infarct the third nerve and should produce other signs of third nerve dysfunction. An intraocular tumor may produce isolated inferior oblique palsy, but the clicking sound heard by the patient is specific for Brown syndrome. A patient with intraocular tumor may also be expected to have proptosis.

41. D. Raymond syndrome is one of medial inferior pontine syndromes characterized by ipsilateral abducens nerve palsy and contralateral hemiparesis. Paramedian midbrain infarction affects third nerve and may cause contralateral hemiparesis. Medial superior and midpontine syndromes commonly cause ataxia. Medial medullary syndromes cause ipsilateral tongue weakness and contralateral hemiparesis.

42. B. Patients in upright position have elevated cerebrospinal fluid pressures. Accurate pressures can be measured only in lateral decubitus position. Although elevated pressure is suggestive of bacterial meningitis, in this situation the pressure may actually be normal. Normal opening pressure for a woman of this age is <150 mm H_2O. Acetazolamide could be administered for increased CSF production (as in pseudotumor cerebri), but in this situation is not indicated. This elevated pressure measurement does not place her at increased risk for herniation.

43. C. This infant has Pelizaeus-Merzbacher disease, an X-linked recessive disorder.

44. A. Depression is the most common psychiatric disorder seen in patients with epilepsy. Mania, psychosis, temporal lobe epilepsy personality, and schizophrenia all occur in patients with epilepsy, but at lower frequencies than depression.

45. C. The right abducens nerve would be expected to produce pure horizontal diplopia greatest in right gaze. Lesions of the oculomotor and trochlear nerves would also be expected to produce vertical diplopia, whereas dysfunction of left abducens nerve would cause horizontal diplopia greatest in left gaze.

46. B. Acoustic neuroma is a tumor of the vestibular portion of cranial nerve VIII. It is located at the cerebellopontine angle, and large tumors may affect cranial nerves VI and VII as well as cranial nerve VIII.

47. C. The posterior cerebral artery, oculomotor nerve, and midbrain are the structures that are most likely to be compressed during uncal herniation. The cerebellar tonsils are susceptible during tonsillar herniation. The sixth cranial nerve can be affected by increased intracranial pressure as a false-localizing sign, but not specifically during uncal herniation. The anterior cerebral artery may be compressed during subfalcine herniation. Basilar artery perforators are torn during central, but not uncal, herniation.

48. A. Most patients with ocular myasthenia gravis develop generalization of their symptoms, if this is to occur, within one year. This patient has had symptoms for 2 years, and it is thus likely to be limited to her eyes. She will probably continue to require treatment with pyridostigmine.

49. C. Demyelination without conduction block would produce normal SNAP amplitude but decreased conduction velocity. An axonal lesion would produce decreased amplitude with normal or slightly slow conduction velocity. Demyelination with conduction block would produce both decreased SNAP amplitude and conduction velocity.

50. C. This man's history is most consistent with REM-sleep behavioral disorder. This disorder is a risk factor for the development of Lewy-body disease, but not the other listed dementias.

51. C. Confusion, bilateral abducens palsies, and limb ataxia is most consistent with Wernicke encephalopathy, which should be emergently treated with thiamine. Although a noncontrast head CT would be valuable, thiamine administration should not be delayed. Lumbar puncture could be useful to evaluate for suspected Guillain-Barré syndrome or meningitis, but these diagnoses are less consistent with this patient's presentation. Benadryl (diphenhydramine) administration can reverse an oculogyric crisis (consider including this in the text), but in an oculogyric crisis, the eyes would be expected to be deviated to the same direction. Neurosurgical consultation may be needed in a patient with this presentation but should follow thiamine administration and a noncontrast head CT.

52. B. The history is most consistent with benign rolandic epilepsy. This diagnosis could be confirmed by EEG showing spikes in central/centrotemporal regions. MRI of the head is indicated in atypical presentations or for children with abnormal neurologic examinations. Benign rolandic epilepsy resolves on its own, and if seizures are infrequent and do not occur during daytime, treatment is not necessary. Hyperventilation can produce absence seizures or their EEG changes, but does not produce seizures of benign rolandic epilepsy.

53. B. Uncal herniation most typically affects the ipsilateral oculomotor nerve. The Kernohan notch phenomenon refers to compression of the contralateral cerebral peduncle against the free edge of the tentorium, resulting in a hemiparesis ipsilateral to the side of the hemiparesis. A pupil that is fixed and dilated on the left and is accompanied by left hemiparesis is most likely secondary to a left-to-right uncal herniation with compression of the left oculomotor nerve and right cerebral peduncle.

54. C. This patient has a history and physical examination most consistent with Whipple disease. Jejunal biopsy will show PAS+ organisms, and is the most sensitive method of establishing a diagnosis. The other listed choices are not likely to yield the correct diagnosis.

55. B. Flaccid paralysis with absent reflexes of acute onset is most consistent with Guillain-Barré syndrome (GBS). Of the choices listed, the laboratory abnormality most associated with GBS is hyponatremia secondary to secretion of inappropriate antidiuretic hormone (SIADH). Elevated white blood count, hyperglycemia, and elevated transaminases are not expected in GBS. The characteristic CSF findings in GBS are normal opening pressure with normal cell count and increased protein.

56. E. *Streptococcus pneumoniae* is the most common cause of bacterial meningitis in immunologically competent adults.

57. D. This infant's history is most consistent with Aicardi syndrome, which is characterized by clinical triad of infantile spasms, agenesis of the corpus callosum, and retinal lacunae. Although hippocampus is a frequent site of pathology in seizure disorders, corpus callosum should be the focus of the evaluation. Imaging of the pineal body, posterior commissure, and thalamus are usually normal in Aicardi syndrome.

58. C. The combination of a pupil that does not react to light but dilates briskly after application of a dilute pilocarpine solution and decreased or absent reflexes is diagnostic of Adie tonic pupil. An aneurysm compressing the left third nerve would lead to a dilated pupil, but the pupil would not be supersensitive to pilocarpine. Horner syndrome produces a constricted pupil. Miller-Fisher variant of Guillain-Barré syndrome would produce external ophthalmoplegia. An Argyl-Robertson pupil is small and unreactive

59. A. Friedreich ataxia characteristically has a preadolescent onset. It is inherited in an autosomal-recessive fashion, so her brother may be affected. Dorsal column sensory loss, areflexia, and upgoing toes are common features of Friedreich ataxia.

60. D. This patient is clearly symptomatic from a subdural hematoma of moderate size. The hypodense appearance on the head CT indicates that the clot has liquefied and can be drained via burr holes rather than an open craniectomy. Repeating the head CT or obtaining further imaging is not indicated, as this subdural hematoma should be drained.

61. C. The patient described in this vignette appears to have had convulsive syncope. This is characterized by asymmetric myoclonic jerks and incontinence without a postictal state. The best treatment for this disorder is management of the underlying cause of his syncope. In this case, he had falls in both blood pressure and heart rate, suggesting that there is an underlying cardiac defect that should be corrected. He does not have epilepsy, so anticonvulsants and epilepsy surgery are not likely to be helpful. β-Blockers will likely increase the chance of recurrence, as the main problem appears to be bradycardia. Salt tablets may help to keep his blood pressure elevated, but it appears that bradycardia is the underlying source of his problems.

62. B. Removal of the anterior temporal lobe may disrupt Meyer loop, resulting in loss of the superior part of the left hemifield of vision. The entire left hemifield would be affected by an occipital lobe lesion; however, there will be macular sparing. The inferior part of the left hemifield would be missing in a parietal lobe lesion. Macula-sparing lesions are characteristic of contralateral posterior cerebral artery infarctions involving the occipital cortex.

63. D. The patient described most likely has cyanotic syncope. The most likely EEG finding is flattening of the background. 2-Hz spikes and waves are seen in Lennox-Gastaut syndrome. 3-Hz spikes and waves are the findings of absence or myoclonic seizures. Hypsarrhythmia is associated with infantile spasms. Background delta rhythm may be seen in the context of an encephalopathy, but is not associated with cyanotic syncope.

64. D. This patient has a right "one-and-a-half syndrome." This is classically caused by a lesion of the right pontine tegmentum. Midbrain lesions that affect eye movements usually also affect vertical eye movements. Left pontine tegmental lesions may produce a one-and-a-half syndrome with no horizontal movements of the left eye and no adduction of the right eye. Left medullary lesions may produce problems with vertical eye movements, but horizontal eye movements are usually preserved.

65. B. The Moro reflex is characterized by arm extension, abduction, and opening of the hands.

66. E. The eighth cranial nerve is the most likely one to be affected as a long-term consequence of bacterial meningitis.

67. B. Cytotoxic edema is due to intracellular accumulation of water produced by injury that damages the capacity of cells to maintain homeostasis. It is most commonly seen as a result of ischemia, trauma, and toxic processes. Cytotoxic edema does not respond to steroid. Vasogenic edema is secondary to increased permeability of the blood–brain barrier and is seen in the setting of abscesses and brain tumors. Vasogenic edema responds to steroids but should not be used in trauma. Interstitial edema is associated with hydrocephalus and does not respond to steroids.

68. B. The most common location of strokes that produce depression is the left frontal lobe.

69. B. Respiratory effort is absent during an apneic episode, which distinguishes central sleep apnea from obstructive sleep apnea. In both conditions, airflow decreases last longer than 10 seconds and are associated with decreased oxygen saturations. The apnea–hypopnea index is a measure of apnea severity, with >5 being classified as mild, >15 as moderate, and >30 as severe. The grading is the same for central and obstructive sleep apneas. Airflow decreases by 90% during an apneic episode, not 50%.

70. A. Olfaction is the only sensation that does not have thalamic relays. The lateral geniculate nucleus contains visual relays, the medial geniculate nucleus contains auditory relays, and the ventral posterior thalamus contains both touch and taste relays.

71. D. This patient's history is most consistent with idiopathic brachial neuritis, also known as Parsonage-Turner or neuralgic amyotrophy. Most likely, this will improve in several months without treatment.

72. C. Fracture of the temporal bone is most likely to produce the vertigo from which this patient suffers. Fracture of the cribriform plate of the ethmoid bone may produce anosmia, but not vertigo. Fracture of the occipital or parietal bones would not be expected to produce vertigo. Fracture of the clivus may damage the sixth cranial nerve.

73. E. Brainstem auditory evoked potentials (BAEPs) produce waves that can localize pathology. Wave I is produced by the eighth cranial nerve; wave II by the cochlear nucleus; wave III by the superior olivary nucleus; wave IV by the lateral lemniscus; and wave V by the inferior colliculus. The principal sensory nucleus of the trigeminal nerve is not involved in the production of BAEPs.

74. B. His change in personality is most consistent with frontotemporal dementia. Alzheimer disease is typically characterized by memory deficits, whereas Lewy-body disease features cognitive fluctuations and visual hallucinations. The age of onset of his symptoms make bipolar disorder and schizophrenia less likely.

Index

A

Abscesses, 163
Acoustic reflexes, 51
Acquired autoimmune myasthenia gravis (MG), 148
Acquired hypercoagulable state, 102
Action tremors, 155–156
Acute ataxia, 110
Acute disseminated encephalomyelitis (ADEM), 135
    CSF findings, 135
Acute glaucoma, 249
Acute hemiplegia, 219–220
Acute meningitis (AM), 163
Acute myelitis, 117
Acute noncompressive myelopathy, differential diagnosis, 134
Acute pain, 188
Acute pyogenic infections, 59–60
Acute spinal cord injury, 117
Acute subdural hematoma (SDH), 256–257
Acute uremic polyneuropathy, 126
Acute viral infections, 61–62
Adaptive pain, maladaptive pain (contrast), 187
Addiction, 188–189
Addison disease (adrenocortical insufficiency), 285
Adie tonic pupil, 249
Adrenoleukodystrophy, 136
Adults
    infratentorial tumors, 74
    supratentorial tumors, 72–74
Afferent fibers, 109
Afferent innervation, interruption, 282
Ageusia, 288
Alexander disease, 136
Allodynia, 186–187
Altered states, 209–211
Alzheimer disease (AD), 201–203
    diagnosis-two criteria, 202
    epidemiology, 201–202
    pathology, 202
    symptoms, 202
    treatment, 202–203
Alzheimer's, pharmacology, 83
Amygdala, 21
Amyloid neuropathies, 126
Analgesia, 186
Ankylosing spondylitis, 119
Anosmia, 288
Anterior cerebral artery, 30
Anterior cerebral artery (ACA) syndrome, 100
Antibiotics/antivirals, 84–85
Anticholinergic/myasthenia gravis, pharmacology, 85
Anticonvulsant therapy, 173
Anti-emetic/motion sickness, pharmacology, 85
Anti-epileptic pharmacology, 87–89
Antihypertensive medication, 102,
Antimicrobials, 127
Antineoplastic drugs, 127
Antiparkinsonian pharmacology, 86
Antiplatelet pharmacology, 86–87
Antithrombotics/anticoagulants, pharmacology, 89
Anxiety, 205–206
    neurosis, 206
Aortic aneurysm, 114
Aqueduct of Sylvius, 66
Argyl-Robertson pupil, 302
Arousal, 21–23
Arsenical polyneuropathy, 127
Astrocytic tumors, 173–174
Asymptomatic carotid artery stenosis (ACAS), 97
Ataxia, 157–160, 217–218
Atherosclerosis, 67–71
Atypical primary Parkinsonian disorders, 152–154
Autoimmune function, 117
Autonomic dysfunction, 282
Autonomic nervous system (ANS), 22–23, 281
    answers/explanations, 287
    study questions, 286
Autonomic neuropathies, 281
Autosomal-dominant cerebellar ataxias, 157
Autosomal recessive ataxias, 159–160
Axonal injury, 79

B

Bacterial infections, 59–61
Bacterial meningitis, 165
Bacterial toxins, 61
Balance, function, 13–14
Basal ganglia, 19–20
    diseases, 75–76
Basilar artery, 31–32
Benign nocturnal myoclonus, 196
Benign Rolandic epilepsy, 244
Benign tumors, 175–176
Bilateral ageusia, 289
Bilateral ophthalmoplegias, 291
Bilateral ptosis, 248
Bilateral pupillary problems, 249
Binswanger disease, 103
Bladder
    dysfunction, 282
    sensory afferents, interruption, 282
Blinking, 249
    inability, 248
Blood electrolytes, 155
Bowel
    ileus, 282
    problems, 282

Brachial mononeuropathies, 125
Brachial plexus neuropathies, 124
Brain
 damage, 78–79
 formation, 2–3
 surface contusions/lacerations, 79
 tumors, pathology, 71–74
Brainstem
 diseases, 76–77
 glioma, 177
Brainstem auditory evoked potentials (BAEPs), 50–51
Burning mouth syndrome, 289

C

Canavan disease, 136
Carbon monoxide, impact, 64
Cardiac embolism, 96
Carotid artery dissection, 27
Cations, 38
Cauda equina syndrome, 118
Central core disease (CCD), 145
Central nervous system (CNS)
 cysts, 74
 myelin, 63
 tumors, 74
  diagnosis, 172
  first-line treatment, surgery (usage), 172
  pathophysiology, 169
Central pontine myelinolysis (CPM), 64, 135
Central/primary facial pain, 182
Central (transtentorial) herniation, 254
Central vestibular disorders, 277
Centronuclear (myotubular) myopathy, 146
Cerebellum, 18–19
 anatomy, 108–110
 answers/explanations, 113
 cells, 109
 clinical features, 110–111
 hereditary functions, 111
 infectious diseases, 110–111
 lobules, 18–19
 neuronal organization, 109–110
 study questions, 112
 vascular syndromes, 110
Cerebral amyloid (congophilic) angiopathy, 104
Cerebral artery syndromes, 99–100
Cerebral concussion, 79
Cerebral contusion, 255
Cerebral edema, 80
Cerebral hypotonia, 216
Cerebral palsy, 219
Cerebrospinal fluid (CSF), 164–165
 appearance, 164
Cerebrovascular disease, 95–96
 answers/explanations, 107
 evaluation/management, 100–102
 study questions, 106
Cervical spondylosis (myelopathy, inclusion), 119
Childhood headaches, 211
Children

infratentorial tumors, 71
supratentorial tumors, 71–72
tumors, impact, 176–178
Chorea, 156-157
 inhibitory output, reduction, 156–157
Chronic ataxia, 217–218
Chronic hemiplegia, 220
Chronic inflammatory demyelinating polyradiculopathy (CIDP), 124
Chronic pain, 187
 management, 188
Chronic progressive external ophthalmoplegia (CPEO), 147
Chronic subdural hematoma, 257
Churg-Strauss/hypereosinophilia, 124
Cigarette smoking cessation, 102
Circadian rhythm disorders, 245
Circumscribed neuropsychiatric syndromes, 268
Closed head injury, 254
Cluster, 183
CmyD, 144
Cochlear nucleus, auditory neurons, 13
Cognitive alteration, 200
 answers/explanations, 208
 reversible causes, 200–201
 study questions, 207
Cognitive impairment, exclusion, 271–272
Colloid cysts, 176
Coma patterns, 48
Complex partial seizures, 193
Complex regional pain syndrome (CRPS), 187
Compound muscle action potentials (CMAPs), 49–50
Compression injury, 118
Computerized tomography (CT)
 scan, appearance, 257
 usage, 224–225
Concentric sclerosis of Balo, 133
Concussion, 254
Congenital malformations, 64–67
Congenital megacolon (Hirschsprung disease), 282
Congenital muscular dystrophies (CMDs), 142
Congenital myasthenic syndrome (CMS), 147
Congenital myopathies, 145–146
Conus medullaris syndrome, 118
Conventional angiogram, 227
Convulsive status, 196–197
Convulsive syncope, 277
Convulsive types, 192
Corpus callosum, agenesis, 65
Cortex, diseases, 75–76
Cortical disorders, 65
Cortical venous thrombosis, 105
Coup/contrecoup contusions, 79
Coup/contrecoup fractures, 79
Cranial nerves, 21
 palsies, 257
Cranial neuralgias, 182
Craniopharyngioma, 177
Creutzfeldt-Jakob disease, 62–63
Critical illness consults, 263–264

Cryoglobulinemia, 125
CSF polymerase chain reaction (PCR), 135
Cushing disease, 285
Cushing syndrome, 284
Cyanotic syncope, 195
Cytology, 35–37
Cytotoxic edema, 80

D

Dandy-Walker malformation, 66
Daytime sleepiness, excess, 242–244
    treatment, 243–244
Deep nuclei, 108–109
Delirium, 200–201
    medical consult, 261
Dementia with Lewy bodies (DLBs), 203
    diagnosis/treatment, 203
    variable time course, 203
Demyelinating diseases, 63–64
Demyelination, 131
    answers/explanations, 140
    study questions, 139
Denatorubropallidoluysian atrophy (DRPLA), 159
Dermatomyositis, 144–145
Detoxification, 188–189
Development, 1
    answers/explanations, 7
    study questions, 6
Diabetes, control, 102
Diabetes insipidus, 283
Diabetic subacute asymmetrical/multifocal polyneuropathy, 128
Dialysis, 262
Diffuse axonal injury, 254–255
Diphtheric polyneuropathy, 124
Discriminative touch, 8–9
Disordered emotional expression, 206
Distal myopathies, 144
Dizziness, 275
    answers/explanations, 280
    study questions, 279
Doppler ultrasound/transcranial Doppler, 227
Drugs, impact, 127
Dural thrombosis, 105
Dysequilibrium, 277–278
Dysesthesia, 186
Dysosmia, 288
Dystonia, 154
Dystrophinopathies, 141–142

E

Efferent innervation, interruption, 282
Elderly, headaches, 185
Electrical status epilepticus, 244
Electroencephalogram (EEG), 44–48
Electromyogram (EMG), 53–54
Emergent noncontrast CT, 257
Emery-Dreifuss muscular dystrophy, 143
Emotional alteration, 200
    answers/explanations, 208
    reversible causes, 200–201
    study questions, 207
Encephalitis, 163
Environment, movement (false sensation), 275
Ependymoma, 177
Epidural (extradural) hemorrhage, 80
Epidural hematoma (EDH), 255–256
    death, 255
Epilepsia partialis, 195
Epilepsy, 192
    answers/explanations, 199
    definitions, 192
    special syndromes, 195
    study questions, 198
Episodic ataxias, 158–159
Ethylene glycol, impact, 64
Evoked otoacoustic emissions, 51
Excitatory receptors, 41
Exogenous modifiers, 38
Eyelid abnormalities, 248–249
    signs, 248–249
Eye movements, 289–291

F

Facioscapulohumeral muscular dystrophy (FSH), 143
Fatigue, 204–205
Febrile seizures, 195
Fibrocartilaginous embolism, 114
Fibromyalgia, 187
Final exam, 295–304
    answers/explanations, 305–313
Fissures, 108
Focal seizures, 194–195
Free running sleep pattern, 245
Frontotemporal lobar dementia (Pick disease), 203–204
Funduscopic examination essentials, 250

G

Generalized idiopathic seizures, 192–194
Germinal matrix lesions, 66
Giant cell arteritis, 102, 185
Gigantism, 284
Glial cells, 36, 38
Global hypothalamic syndromes, 283
Glutamine receptor, 41
Glycogen storage myopathies, 146
Gold standard radiographic test, 171
G-protein receptors, 42
Growth abnormalities, 284
Guillain-Barré syndrome (acute inflammatory polyneuropathy / acute inflammatory demyelinating polyneuropathy), 123–124, 136–138
    clinical features, 137
    diagnosis, 137
    epidemiology, 136
    pathogenesis/pathophysiology, 136
    physical examination, 137
    prognosis, 138

Guillain-Barré syndrome (contd.)
   risk factors, 136
   treatment, 137–138
   variants, 138
Gunshot wounds, 257

H

Hair cells, 14
Hallucinations, 289, 292
HD neurodegenerative character, 157
Headaches, 181, 211–212
   acute treatment, 184
   answers/explanations, 191
   childhood features, 211
   emergencies, 185–186
   epidemiology, 181
   nonpharmacologic management, 183
   pathophysiology, 183
   pharmacologic management, 184
   preventive treatment, 184
   prominence, 185–186
   study questions, 190
Head injury, penetration, 257
Head trauma, precipitation, 257
Hearing, 291–292
   function, 13
   loss, 291
Hemorrhagic strokes, 104–105
Hepatology, 262–263
Hereditary disorders, 136
Hereditary immunodeficiency syndromes, 170
Hereditary metabolic neuropathies, 221
Hereditary sensory and autonomic neuropathies (HSANs), 220
Herniation syndromes, 254
Hiccup, 283
Higher functions, localization, 23–24
High-grade diffuse astrocytic tumors, 174
Histology, 35–37
Holoprosencephaly, 65
Homeostasis, 21–23
Homocysteine lowering, 102
Homosysteins, increase, 102
Horner syndrome, 281
Hydranencephaly, 66
Hyperosmia, 288
Hyperpathia, 186
Hypertensive encephalopathy, 103
Hypertensive ICH, 104
Hyperventilation, 283
Hypogeusia, 289
Hypothalamic function, loss, 283
Hypothalamus, 281
   answers/explanations, 287
   study questions, 286
Hypotonic infant, 216–217
Hypoxia, 209

I

Iatrogenic function, 118
Idiopathic eosinophilic syndrome, 124

Idiopathic hypersomnia, 243
Immune disorders, 147–148
Immunosuppressive therapy, 211
Impotence, 283
Indolent headache, 185
Infection, 163
   answers/explanations, 168
   history/examination, 163–164
   study questions, 167
Infectious diseases, 59
Inflammation, 115–116
Inflammatory myopathies, 144–145
Inherited mixed polyneuropathies, 126
Inherited polyneuropathies (metabolic disorders, inclusion), 126
Inherited sensory polyneuropathies, 125–126
Inhibitory postsynaptic potentials (IPSPs), 42
Inhibitory receptors, 41–42
Initial GCS, predictor, 257
Inner ear, 13
Internal carotid artery (ICA), 99–100
Internal carotid segments, 27
Internal medicine, 260
   answers/explanations, 266
   study questions, 265
International Headache Society classification/diagnosis, 181–182
Interstitial/hydrocephalic/pressure edema, 80
Intracranial hemorrhage, 97
Intracranial pressure (ICP), increase, 211–212, 254
Ion channels, 38–39
Ipsilateral relative afferent pupillary defect (RAPD), 133
Ischemic stroke, 96
Isoniazid (INH), 127

J

Jet lag, 245
Jitteriness, 195

K

Kearns-Sayre syndrome, 147
Kindling, 187
Klein-Levin syndrome, 243
Krabbe's globoid cell leukodystrophy, 136

L

Laboratory tests, usage, 267
Lacunar infarcts, 103
Lacunar strokes, 97
Landau-Kleffner syndrome, 245
Lead neuropathy, 127
Leukodystrophies, 63–64
Levator muscle, paralysis, 248
Lightheadedness, 278
Limb-girdle muscular dystrophies (LGMDs), 142–143
Limbic system, emotion (relationship), 206
Lipid lowering, 102
Longitudinal (sagittal) zones, 108
Lumbar puncture, 164

Lumbar stenosis, 119
Lumbosacral plexus, 125
Lupus, 125
Lyme disease, 123

M

Macroglobulinemia, 127
Magnetic resonance imaging (MRI), 96
    unavailability, 171–172
    usage, 225–227
Major neuropsychiatric syndromes, 269–270
Maladaptive pain, 187
Marcus-Gunn pupil, 249
Medical consults, 261–264
Medications, 91–92
Medulloblastoma, 177
Membrane potential, 38–39
Meningiomas, 175
Menstrual related hypersomnia, 243
Mental status examination, 267
Metabolic disorders, 64
Metabolic function, 117
Metabolic myopathies, 146
Metachromatic leukodystrophy, 136
Metastatic lesions, 171
Metazoal infections, 61
Methanol intoxication, 64
Midbrain injury, 255
Middle cerebral artery, 30–31
Migraine, 183, 211
    aura, inclusion, 185
    pharmacology, 89–90
    stroke, 102
    variants, 211
Migrant sensory neuritis of Wartenberg, 123
Mild cognitive impairment (MCI), 201
Mitochondrial myopathies, 146–147
Mitochondrial myopathy encephalopathy lactic acidosis and strokelike episodes (MELAS), 147
Mixed type neurogenic bladder, 282
Modalities, 50–53
Monoclonal gammopathy, undetermined significance, 127
Monocular visual loss, differential diagnosis, 134
Monophasic inflammatory demyelinating disorder, 135
Monoplegia, 219
Motor development, 213
Motor function, 216
Motor neurons, 40–41
Motor systems, sensory systems (integration), 21
Motor tics, 156
Movement, 15–21
Movement disorders, 151
    answers/explanations, 162
    characterization, 151
    study questions, 161
Multicystic encephalomalacia, 66
Multiple sclerosis
    variants, 133
Multiple sclerosis (MS), 131–133
    acute exacerbations, treatment, 132
    attacks, prevention, 132–133
    clinical types, 132
    diagnosis, 131–132
    epidemiology, 131
    Marburg/tumefactive variant, 133
    pathogenesis, 131
    pharmacology, 90
    progression, prevention, 133
    Schilder variant, 133
    symptoms, 131
Multiple sensory deficits, 278
Muscles, 141
    answers/explanations, 150
    contractions, 154
    genetics, 154
    study questions, 149
Muscular dystrophies, 141–144
Myasthenia gravis (MG), diagnosis/treatment, 148
Myasthenic disorders, 147–148
Mycotic (fungal) infections, 61
Myelin, basics, 131
Myelomalacia, 114
Myoclonic epilepsy with ragged red fibers (MERRF), 147
Myoclonic seizures, 193–194
Myoclonus, 154–155
Myotonic muscular dystrophy, 144

N

Nap testing, 241–242
Narcolepsy, 242–243
Neck, recoil injury, 80
Nemaline myopathy (NEM), 145–146
Neoplasm, 110, 169
    answers/explanations, 180
    diagnosis, 172–173
    epidemiologic considerations, 170
    genetics, 170–171
    pathophysiology, 169–170
    presentation, 171
    study questions, 179
Neoplastic function, 118
Nerve cells divisions, 35–36
Nerve conduction velocity (NCV), 48–49
    utility, 49
Nervous system
    embryonic/fetal development, 1–4
    origin, 155
Neural crest, 4
Neuralgia, 186
Neural plate (ectoderm)
    development, 1
    differentiation, 1–2
Neural synaptic transmission, 41–42
Neural tube
    defects, 65
    formation, 2
Neurocardiogenic syncope, 278
Neurodegenerative diseases, 74–78

Neuroimaging, usage, 267
Neurologic conditions, 270–271
Neurology patients, complications (medical issues), 260–261
Neuromuscular junction (NMJ), diseases, 147–148
Neuromyelitis optica (NMO)/Devic disease, 133
Neurons, myelitis, 115
Neuroophthalmology, 248
    answers/explanations, 252
    study questions, 251
Neuropathic pain, 186
Neuropathy, 123
Neurophysiologic testing, 35
    answers/explanations, 57–58
    study questions, 55–56
Neuropsychiatric disorders
    nonpharmacologic treatments, 271
    pharmacologic treatments, 271–272
    treatment, 271–272
Neuropsychiatric syndromes, 268–271
Neuropsychiatry, 267
    answers/explanations, 274
    study questions, 273
Neuropsychological testing, 267
Neuroradiology, 224
    answers/explanations, 239–240
    approach, 224
    imaging modalities, 224–228
    study questions, 229–238
Neurosurgery, 253
    answers/explanations, 259
    management, 253–254
    study questions, 258
Neurosyphilis, 102, 116
Neurotransmitters,, 44
    release, protein involvement, 43–44
NF-2 gene, 175
Night-time involuntary limb movements, 242
Nocturnal seizures, 244–245
Nonatherosclerotic ischemic stroke, 102–103
Noncontrast CT scan, 255
Nonconvulsive types, 193
Nonfocal intracranial lesions, 48
Non-rapid eye movement (Non-REM), 244
Nonsystemic vasculitic neuropathy, 123
Nutritional deficiency, 127

O

Obsessive compulsive disorder (OCD), 156
Obstructive sleep apnea, 243
Oculaopharyngeal muscular dystrophy, 143
Ocular motor systems, 20–21
Oligodendrogliomas, 174
    biopsy, 174
Ondine curse, 283
Ophthalmoplegias, 290
Optic neuritis, 133–134
    funduscopic examination, 133–134
Orthostatic hypotension, autonomic causes, 281

P

Paget disease (osteitis deformans), 119

Pain, 181
    acute treatment, 184
    answers/explanations, 191
    definition/clarification, 186
    evaluation, 187–188
    management, 188
    nonpharmacologic management, 183
    pathophysiology, 183
    pharmacologic management, 184
    pharmacology, 90–91
    preventive treatment, 184
    sensation, 9, 15
    study questions, 190
    transmission, pathways, 15
Pallid syncope, 196
Panic attacks, 205
Papilledema, 289
PAPLA syndrome, 102
Parahippocampal gyrus, 21–22
Paraneoplastic problem, 127
Paraproteinemia neuropathy, 127
Parasitic infections, 61
Parasomnias, 244
Parkinson disease (PD), 151–152
Parosmia, 288
Partial focal seizures, 194–195
Partial hypothalamic syndromes, 283–285
Pathologic EEG, 46
Pathologic laughing/crying, 206
Pathology
    answers/explanations, 82
    definition, 59
    study questions, 81
Pediatric headaches, 185
Pediatrics, 209
    answers/explanations, 223
    developmental delay, 212–215
    global delay, 213
    infection, 209–210
    milestones, loss, 214–215
    screening tests, 212
    study questions, 222
Pelizaeus-Merzbacher disease, 136
Perception, 8–15
Periodic limb movement disorder (PLMD), 242
Peripheral nerve diseases
    autonomic signs, 123
    motor signs, 122
    sensory signs, 122
    symptomatology/definition, 122–123
Peripheral nerves, 122
    answers/explanations, 130
    autoimmune problems, 125
    iatrogenic problems, 127
    inflammatory/infectious problems, 123–124
    metabolic problems, 125–126
    neoplastic problems, 127
    study questions, 129
    systemic problems, 127–128
    trauma, 124–125
Peripheral vestibular disease, 276–277
Periventricular leukomalacia, 66

Phantosmia, 288
Pharmacology, 83
    answers/explanations, 94
    study questions, 93
Physiologic derangements, 96
Physiology, 35
    answers/explanations, 57-58
    study questions, 55-56
Pilocytic astrocytoma, 177
Pineal tumors, 177-178
Pituitary adenoma, 175
Placebo effect, 186
Placidity/apathy, 206
Plain films, usage, 224
Plasticity, 44
Plegias, 219-220
PNS disease, neurophysiologic testing (role), 128
Polyarteritis nodosa, 123
Polymyositis, 145
Polysomnography, 241-242
    indications, 241
Porphyric polyneuropathy, 126
Posterior cerebral artery, 31, 32
Posterior cerebral artery (PCA) syndrome, 100
Postmenopausal women, 185
Post myelogram CT, 227-228
Postsynaptic responses, 43
Posttraumatic headaches, 185-186
Posture, 17-18
Precocious puberty, 284
Pregnancy, medical consults, 263
Presyncope, 277
Primary central nervous system (CNS), tumors, 171-172
Primary headache categories, 181-182
Primary Parkinsonian disorders, 151-154
Prion diseases, 62-63
Progressive multifocal leukocephalopathy (PML), 135
Prolonged/chronic pain, neurophysiology, 186-187
Proteins, 36-37
Protozoal infections, 61
Proximal myotonic myopathy (DM2 / PROMM), 144
Pseudo-addiction, 188
Psychiatric/overdose pharmacology, 91
Psychogenic deafness, 292
Psychogenic seizures, 196
Psychological pain, 188
Pupillary defects, 289
Pupils, 249
    noncircular shapes, 249

R

Radiographic imaging, 171
Rage, 206
Rapid eye movement (REM), 244
Raynaud syndrome, 282
Recurrent ataxia, 217
Reflex epilepsy, 195
Reflexes, presence, 4-5
Reflexive swallowing, 283
Renal medical consult, 261-262

Respiration, 283
Respiratory arrest, 255
Restless leg syndrome (RLS), 242
Rest tremors, 155-156
Reversible ischemic neurologic deficit (RIND), 98
Rheumatoid arthritis (RA), 125
Riley-Day syndrome, 281
Rolandic epilepsy, 195

S

Saccular arterial aneurysm, 104
Secondary headache categories, 182
Second messengers, 42-43
Seizures
    age-dependent mimicking syndromes, 195-196
    break, 196-197
    definitions, 192
Sensation, 8-15, 220-221
Senses, 288
    answers/explanations, 294
    study questions, 293
Sensory nerve action potentials (NAPs), 48-49
Sexual function disorders, 283
Shift work sleep disorder, 245
Sickle cell disease, consideration, 102
Simple ophthalmoplegias, 290
Simple partial seizures, 194
Sjögren-sicca syndrome, 123
Skull base fractures, 257
Sleep, 46, 241
    answers/explanations, 247
    pattern
        advancement, 245
        delay, 245
    study questions, 246
Small/medium-sized vessels, vascular arteritis, 123
Smell, 288
    function, 14
    loss, 288
Somatic sensation, 8-9
Somatosensory evoked potentials (SEPs), 50
Speech, developmental delay, 212
Spinal arachnoiditis (chronic adhesive arachnoiditis), 115
Spinal cord, 114, 216
    answers/explanations, 121
    diseases, 77-78
    formation, 3-4
    hemorrhage, 114
    infection, 116
    lesions, 282
    study questions, 120
    vascular malformations, 114
Spinal cord injury (SCI), clinical effects, 116
Spinal MRI, usage, 134
Spinal reflexes, 16-17
Spinal subdural/epidural hemorrhage, 114
Spinal tumors, 175-176
Spinocerebellar ataxias, 158
Stress syndrome, 206
Stroke
    complication, 260-261

Stroke (*contd.*)
    deterioration, 99
    pathogenesis, 96–97
    patients, 104
Structural anatomy, 8
    answers/explanations, 26
    study questions, 25
Subacute bacterial infections, 60–61
Subacute infections, chronic infections (contrast), 163
Subacute sensorimotor paralysis (symmetrical), 127–128
Subacute viral infections, 62
Subarachnoid hemorrhage (SAH), 97, 104
Subdural hematoma (SDH), outcomes, 256
Subdural hemorrhage, 80
Subfalcine herniation, 254
Sudden onset headache, 185
Suicide attempts, 257
Swallowing, 283
Symmetrical noninflammatory demyelination, 135
Sympathetic storm, 282
Synapses, 13, 39–40
Synaptic bouton, 40–41
Synaptic connections, 41
Synaptic transmission, 39–40
Syncope, 277
Syndrome of inappropriate ADH (SIADH) secretion, 284–285
Syringomyelia, 221
Systemic function, 119

T

Taste, 288–289
    function, 14–15
Temperature regulation, disorders, 284
Tension-type headache (TTH), 182
Third nerve dysfunction, 249
Tics, 156
Tinnitus, 291
Tissue diagnosis, 174
Todd paralysis, 220
Tonsillar herniation, 254
Toxic myasthenic syndrome, 147
Transient ischemic attack (TIA), clinical features, 96–97
Transient motor/vocal tics, 156
Transient neonatal MG, 148
Transmitter release, 43–44
Transverse myelitis, 134–135
    CSF analysis, 134
    prognosis, 135
Trauma, 116–117
    basics, 253–254
Traumatic brain injury (TBI), 78–80

Traumatic ICH, delay, 255
Traumatic subarachnoid hemorrhage, 255
Tremors, 155–156
Triphasic waves, 48
Tumors, 118
    suppressor genes, 170–171

U

Unbalance, sensation, 278
Uncal herniation, 249, 254
Uncontrolled hypertension, 103
Unilateral ageusia, 289
Unilateral ptosis, 248
Uremic neuropathy, 262

V

Vacuolar myelopathy (AIDS, inclusion), 115
Vascular anatomy, 27
    answers/explanations, 34
    study questions, 33
Vascular cognitive impairment, 204
Vascular diseases, pathology, 67–71
Vascular Inflammation Trauma Autoimmune Metabolic Iatrogenic Neoplastic Systemic(VITAMINS), 114–119
Vasogenic edema, 80
Venous sinus thrombosis, 102
VEPs, 134
Vertebrobasilar cerebral artery, 31
Vertebrobasilar syndromes, 100
Vertigo, 275–277
    anatomy/physiology, 275
    answers/explanations, 280
    sensation, 275
    study questions, 279
Viral infections, 61–62
Viral inflammation, 115
Vision, 250, 289
    function, 9–13
Visual defects, 250
Visual evoked potentials/responses, 53
Vitamin B12 deficiency, 117
Vitamin deficiency disorders, 64
Vitamin E deficiency, 117
Voluntary movement, 15–16
Voluntary swallowing, 283

W

Wegener syndrome, 124
Weight alterations, hypothalamic disease (association), 284
Whiplash, 80
Wind-up, occurrence, 186
World Health Organization (WHO) grades, 173